Ethics and Chronic Illness

This book provides an account of the ethics of chronic illness. Chronic illness differs from other illnesses in that it is often incurable, patients can live with it for many years, and its day-to-day management is typically carried out by the patient or members of their family. These features problematise key distinctions that underlie much existing work in medical ethics including those between beneficence and autonomy, between treatment and prevention, and between the recipient and provider of treatment.

The author carries out a detailed reappraisal of the roles of both autonomy and beneficence across the different stages of treatment for a range of chronic illnesses. A central part of the author's argument is that in the treatment of chronic illness, the patient and/or the patient's family should be seen as acting with healthcare professionals to achieve a common aim. This aspect opens up unexplored questions such as what healthcare professionals should do when patients are managing their illness poorly, the ethical implications of patients being responsible for parts of their treatment, and how to navigate sharing information with those directly involved in patient care without violating privacy or breaching confidentiality. The author addresses these challenges by engaging with philosophical work on shared commitments and joint action, responsibility and justice, and privacy and confidentiality.

The Ethics of Chronic Illness provides a new, and much needed, critical reappraisal of healthcare professionals' obligations to their patients. It will be of interests to academics working in bioethics and medical ethics, philosophers interested in the topics of autonomy, responsibility, and consent, and medical practitioners who treat patients with chronic illness.

Tom Walker is Senior Lecturer in Ethics and Director of the Centre for the Study of Risk and Inequality at Queen's University Belfast, UK.

Routledge Research in Applied Ethics

Hobbesian Applied Ethics and Public Policy
Edited by Shane D. Courtland

Does the Pro-Life Worldview Make Sense?
Abortion, Hell, and Violence Against Abortion Doctors
Stephen Kershnar

The Injustice of Punishment
Bruce N. Waller

Friendship, Robots, and Social Media
False Friends and Second Selves
Alexis M. Elder

The Capability Approach in Practice
A New Ethics for Setting Development Agendas
Morten Fibieger Byskov

The Ethics of Counterterrorism
Isaac Taylor

Disability with Dignity
Justice, Human Rights and Equal Status
Linda Barclay

Media Ethics, Free Speech, and the Requirements of Democracy
Edited by Carl Fox and Joe Saunders

Ethics and Chronic Illness
Tom Walker

For more information about this series, please visit: www.routledge.com/Routledge-Research-in-Applied-Ethics/book-series/RRAES

Ethics and Chronic Illness

Tom Walker

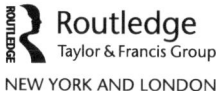
NEW YORK AND LONDON

First published 2019
by Routledge
52 Vanderbilt Avenue, New York, NY 10017

and by Routledge
2 Park Square, Milton Park, Abingdon, Oxon OX14 4RN

Routledge is an imprint of the Taylor & Francis Group, an informa business

© 2019 Taylor & Francis

The right of Tom Walker to be identified as author of this work has been asserted by him in accordance with sections 77 and 78 of the Copyright, Designs and Patents Act 1988.

All rights reserved. No part of this book may be reprinted or reproduced or utilised in any form or by any electronic, mechanical, or other means, now known or hereafter invented, including photocopying and recording, or in any information storage or retrieval system, without permission in writing from the publishers.

Trademark notice: Product or corporate names may be trademarks or registered trademarks, and are used only for identification and explanation without intent to infringe.

Library of Congress Cataloging-in-Publication Data
Names: Walker, Tom, 1965– author.
Title: Ethics and chronic illness / Tom Walker.
Description: 1 [edition]. | New York : Taylor & Francis, 2019. |
　　Series: Routledge research in applied ethics ; 14 | Includes
　　bibliographical references and index.
Identifiers: LCCN 2019006703 | ISBN 9780367210205 (hardback)
Subjects: LCSH: Medical ethics—Case studies. | Physician and patient.
Classification: LCC R724 .W29 2019 | DDC 174.2—dc23
LC record available at https://lccn.loc.gov/2019006703

ISBN: 978-0-367-21020-5 (hbk)
ISBN: 978-0-429-26486-3 (ebk)

Typeset in Sabon
by Apex CoVantage, LLC

Contents

Preface   viii

1   **The Problem: Ethics and Chronic Illness**   1
    1.1 Introduction 1
    1.2 What Makes Chronic Illness Different? 3
    1.3 The Importance of 'When?' 7
    1.4 Choosing 13
    1.5 Acting 17
    1.6 Helping Others Act 22
    1.7 Advising and Preventing 28
    1.8 Conclusion 30

2   **Working Out What Will Benefit Patients**   34
    2.1 Introduction: The Epistemic Argument 34
    2.2 What Is It Exactly That the Healthcare Professional Is Attempting to Determine? 37
    2.3 Should Healthcare Professionals Always Use the Most Reliable Methods? 45
    2.4 Interim Conclusion 49

3   **Is an Informed Patient's Choice Good Evidence That the Option Chosen Is What Is Best for Him?**   53
    3.1 Introduction 53
    3.2 Where Patient Involvement Is Not Needed to Determine What Is Best for the Patient 55
    3.3 How Are Patients Making Decisions When Asked to Make Them? 60
    3.4 The Problem of Risk and Uncertainty 67
    3.5 Conclusion 71

Contents

4 'It should be up to the patient what happens to her'   74
    4.1 Introduction 74
    4.2 The Capacity to Choose and the Value
        of Choice 78
    4.3 Choice and the Autonomous Life 80
    4.4 The Symbolic Value of Choice 88
    4.5 Conclusion 95

5 Consent and the Treatment of Chronic Illness   99
    5.1 Introduction 99
    5.2 Regulatory Consent 102
    5.3 When Is Non-Regulatory Consent Needed and Who
        Is It Needed From? 107
    5.4 The Constitutive Rules for Non-Regulatory Consent
        and What They Mean for Healthcare Professionals'
        Obligations 113
    5.5 Conclusion 128

6 How to Respond to Non-Adherence   131
    6.1 Introduction 131
    6.2 Clarifying the Benefits of Treatment for Chronic
        Illness 132
    6.3 Two Reasons for Non-adherence 136
    6.4 Is Intervention in the Face of Non-Adherence
        Permissible? 141
    6.5 Patient Responsibility and the Obligations of
        Healthcare Professionals 151
    6.6 Conclusion 159

7 Broadening Our Vision: The Role of Families and Others   163
    7.1 Introduction 163
    7.2 Other People as Helpers or Obstacles 166
    7.3 Privacy and Confidentiality 177
    7.4 Conclusion 192

8 Changes Over Time   194
    8.1 Introduction 194
    8.2 When What Healthcare Professionals
        Can Do Changes 195
    8.3 When the Patient's World Changes 199

    8.4 *When the Patient Plans to Do Something Different* 205
    8.5 *Conclusion* 219

9 **Conclusion**   221

References   227
Index   240

Preface

Healthcare ethics is now a well-established and vigorously growing field. Like any discipline there are some topics and questions that receive considerable focused attention, and others that are comparatively neglected. This book is an attempt to shed light on one of the more comparatively neglected topics: the obligations of healthcare professionals when treating patients with chronic illness. The kinds of activities healthcare professionals engage in when treating such patients are different from, though they overlap with, the activities they engage in when treating patients with acute conditions. Those activities are also different from, though again they overlap with, the activities of public health professionals. As such, healthcare professionals working in this area face distinct ethical challenges. That this is the case was first brought home to me by my students on Master's courses in medical ethics at both Keele University and Queen's University Belfast (many of whom had considerable practical experience in healthcare). The ethical challenges they reported facing in their work did not always fit well within the frameworks established in the discipline. That those frameworks had little to say about the distinctive and serious ethical challenges healthcare professionals face when treating patients with chronic illness, particularly in connection to non-adherence, also became clear while working with Professor Liam Heaney on patient responsibility in asthma care. I would like to thank the students on these courses and Professor Heaney for opening up this area for me, and helping me to understand the nature of the ethical problems involved.

This book has been several years in the making. During that time various parts of it have been presented to audiences at the University of Bristol, the Chinese University of Hong Kong, the University of Copenhagen, the Hastings Center, Keele University, Oxford University, NUI Galway, Queen's University Belfast, and the University of Sydney. I would like to thank the audiences at all these places for their very helpful comments and criticisms of my ideas as they developed. I would also like to thank the Arts and Humanities Research Council (grant number: AH/P007619/1) and Queen's University Belfast for funding periods of research leave without which the work could not have been completed.

1 The Problem
Ethics and Chronic Illness

1.1 Introduction

Suppose someone turned to either medical ethics or healthcare ethics as a way to learn what doctors, nurses, and other healthcare professionals do. What would they find? They would learn a lot about interventions at the start of life (new reproductive technologies, abortion, genetic modification), and at the end of life (assisted dying, euthanasia, palliative care). They would learn a lot about medical research. They would learn a lot about procedures to protect patients, such as those governing informed consent. They would learn about the things healthcare professionals do with information obtained from both patients and the samples taken from them—and about the challenges of protecting privacy and maintaining confidentiality when doing so. They would learn about public health policy and how to prevent illness.

That would all be very useful. But the resulting picture would be incomplete. They would find out little, if anything, about the treatment of incurable conditions that patients generally live with for months or years: things like diabetes, asthma, arthritis, Parkinson's disease, and some cancers. They might end up unaware that much of medicine is delivered by the patient him or herself, rather than directly by a doctor or other healthcare professional. They might not notice the ways healthcare professionals support and assist those patients to treat themselves. They might end up with only a limited understanding of the work frontline healthcare professionals do in preventing illness, and in advising their patients. They might not understand that respecting patients' privacy is not simply a matter of data protection. These are things that ethicists have not said much about.

They are, however, important in healthcare delivery. For example in England and Wales, the Department of Health reported in 2010 that patients with long term conditions accounted for over 50% of all General Practitioner appointments, over 65% of outpatient appointments, and over 70% of both inpatient bed days and the total health and social care budget (Department of Health, 2010, p. 4). This is not just a feature of high income countries. Globally, non-communicable or chronic diseases are the leading cause of death (with cardiovascular diseases, cancers, respiratory diseases [including asthma], and diabetes playing by far the largest role) (World Health Organization, 2014, p. 9). The prevalence of diabetes, for example, has increased significantly over the past three decades—up from 4.7% of adults globally in 1980 to 8.5% in 2014 (World Health Organization, 2016, p. 25). This increase has occurred in all WHO regions, and means that in 2014 an estimated 422 million adults worldwide were living with diabetes. Diabetes is not equally prevalent in all regions. But even in Africa, the WHO region with the lowest prevalence, an estimated 25 million adults were living with diabetes in 2014—a prevalence of 7.1% (up from 3.1% in 1980). This is not significantly lower than the prevalence in either Europe (7.3%) or the Americas (8.3%) (World Health Organization, 2016, p. 25). Even though not everyone with diabetes is receiving treatment, these figures indicate that around the world considerable healthcare resources are being used to do just that. The same is true for other chronic illnesses.

While the proportion of both healthcare professionals' time and health service budgets devoted to treating those with chronic illness is already high, it can reasonably be expected to grow over the coming years. There are two reasons for this. First, in 2013 member states of the World Health Organization agreed that a set of basic technologies and medications should be available in 80% of cases by 2025. These technologies and medications include (among other things) aspirin, a statin, insulin, a steroid inhaler, a bronchodilator, and equipment to measure blood pressure, blood sugar levels, and blood cholesterol (World Health Organization, 2014, p. 105). As progress is made towards meeting this target healthcare professionals worldwide will have the resources to treat patients with chronic conditions who would currently go untreated.

Second, chronic diseases are, in most cases, more common among older adults than among those who are younger (though of course people can experience them at any age). A significant proportion (40%) of the increasing prevalence of diabetes between 1980 and 2014, for example, was directly attributable to population ageing (with another 32% attributed to interaction effects between population ageing and increasing age-specific prevalences) (World Health Organization, 2016, p. 25). Conditions such as osteoarthritis are also much more prevalent among older age groups (Martin and Buckwalter, 2002). Worldwide the population is continuing to age (World Health Organization, 2015). It is thus foreseeable that the number of people living with chronic disease, and hence with chronic illness, will increase. Furthermore, those people are also likely to live longer once they have contracted those diseases—something made possible by improved access to treatment. All of this means that while treating and caring for those with chronic illness is already an important part of healthcare provision worldwide, it will become even more significant in the future.

What then explains the mismatch between what ethicists spend their time looking at, and what healthcare professionals increasingly spend their time doing? One possible explanation is that ethicists focus on those areas of healthcare that raise challenging ethical problems, and not all areas do. There is something to be said for this. If we trace the development of healthcare ethics as a discipline, we see it responding to new technologies, contentious social issues, and ethical malpractice (Jonson, 1998). The most pressing ethical problems have arisen in particular areas and those needed to be dealt with first. But that does not explain the continuing neglect of chronic illness. Healthcare professionals treating those with these illnesses face distinctive, inherently ethical, challenges. Were they to turn to either medical ethics or healthcare ethics to help them resolve these challenges they would largely look in vain. This book aims to fill that gap.[1]

1.2 What Makes Chronic Illness Different?

You might, however, wonder whether there is much of a gap to be filled. There exists a considerable body of work on the ethics of treating those whose condition is either curable or terminal. And, you might think, this work can be fairly easily adapted to cover the treatment of those with chronic illnesses. The aim of this chapter is to show that it cannot. In order to do that I need to start by saying something about what chronic illnesses are, and how they might differ from other types of illness. Doing so is not straightforward. Within the medical literature there are different accounts of what makes a disease, or an illness, chronic (for an overview see Bernell and Howard, 2016). Some of these attempt to provide a definition, others are a list of conditions that count as chronic. In this book I will be taking it that chronic illnesses share three features: 1. they are currently incurable, 2. they are not immediately life threatening when appropriate treatment is given, and 3. they are long lasting. That is, as I will be using the term chronic illnesses are ones that people live with, not those from which they are cured.[2] In this section I want to say a bit more about these illnesses and what can be done for those with them. This is necessarily selective. It does not, and does not attempt to, give a comprehensive account of either chronic illness or chronic disease. The aim is rather to highlight those features that will be important for the ethical analysis in the rest of the chapter.[3]

In thinking about both chronic disease and chronic illness it is useful to draw a distinction between the patient as an organism (a body) and the patient as a person (see Richman, 2004; Parens, 2017). To say that chronic diseases cannot be cured is to say that they involve an irreversible change in the organism that affects its functioning.[4] In diabetes, for example, the process by which insulin moves glucose (obtained from food) out of the blood into cells where it is broken down to produce energy ceases to operate effectively. This can happen for three reasons: 1. the body's immune system attacks the insulin producing cells in the pancreas meaning no insulin is produced (type 1 diabetes), 2. the pancreas does not produce enough insulin (type 2 diabetes), or 3. the body cannot effectively use the insulin it does produce (type 2 diabetes). In Parkinson's disease the loss of dopamine producing nerve cells in the substantia nigra (a part of the brain) means that less dopamine is available for the parts of the brain that control movement. That, in turn, means those parts cannot operate as well as they used to. In asthma, inflammation of the tubes that carry air into and out of the lungs can cause them to temporarily narrow. When that happens breathing becomes more difficult. In osteoarthritis the cartilage lining the joints (most commonly those in the hands, spine, knees, or hips) thins and roughens. And, in rheumatoid arthritis the body's immune system targets the joints, which over time can lead to the joint breaking down. None of these physical changes can currently be reversed. It is not possible, for example, to 'fix' the pancreas or replace lost cells in the substantia nigra.[5]

That it is not possible to reverse these changes in the organism, however, does not mean that nothing can be done for the patient as a person. Without treatment many chronic diseases, including asthma and diabetes, can kill. This can happen, for example, when a diabetic's body breaks down fat to obtain energy, releasing ketones, because too much glucose remains in the blood over a long period (known as diabetic ketoacidosis). In these cases emergency interventions are needed to keep the patient alive. But treatment can also mean these life-threatening situations do not occur in the first place—for example, by keeping the diabetic patient's blood glucose levels close to normal. So one thing that can be done for patients with chronic illness is to prevent the underlying disease killing them (or at least make it less likely that it will do so). Even where untreated chronic illness does not directly threaten a patient's life, it can increase their chances of getting other conditions (some of which are themselves life threatening). Diabetes again provides a good example. In most cases untreated type 2 diabetes will not cause diabetic ketoacidosis. But it will increase, sometimes substantially, the risk of (among other things) heart disease, stroke, nerve damage, kidney disease, foot ulcers, sexual dysfunction, and diabetic retinopathy (damage to the retina that can lead to blindness). By keeping a patient's blood glucose levels close to normal these increased risks can be avoided. Doing so does not mean a patient will avoid these problems, but it does prevent their diabetes making them more likely. Here again is something that can be done for at least some patients with chronic illness.

Not all chronic illnesses are life-threatening even if left untreated. Untreated osteoarthritis, for example, will not kill anyone in either the short or long term. But this does not mean nothing can be done for those with these conditions. The symptoms of chronic disease can be debilitating and interfere with the patient's ability to live their life as they choose. Osteoarthritis is painful and makes movement difficult. Asthma causes breathlessness. Parkinson's disease causes tremors, slow movement, and muscle stiffness. In all these cases the patient's illness makes it harder for them to move around, perform everyday tasks, and do the things other people do—things like going to work, visiting friends and family, and living in their own home. Which things it makes harder, and how much harder it makes them, will vary depending on the type of illness and its severity. Whether we are concerned with arthritis, Parkinson's disease, or asthma, the right treatment can (at least to some extent) prevent, alleviate, or minimise these effects. That will not cure the patient as an organism, but may well benefit them as a person. Furthermore, many chronic illnesses—including Parkinson's disease, type 2 diabetes, and rheumatoid arthritis—are progressive, with symptoms getting worse over time. In some cases appropriate action can slow the rate of progression. While that will not benefit the patient in the short term, it may well do so in the long term. Their life in the future will not be as compromised by their illness as it would otherwise have been.

We can now see one way chronic illnesses differ from other conditions—the aims of treatment. With chronic illness the aim is not to cure the patient, nor necessarily to prolong their life. It is to prevent future illness and/or manage the patient's symptoms. Which of these plays the biggest role, and the balance between them, will vary from case to case. For example, prevention may be the main aim when treating a patient with type 2 diabetes, whereas symptom management may be the focus where the patient has asthma. Recognising these different aims should affect how we think about two things: what it is to benefit a patient, and how prevention fits into clinical ethics. Symptom management, as we will see in more detail later, often benefits the patient by making it easier for them to live their life despite being ill. That is, treatment benefits the patient by enhancing their autonomy (on some accounts of autonomy). Linking benefits and autonomy in this way, however, may seem problematic—particularly given the prevalence of accounts, such as the four principles approach, that categorise these as independent and distinct values (Beauchamp and Childress, 2009; Gillon, 2003). In healthcare ethics, accounts of the benefit of treatment have also tended to focus on the short term, rather than on the long term, benefits of preventing future ill health. Discussion of ethics and prevention has to date largely been the preserve of public health ethics (with its focus on healthcare policy). But where treatment *is* prevention a different approach is needed. To date that is not something that ethicists have provided.

If its aims distinguish the treatment of chronic illness, so too does the way it is delivered. While the details vary considerably, in many cases regular (often daily) action is needed over a long period. Much of this action is performed, not by a healthcare professional, but by either the patient or members of the patient's family. A couple of examples will help to illustrate this point. As we have seen treatment for diabetes aims to keep blood glucose levels close to normal. What that requires varies with the type of diabetes, and (in the case of type 2 diabetes) its severity. The amount of glucose in a patient's blood is affected by what they eat and how much exercise they take. For this reason controlling diet (reducing the amount of fat and sugar, increasing the amount of fibre) and exercise have an important role to play in managing diabetes. For some patients with type 2 diabetes they are all that is needed. Where they are not, medication will also be required. While diet and exercise are also important for patients with type 1 diabetes, they also require insulin—delivered either by daily injections or by a pump that allows insulin to flow continuously into the bloodstream. All this requires action and monitoring on a day by day basis. For practical reasons that has to be done by either the patient or members of their family. That does not mean there is no role for healthcare professionals. Both insulin and the medications used to control type 2 diabetes are typically prescription only, and so must be supplied by them. Typically they will also both carry out regular blood tests to monitor how stably blood glucose levels are being maintained, and provide advice and support for patients who are managing their own condition. Finally, they have an important role when things go wrong. If the patient has diabetic ketoacidosis, they will usually need hospital treatment. Where blood glucose levels fall too low (hypoglycaemia) because too much insulin has been injected, immediate action is also needed. While in this case the necessary action will normally be performed by the patient or those close to them (such as family and friends), explaining what to do when this happens is part of the healthcare professional's' role.

As with diabetes the treatment of asthma involves coordinated action by healthcare professionals and patients. And, also as with diabetes, what is required will vary depending on the details of the case, including the severity of the condition. Treatments for asthma aim at either relieving or preventing symptoms (or both). While short-acting reliever inhalers as the name suggests relieve symptoms at the time they occur, prevention requires a different response. The symptoms of asthma, such as breathlessness, are often experienced in response to triggers (things like fur, pollen, cigarette smoke, and sudden changes in the weather). Where a patient's triggers can be identified, avoiding them can help prevent these symptoms. But that is not always possible, and where it is possible it is not always sufficient (even when combined with the use of a short-acting reliever inhaler). In these cases a different type of inhaler, a preventer inhaler or combined preventer and long-acting reliever inhaler, may be needed. Avoiding triggers and using the inhaler are things the patient must do themselves, though the inhalers must be provided by healthcare professionals. For some patients even these methods are not enough. As such, other forms of treatment are needed. Depending on the details these may involve the patient taking tablets every day, being given injections every few weeks, or in a few cases having an operation (bronchial thermoplasty—where some of the muscles around the airways are intentionally damaged by inserting a tube, which is then heated, into the lungs via the mouth or nose).

This brief overview of treatments for two different conditions highlights that treating chronic illness requires a variety of approaches (and we might have seen even more if we had looked at other conditions—for example, physiotherapy is sometimes part of the treatment for Parkinson's disease and rheumatoid arthritis). Some of these—taking blood samples and performing operations—are familiar within both medical and healthcare ethics. Others—enabling and supporting the patient to treat him or herself—are not. It should be possible to slot the former into existing ethics frameworks without too much difficulty. But what about the latter? Can they also be incorporated into those frameworks? As John Harris has pointed out we should not assume that what we say about one type of treatment can be extended to cover other types of treatment (Harris, 1985, p. 63). Furthermore do these different types of treatment even raise any ethically interesting or challenging questions? It is to these questions that we must now turn.

1.3 The Importance of 'When?'

So far I have merely described some features of chronic illnesses. While that was important it does not in itself show there is a gap in the ethics literature. Doing that requires more direct engagement with that literature. For that reason I want to start by looking at a topic that is very familiar in healthcare ethics—consent (or as it is more normally called, 'informed consent'). However I want to approach it from a somewhat unusual angle. My reason for doing so is to highlight some of the problems that occur when we take tools developed to deal with ethical challenges arising in the treatment of acute conditions (where consent is of great importance) and apply them to other areas of healthcare. Doing this will reveal that specific ethical questions and challenges arise when treating patients with chronic illness—ones that can be hard to see with more conventional approaches. It is useful to begin by noting that all medical treatment, whether for acute or chronic conditions, takes place over time and usually involves multiple steps. In both healthcare ethics and medical ethics this process is rarely considered in its entirety. Instead, ethicists jump in at what appear the most ethically salient points. One such point is that at which consent (or informed consent) is obtained. Much work has been done both on why consent (or informed consent) is needed and what is needed for consent (we will look at this in detail in chapter five). But what if we ask instead 'when is consent (or informed consent) needed?'

To answer this question we need to look at what consent does. When I consent to you doing something (as opposed to consenting to do it myself), I make it permissible for you to do it. More formally, for S to consent to T doing X, is for S to have made it permissible for T to do X (Feinberg, 1986, p. 177; Raz, 1986, p. 81; Manson, 2007, pp. 297–298; Owens, 2012, p. 165). While this is the normal way of characterising 'consent', it might be thought to imply that if S has consented to T doing X, it is all things considered permissible for T to do X. That, however, would be a mistake. Suppose Bill has promised Mary that he will not have sex with Sue, and subsequently Sue consents to Bill having sex with her. Sue has genuinely consented, but that does not mean it is morally permissible for Bill to have sex with her. Were he to do so he would be breaking his promise to Mary and that is something he should not do. It is relatively easy to tighten up the definition to avoid this implication. When we do so we get the following: for S to consent to T doing X is for S to have changed the situation from one in which it would be wrong for some reason, R, for T to do X to one in which T's doing X would not be wrong for that reason. This leaves it open whether or not doing X would nevertheless still be wrong all things considered. It is this definition of 'consent' that I will be using in what follows.

If this is what consent is, a person only needs consent when they already have a reason to act—they do not need other people to make it permissible for them to do things they are not going to do anyway. For example, a nurse only needs consent to take a blood sample if she is going to take a blood sample; and a surgeon only needs consent to replace a hip if she is going to replace a hip (something that might be required in the treatment of osteoarthritis).[6] So before healthcare professionals even get to the point of needing consent a decision about what to do must have been made. Who makes that decision—healthcare professional, patient, or both—is itself morally important. If our focus is on consent, the only way to take account of this is to squeeze the issue of who chooses in with consent. Where we are interested in informed consent, rather than simply consent, this may not matter. The term 'informed consent' is frequently used to refer to a particular type of institutional process or procedure (Faden and Beauchamp, 1986, pp. 276–287; Beauchamp, 2011, pp. 517–518).[7] If both choice and consent are important it may make sense for those procedures to aim both at ensuring the patient has a choice over what treatment to have, and at ensuring he has consented to any treatment he is given. To the extent that they have this dual role 'informed consent' covers both choice and consent. But we should not let the terminology here confuse us. In this context 'informed consent' is simply the name of a set of institutional rules. It is neither a particular form of consent (consent that is informed rather than uninformed), nor solely concerned with consent. Because of this, and to avoid possible confusion, I will where possible avoid the term.

Whatever the value of combining consent and choice into one procedure in other contexts, when it comes to chronic illness they must be kept apart. There are two reasons for this. First, as David Owens has argued choosing and consenting perform different tasks (Owens, 2011, 2012). When choosing, a person attempts to determine what will be done (for example, does he have hip replacement surgery or not). To the extent that his choices are enacted they directly affect what happens. In contrast, when he consents he only directly affects what is permissible. Consenting changes the normative landscape so that what was previously wrong for some reason is no longer wrong for that reason. While that might affect what happens, it does so indirectly—removing a normative barrier that prevents the other person doing what the person consenting wants. One of the reasons patients give consent is to remove barriers of this type. For example, when I consent to my doctor giving me a painkilling injection I do so because I want her to give me that injection, and I realise that she will not do so unless I consent.[8] Simply removing that barrier, however, does not mean that what I want to happen (the thing that I have consented to) will happen. All I have done is make it permissible to act, and that something is now permissible does not mean that anyone will do it (and certainly does not mean that anyone has an obligation to do it). That is, while consenting is a way in which patients sometimes attempt to enact their choices, it is distinct from those choices.

The second reason it is important to keep choice and consent apart when thinking about chronic illness is that a person can have chosen a course of action but not consented to it, or consented to it but not chosen it. It might seem odd for someone to consent, to make permissible, an act that they have not chosen (and perhaps do not want the other person to perform). But it need not be. To see how this might happen, consider the following non-medical example. I consent to you taking all the books in the front room but have temporarily forgotten that I left a book I want to keep in that room (I do not remember something that in a sense I know perfectly well, and could have recalled with a little effort).[9] In this case you will have done nothing wrong if you take the book. When I find out what you have done I may kick myself for not thinking before speaking, but it would be inappropriate for me to claim that I did not consent. There is no failure of understanding here of the type that might invalidate my consent—I understand perfectly well that the book is in the front room, I just did not take account of that fact when giving my consent. Something similar is certainly possible when patients make decisions. We need to distinguish between an informed patient (one who understands relevant information) and an informed choice (one made taking account of that information). Informed patients may not always make informed choices, and it is this that leads to the possibility of their consenting to something they have not chosen.

Far more common in healthcare (particularly when it comes to chronic illnesses) are cases where a patient has chosen a certain treatment but not, or not yet, consented to it. Sometimes when a patient visits a healthcare professional the choices he, or they, make are acted on straight away. For example, if in a meeting with the local nurse it is decided to test the patient's blood pressure, she may well carry out that test there and then. In such cases both the choice to have the test, and consent to the actions involved in performing it, happen during the same consultation. Things are different where the illness, or the treatment, is more complex or time consuming. If in a consultation with his oncologist a patient decides to have surgery,[10] he will not get the surgery there and then. Instead a process is initiated that will result in him having surgery at some later date. Furthermore, it is unlikely that the patient's oncologist will perform the surgery. Instead this will be done by a specialist surgeon. It is this surgeon who needs his consent—she (not the oncologist) would be acting wrongly if the surgery were performed without it. In practice, therefore there will be a period during which the patient has chosen surgery but has not yet consented to it. The nature of the interactions the patient has with his oncologist and his surgeon are also different. In his meetings with the former, healthcare professional and patient are concerned with what is to be done. In contrast, by the time the patient arrives for surgery he has already decided what treatment to have—if he had not, or he had decided on something other than surgery, he would not be there. The focus now is on obtaining consent for the proposed surgery. In this example, although the patient has chosen he has not yet consented and his consent is needed. We also need to recognise, however, that sometimes given the nature of the choice made, no consent will be needed. This is easiest to see where the choice is to have no treatment. In general healthcare professionals do not need permission to do nothing. There are, of course, circumstances where doing nothing is wrong. Healthcare professionals have positive obligations (for example to benefit their patients) and doing nothing can mean they are not fulfilling those obligations. But in these cases the reason doing nothing is wrong is not that they do not have the patient's consent.

As we have just seen, focusing on when consent is needed reveals that we need to keep apart two topics that are sometimes conflated: choosing what treatment to give, and consenting to that treatment. This is particularly important when our focus is on chronic illness. That is because consent changes what it is permissible to do. As such, healthcare professionals only need consent for those things that 1. they are going to do, and 2. would be wrong if done without that consent (but not if done with it). While invasive treatments like surgery fit these conditions, the same is not true of all treatments for chronic illnesses. As we have seen, where patients are living with a condition it is common for treatment to be delivered either by the patient himself, or by members of his family.[11] A type 1 diabetic, for example, will need to monitor his blood glucose level, decide how much insulin is needed (taking account of his plans for the day), give himself that insulin, and manage his diet. All on a day to day basis. If he is unable to manage this himself, family members will need to do much of it for him. Family members may also play a role in helping him control his diet (something that is easier if those living with him support his attempts to change; see Vogel, 2016), or as the first line of response if his blood glucose level falls too low. In cases like these healthcare professionals do not need consent because someone else is the one acting, though important questions about treatment choice remain.

Even where a healthcare professional is the one acting, she may not be doing anything for which consent is needed. Suppose a patient's doctor prescribes medication for him to take at home (as will often happen in the treatment of patients with chronic illnesses). In doing so she opens up an opportunity for the patient to treat himself that he did not previously have. This is not a failure to respect his autonomy (on any account of autonomy). So, if (as is standardly held) consent is needed to avoid the wrong of failing to respect autonomy, no consent is needed here. Indeed, if (as writers such as Tom Beauchamp and Neil Levy have argued) respect for autonomy has a positive element, incorporating a requirement to enable or promote autonomy, her actions are precisely what is needed to respect her patient's autonomy (see Beauchamp, 2010b, p. 37; Levy, 2014).[12] This is another case where choice and consent come apart—the patient may have chosen this course of treatment but he has not (indeed, cannot) have consented to it.

In all these cases consent is not needed (though institutional 'informed consent' procedures may still apply). That does not, however, mean they are ethically unproblematic. They can, and often will, pose ethical challenges for healthcare professionals—particularly when treating patients with chronic illnesses. One such challenge, as we have already seen, concerns who makes treatment decisions. Another stems from the fact that patients do not always adhere to agreed treatment plans. This non-adherence can be either intentional or non-intentional—examples of the latter include the patient 1. forgetting to take his medication, 2. using equipment (such as an asthma inhaler) incorrectly, or 3. misunderstanding what he needs to do. It is also common (see, Osterberg and Blaschke, 2005; Ho, Bryson, and Rumsfeld, 2009; Tamblyn et al., 2014). To take just one example, Jackevicius, Li, and Tu found that fewer than a quarter of patients were taking all their cardiac medication just seven days after being discharged from hospital after an acute myocardial infarction (Jackevicius, Li, and Tu, 2008). If a healthcare professional suspects non-adherence and does nothing about it she may be criticised for neglecting her patient. On the other hand, if she tries to intervene to improve adherence she runs the risk of failing to respect his autonomy. So what should she do? And what are the limits to her obligation to try to help her patient here? These are ethical questions. But they only arise in cases where the patient is largely treating himself (or being treated by family members), as is the case with many chronic illnesses. As such, accounts of what healthcare professionals should do developed in response to other types of treatment say nothing about them.

The two topics we have just been looking at (patient choice and helping patients treat themselves) are apt to get missed if we focus only on acute illnesses (and only on consent). However, dealing with them is necessary if we want to know what healthcare professionals should do when treating those with chronic illnesses. While values like beneficence and respect for autonomy will be important when doing this, it will be necessary to rethink what these require. For example, to date medical ethicists (in particular) have characterised what is needed to respect autonomy almost entirely in terms of informed consent (Lysaught, 2004, p. 678). That is not surprising—acting without consent can be a serious wrong—but it is also inadequate. There is more to respecting autonomy than obtaining consent before giving treatment. In addition to those topics already mentioned, it, along with other values, is important when it comes to assessing healthcare professionals' role in giving advice about how to avoid getting or exacerbating chronic illnesses. A person's chances of becoming ill are influenced by what they do. For example, things that increase their weight affect their chances of developing type 2 diabetes (among other things). As we have already seen, prevention is often characterised as a public health issue, and work in public health ethics on behaviour change has for good reasons focused on public policy. But we should not forget the role that frontline healthcare professionals have here, nor the importance of prevention as part of the treatment of at least some chronic illnesses. To fulfil that role healthcare professionals need to provide information and guidance to their patients, but what information should they provide? Existing work in either medical ethics or healthcare ethics is of limited use in answering this question. In general medical ethics texts, for example, it is not unusual to find discussion of what healthcare professionals should tell their patients located in a chapter focused almost entirely on informed consent (see, for example, Harris, 1985, ch.10; Gert, Culver, and Clouser, 2006, ch.9; Beauchamp and Childress, 2009, ch.4). But when it comes to advice, consent is simply not an issue—these are not cases where permission is being either sought or given. It is true that other cases have not been entirely ignored. There has, for example, been extensive discussion about the provision, or withholding, of information about a terminal diagnosis (see, for example, Harris, 1985, pp. 208–212; Beauchamp and Childress, 2009, p. 105). Arguments in favour of providing this information have largely relied on the idea that withholding it would be a failure to respect the patient's autonomy. But that healthcare professionals ought not to withhold certain information does not tell us everything we need to know about what information they ought to provide.

In this section I have identified four types of activity healthcare professionals need to engage in when treating patients with chronic illnesses:

choosing, acting, helping others act, and advising. Some, but not all, are activities they also engage in when treating other types of illness. In the chapters that follow I will take these four activities in this order. It is important, however, to remember two things. First, each activity may recur multiple times during the course of treatment. Second, which of these activities is required will vary depending on the nature of the illness, the patient, and the available treatments. Because some of these topics are familiar from discussions of other areas of healthcare ethics, I will sometimes use examples from those areas to make my point—particularly in chapters two, three, and four. Before we get into the first topic, however, I want to spend the rest of this chapter explaining a bit more about each type of activity and how it will be dealt with in this book.

1.4 Choosing

Choosing comes first. Before a treatment plan can be implemented it must be produced. But who should choose? And what weight should healthcare professionals give to their patients' choices? How we answer these questions depends on our starting point. We could start from healthcare professionals' obligations to benefit, and not to harm, their patients (that is from their obligations of beneficence and non-maleficence). They have to design a plan that will ensure they can fulfil these obligations. Alternatively we could start from the importance of respecting patient autonomy, and argue that it should be up the patient what treatment (if any) he receives. I will take these in turn.[13]

It is uncontroversial that healthcare professionals should not harm their patients. It is equally uncontroversial that they should benefit their patients. To fulfil these obligations healthcare professionals must first work out, for each patient, which of the things they can do would benefit him, and which would harm him. Doing this is not easy when it comes to the treatment of chronic illnesses for three reasons (only one of which has been extensively investigated by healthcare ethicists). First, what happens is not entirely within their control. Whether scheduling surgery will benefit a patient depends both on how well the surgical team perform the operation, and on whether the patient turns up for it at the right time. Similarly, prescribing a course of medication to be taken at home will only benefit a patient if the pharmacist correctly prepares the medication and the patient takes it. As Everett Koop points out, "Drugs don't work in patients who don't take them" (quoted in Ho, Bryson, and Rumsfeld, 2009, p. 3028). So to work out what will benefit her patient a healthcare professional must take account of what other people will do. It may be reasonable for her to assume that other healthcare professionals (the surgical team, the pharmacist) will perform their parts well—the healthcare system will have checks and procedures in place to ensure this. But what the patient will do is a different matter. In most situations the healthcare professional involved can attempt to find this out by asking her patient, or by seeking his agreement that he will do what is required (Walker, 2017).[14] For that to be effective she would also need to tell him what he needs to do, and why he needs to do it (he is unlikely to agree without being given some reason to do so). The requirement to do this is independent of the need to obtain consent as this is conceptualised in healthcare ethics. What is being sought is the patient's agreement that he, the patient, will do certain things—not, as is the case with consent, his permission for someone else to do them.[15] Healthcare professionals also need to remember that, as we saw above, the mere fact that a patient has agreed to a treatment plan does not mean that he will follow that plan. As such, his agreement cannot be taken at face value. How much weight it should be given depends on two things: general evidence about patient behaviour, and information gleaned from past experience with each particular patient. If someone always agrees but rarely does what he says, then his agreement provides little evidence that he will take the steps necessary for his treatment to be effective. On the other hand, if he virtually always does what he says he will, his agreement may be very strong evidence that he will take those steps.

The second source of difficulty is that treatments affect different people in different ways. For example, many, if not most, medications come with possible side effects. Some patients will experience these side effects and others will not. Similarly, how effectively a treatment deals with an underlying medical problem can vary from patient to patient. As such, there will frequently be some uncertainty about how a proposed treatment will affect a given patient. The only way to resolve this uncertainty is to start the treatment, and see what happens (a task that will normally require input from the patient). Because of this, where treatment is ongoing over a reasonable period of time, as it often is in the treatment of chronic illnesses, treatment may be initiated on a provisional basis—doing so is part of the process of determining what is best for the patient. In such cases the decision about what will benefit a patient, and what might harm him, is not a one off. To fulfil her obligations of beneficence and non-maleficence the healthcare professional will need to keep an eye on the effects of treatment and, where necessary, adjust it in response to any new information that arises from the process of delivering it. Doing this can create challenges for the healthcare professionals involved, at least in part because patients may be reluctant to change treatments, preferring the familiar (in part because it is familiar). How healthcare professionals should deal with this depends on what they should do in cases where the patient is treating himself (something that will be covered in chapters six and eight).

Finally, the third source of potential difficulty, and the one that has been more widely discussed in the literature to date, is that while healthcare professionals have expertise in the effects of different treatments on the body, what really matters is how those treatments affect the patient as a person (Richman, 2004, p. 28; Veatch, 2006; Molyneux, 2009). This is not easy for the healthcare professional to assess, and her medical training gives her no special expertise in doing so. The problem is that how treatment affects someone as a person depends on how it affects their way of life, interferes with or promotes their aims, and aligns (or fails to align) with their values. Because these all vary from person to person the effect of treatment on a patient's well-being also varies from person to person. Even something that would completely alleviate the symptoms of a patient's illness can in some circumstances harm him all things considered. For example, in his memoirs Stefan Zweig reports that while living with cancer of the jaw Sigmund Freud,

> did not want the clarity of his mind to be impaired for a single hour by [sleeping pills or pain-killing injections], he preferred to suffer and stay fully conscious, he would rather think while in pain than not think at all.
>
> (Zweig, 2009, p. 449)

While avoiding painkillers might have been best for Freud, having them may well have been best for others. As with the first problem described above, it looks like healthcare professionals have a way around this problem—they should get their patient's input. The patient both knows what is important to him (his goals, his values, and his commitments), and has a lifetime of experience in using that knowledge to make decisions about what to do. He thus appears to have the expertise she lacks. However, he will only be able to effectively use that expertise if he also understands what the treatment involves and the potential consequences of taking it. Without that information he is in no position to accurately assess how taking it would affect him. If this is right, then healthcare professionals have a way to solve the epistemic problem they face. They can provide their patients with relevant information in an understandable form and let them choose what treatment to have. Outsourcing the decision-making process in this way would, on this line of argument, be the most reliable method healthcare professionals have of working out what they should do if they are to satisfy their obligations to benefit, and not harm, their patients.

The argument sketched out here, and I will consider it in much more detail in chapter two, does not rely on the idea that healthcare professionals should respect their patient's autonomy—though it might lead to the same conclusions as arguments based on that requirement. Instead it relies on the idea that a patient, when suitably informed, is a better judge of what will benefit, and what might harm, him than the healthcare professionals treating him. As such, it is related to arguments for informed consent based on the idea that the patient is the best judge of his own interests (see, for example, Molyneux, 2009; Ross, Capozzi, and Matava, 2012; Taylor, 2005a), though it is not itself an argument about consent. All arguments of this type face significant challenges. First, to support the argument we would need to be much clearer about what the relevant decision is—what is it that the healthcare professional is trying to determine, and what is it that the patient is supposed to have more expertise in than her. Second, it relies on the empirical claim that the patient is a better judge of his own interests than the healthcare professional, and this claim has come under sustained assault on the basis of work in the social sciences (for an overview see Kahneman, 2011; or Thaler, 2015). Whether these challenges can be met will be the topic of chapters two and three. There I will argue that sometimes they can, and sometimes they cannot. What is true of some types of medical treatment is not true of others, and we need to recognise this complexity when thinking about what healthcare professionals should do rather than applying a 'one size fits all' approach.

The above argument assumes that the decision about what to do next is the responsibility of the healthcare professional. While it may be that she ought to involve her patient, she is the one who needs to decide what to do. This account of the relationship between healthcare professional and patient has, however, been challenged (see, for example, Veatch, 2006). The decision, it might be argued, is in fact the patient's to make. It should be up to him, not the healthcare professional, what treatment (if any) he receives. The core value at stake here is neither beneficence nor non-maleficence. It is respect for autonomy. While being the one to choose can be instrumentally valuable for patients, for example where they are (or think they are) more likely than anyone else to make the best choice (Dworkin, 1988, p. 112; Scanlon, 1998, pp. 251–252), it is not only valuable for this reason. For those who are autonomous, choice might also be valuable for one or both of two other reasons (one widely discussed in the existing literature and the other not): 1. choice is how we make our lives our own, and 2. being allowed to choose is symbolically important.

As is well known the word 'autonomy' has a variety of meanings (Dworkin, 1988, pp. 3–6; Arpaly, 2003, pp. 117–148; Taylor, 2005b; Stoljar, 2007; Wilson, 2007, pp. 353–356). At its most basic an autonomous individual is one who governs him or herself (Christman and Anderson, 2005, p. 3; Harris, 1985, p. 195; Levy, 2014, p. 298). People exercise this autonomy, to a large extent, by making choices and acting on them. Being the one to choose enables an individual to shape their life in accordance with what matters to them (including their goals, values, and commitments). It means that they are governing themselves, rather than being governed by others; and making their own decisions, rather than other people making decisions for them. It is also the way, according to Gerald Dworkin, that people give meaning to their lives (Dworkin,

1988, p. 108). For all these reasons having an opportunity to choose is valuable—even if people do not always want to exercise it. Suppose this is right. That in itself will not tell us what healthcare professionals ought or ought not to do. Being the one to choose may matter to the patient, but does that mean the choice should be his to make? It is not clear that it does. In choosing a treatment the patient is frequently choosing not only what he will do, or even what will be done to him, but what someone else will do. When he chooses hip replacement surgery, he is choosing that the surgeon (and her team) perform that surgery; when he chooses to have a course of medication, he is choosing that his doctor write the prescription and his pharmacist fill it. More generally, for his choices to be enacted someone else must do as he chooses. It is, however, far from clear that the requirement to respect autonomy, or the recognition that this is important to the patient, requires healthcare professionals to do this. Indeed if our concern is with autonomy as a value such a conclusion would be odd—it requires healthcare professionals to think that their life should be shaped by the decisions of their patients, and thus may require them to subvert their own autonomy in order to respect that of their patients.

There is much to investigate here, and this will form the topic of chapter four. There I will argue that the value of autonomy does not mean that healthcare professionals should allow their patients to choose what treatment (if any) they have. If we want to defend the claim that patients should be allowed to make such choices, we need to turn to a different account of why having a choice is valuable—one based on what Thomas Scanlon calls the symbolic value of choice (Scanlon, 1998, pp. 253–256). To date this account has played little, if any, explicit role in arguments within healthcare ethics. As we will see in chapter four when it comes to the symbolic value of choice what matters is not that choice is a way in which people shape their lives, it is that not allowing people to make choices (particularly where others are allowed, or expected, to do so) sends a message about how they are seen. That message will frequently be demeaning—communicating that they are not thought to be able (or important enough to be allowed) to do what everyone else does. It is because of this, or so I will argue, that patients should have a choice over what treatment they receive.

1.5 Acting

Having chosen someone must act. Who that is will vary from case to case. It might be a healthcare professional (though not necessarily the one who made the choice), the patient, a member of the patient's family, or a volunteer caregiver. Frequently several people will need to act—the patient must turn up for surgery and the surgical team must do their job; the pharmacist must make up the medications and the patient must take them. But even in these cases we can split what needs to be done into things healthcare professionals need to do, and things other people need to do. Where a healthcare professional needs to act she should do so diligently and with due care and attention. Merely doing that, however, is not always enough to avoid wrongdoing. Sometimes to do what she, or her patient, has chosen she needs to do something that would be wrong if done without his consent—this will be the case, for example, where the healthcare professional is going to carry out hip replacement surgery for a patient with osteoarthritis, or take a blood sample from a diabetic patient to test his blood glucose levels.

The literature on consent in healthcare is voluminous. It is also sometimes confusing—at least in part because the focus is usually on informed consent and, as we have seen, that term can refer to either an institutional procedure or an autonomous authorisation. In practice much of the discussion concerns the former. When used in this way 'informed consent' refers to procedures that, at a minimum, require two things: 1. that healthcare professionals obtain the voluntary agreement of a competent patient before acting, and 2. that they obtain this agreement after explaining "the nature, risks, costs, benefits, [and] side-effects" of the proposed treatment to him (Manson, 2007, p. 299). Where these procedures have been complied with the resulting consent is referred to as 'valid' or 'effective' (Beauchamp, 2011, p. 518).

Criticisms of informed consent (in this sense) fall into one of two categories. The first draws on evidence that patients frequently misunderstand what they are told, to argue that it is much harder to get informed consent than might be thought (see, for example, Corrigan, 2003; Dawson, 2004; Iltis, 2006; Hoffman and Del Mar, 2015)—these criticisms will be assessed in chapter three. The second argues that existing informed consent procedures fail to achieve their aims. Their role is to ensure autonomy is respected, and they are flawed given that role. This could be because they protect non-autonomous choices and actions just as much as autonomous ones (O'Neill, 2003, p. 5; Wilson, 2007, p. 354), that they are not sufficient to ensure autonomy is respected (Beauchamp, 2011; Levy, 2014), or that they rule out things that are not wrong on the grounds of failing to respect autonomy (Taylor, 2005a). These critics then either propose ways to improve informed consent procedures (Levy, 2014), or argue that we should rethink what they are for. For example, Onora O'Neill argues that informed consent procedures should aim at ensuring patients are not coerced or deceived (O'Neill, 2003). In contrast, James Stacey Taylor argues that we should think of their purpose as being to promote well-being (Taylor, 2005a). However, that in turn has been challenged on the grounds that informed consent procedures sometimes prevent healthcare professionals doing what would benefit their patients (Dworkin, 2006, pp. 359–360; Sutrop, 2011, p. 376).

I am not going to assess the details of these arguments here (that would take us too far from my aims). But I do want to draw out two points that will be important for later chapters. First, these critics all take informed consent procedures to have an aim—to promote well-being, or to ensure autonomy is respected—though they disagree about what that aim is. In practice, however, procedures can have more than one aim. Informed consent procedures could, for example, aim both at promoting well-being, *and* at ensuring autonomy is respected (Molyneux, 2009; Ross, Capozzi, and Matava, 2012). What those aims are is not only determined by morality. In the development of informed consent procedures the law has played an important role. So much so that, as Tom Beauchamp puts it,

> The law of informed consent has been more influential as an authoritative set of statements and source of reflection than any other body of thought on the subject. "The doctrine of informed consent," as it is sometimes called, *is* the legal doctrine; and "informed consent" has often been treated as synonymous with this legal doctrine . . .
> (Beauchamp, 2010a, p. 66)

Because of this it is not unusual to find that informed consent procedures are shaped so as to help healthcare professionals comply with the law (for a detailed account see Faden and Beauchamp, 1986; and for a more concise summary see Beauchamp, 2010a; or Beauchamp, 2011). As Neil Manson has pointed out one aim of such procedures is to protect healthcare professionals (Manson, 2007, p. 301), and this is how they achieve that aim.

Because the law has been so closely woven into informed consent procedures they cannot safely be transferred either to different jurisdictions (where the law may be different) or to different contexts (where again the law may be different). This can be obscured by claims that consent is needed to respect autonomy, as it might be thought that autonomy should be respected in these other areas too. What all this means is that, given our purposes, entering debates about informed consent is unlikely to be very useful. Informed consent procedures have largely developed in response to cases where healthcare professionals do something to the patient—for example, act directly on his body, use samples obtained from him, or use information about him (see Faden and Beauchamp, 1986; Beauchamp, 2010a). Our concern, however, is with the treatment of chronic illness. While some aspects of that treatment may involve doing something to the patient, and so fall within the scope of the current law, much of it does not. Even where treatment does fall under the law incorporated into informed consent procedures, focusing on those procedures may not be helpful. To uncover what is morally important we would need to untangle the strands of law and morality. Doing that is likely to be more time consuming than addressing the moral issues directly, particularly given that what the law requires varies from country to country.

Second, it is not unusual to conceptualise informed consent procedures as being a source of guidance for healthcare professionals. However, at least some of these procedures have penalties for non-compliance built into them. Those penalties can be severe—extending to losing one's job, one's licence to practice, or both. As we have also seen informed consent procedures often incorporate legal requirements, and there are penalties for not complying with the law. I will refer to those procedures, or parts of procedures, that have penalties attached as 'regulations', and those that do not as 'guidelines'. Whether informed consent procedures are regulations or guidelines matters. If they are the latter, the reasons healthcare professionals should comply with them are independent of their existence. The actions they forbid would be morally impermissible even if they did not exist. Regulations, on the other hand, not only *tell* people what they should do, they *affect* what they should do. If a regulation says that patients must be adequately informed and their consent sought before giving treatment, that itself gives healthcare professionals reason both to provide that information to their patients and seek their patients' consent. They will, for example, have a prudential reason to do so—to act otherwise would be to expose themselves to potentially severe penalties. But they may also have a moral reason to do what the regulation requires. This will be the case if they have voluntarily agreed to be bound by it (as with many institutional and professional codes of conduct). It will also be the case if the regulation incorporates a legal requirement, and healthcare professionals ought morally to obey the law. These reasons are independent of whether or not the things proscribed by the regulations would be morally impermissible in their absence.

Because of this, healthcare professionals may find that in practice they need consent for two distinct reasons. Giving their patients treatment without consent would be wrong both because it fails to respect the patient's autonomy, and because it is forbidden by regulations they (the healthcare professional) should comply with. As such, if they are to avoid wrongdoing they need their patient to make two changes to the normative landscape: he must bring it about that in giving treatment they are not acting wrongly by 1. failing to respect his autonomy, or 2. failing to comply with regulations they ought to comply with. I will refer to these as 'non-regulatory consent' and 'regulatory consent' respectively. The requirements for regulatory consent and those for non-regulatory consent need not be the same (that they are not is behind many of the criticisms of informed consent outlined earlier). What is needed for the former is in many cases laid down in informed consent regulations (however as we will see in chapter five these are not the only regulations governing what healthcare professionals do, nor the only ones that impose a requirement to obtain consent on them). Standardly, this means that for a patient to give regulatory consent he must be competent, be acting voluntarily, and have substantial understanding of what is to be done and the risks and benefits of doing it. One reason for thinking that things are different when it comes to non-regulatory consent is that these requirements are too easy to meet. A patient's doctor is both competent and likely to have the specified level of understanding. But when she voluntarily agrees to that patient having treatment she is not consenting. She cannot. And the reason she cannot has nothing to do with her competence, her understanding, or the voluntariness of her actions. Something else is needed. In the case of regulatory consent this is provided by the way the regulations are written. They specify who consent is needed from—for example, they may specify that it is needed from the patient if he is a competent adult, or his parents if he is a child. As such, these people, and only these people, can make the required change in the normative landscape. This explanation is not available in the case of non-regulatory consent (as by definition there is no written regulation). So we must look elsewhere. What we need to explain is why, if the patient is autonomous, he alone can make it permissible to give him treatment. If we stick with the idea that consent is needed to avoid the wrong of failing to respect autonomy, then doing so requires adopting something like a sovereignty account of autonomy (as argued for by Joel Feinberg [Feinberg, 1986, pp. 49–51] and Arthur Ripstein [Ripstein, 2006]). On such accounts for someone to be autonomous is precisely for them to have authority over things—like what is done to their body and with their information—that others do not. In contrast accounts of autonomy that conceptualise it in terms of a capacity will not make the required distinction between the patient and his doctor—she has that capacity just as much as he does.

Recognising that patients, at least when autonomous, have an authority others lack affects what healthcare professionals should do when treating those with chronic illness. As such, we need to determine what it is that patients have this authority over. That is no easy task. But as we will see in chapter five it is unhelpful to think of their authority as relating specifically to treatment—it is both wider and narrower than that. Thinking about patients' authority to make things permissible also raises other questions that need to be answered. Is that authority absolute, as Joel Feinberg argues (Feinberg, 1986, pp. 47–97)? And does a person need to understand the risks and benefits of a treatment in order to exercise his authority to make it permissible? At first sight it is not clear that he does. If he has this authority, he should be able to exercise it however much or little he understands. But perhaps he only has the required authority if he has sufficient understanding. Given that to be autonomous is simply to have this authority, that would mean he is not autonomous unless he has that understanding. But if he is not autonomous, then it would not be wrong on the grounds of failing to respect his autonomy to give him treatment without his consent. As such, those treating him would not need his consent anyway (except to comply with regulations). Something has gone wrong here. In chapter five I will set about untangling it as part of working out when healthcare professionals treating those with chronic illnesses need consent and what they need consent for.

1.6 Helping Others Act

Where the patient is the one who must act, consent is not an issue. A diabetic, for example, does not need anyone to make it permissible for him to give himself an injection. However, that it is the patient who must act does not mean those treating him have no obligations. New obligations will arise when either 1. the treatment plan is not working as effectively as hoped, or 2. changing circumstances mean the current treatment might no longer be the right treatment.

As we saw earlier, because both a treatment's effectiveness and its side effects can vary from person to person, it does not always produce as much benefit as anticipated. Detecting this frequently requires patient input. However, patients do not always know what indicates something is wrong, and what is normal given the treatment they are on. As such, healthcare professionals need to ensure their patients know this. Doing so is part of ensuring that their actions (the treatment plan they have initiated) benefit, and do not harm, their patients. Another reason treatment might not be producing the anticipated benefits is that the patient is not following the agreed treatment plan. Where this is intentional he will know that he is not doing so (though he may not have told those involved in his treatment); where it is unintentional he might not. He thinks he is taking his medication at the times and in the doses required, but he is not. He thinks that he is using his asthma inhaler correctly, but he is not. He thinks that he is adjusting his insulin levels adequately to take account of the amount of exercise he is doing, but he is not. As such, he is not in a position to explain to his doctor the cause of the problem. He is as much in the dark about that as she is. In some cases there are things that healthcare professionals can do to minimise the chances of this happening. They could, for example, check that the asthma patient can use his inhaler properly before he starts using it (and repeat this any time he moves to a new type of inhaler). But it is very unlikely that unintentional non-adherence can be completely avoided in this way.

How then should the healthcare professional proceed? If she becomes aware that the treatment plan is not working as well as expected, she cannot simply ignore it. Doing so would be incompatible with her obligation to benefit her patient. But equally she cannot forcibly intervene in his life. Attempting to take over from him, or to micromanage his treatment, can express a view that the patient is just not up to it (particularly if done with an exasperated 'oh, just let me do it' attitude). It both tells him that he is not good enough and interferes with his freedom to live his life on his own terms. And that is not compatible with treating him with the respect he is owed. Resolving these conflicting pressures is challenging.

One reason for this is that, as we have seen, untreated chronic illness can make it harder for people to pursue their goals, fulfil their commitments, and live their life in the way they would choose. It is tempting to describe this by saying that their illness compromises or diminishes their autonomy, and that is how many writers do describe it. However, it is important to see that in this sense, 'autonomy' (what is sometimes called 'personal autonomy') does not mean the same as it did when we were talking about consent in section 1.5 above. Being ill does not (except where it renders a person incompetent) compromise or diminish anyone's authority to make things permissible. Their standing to consent, and the need to obtain their consent, are not affected by the fact that they are ill. The term 'autonomy' here refers to a person's capacity, or ability, to shape their life in accordance with what matters to them. There is nothing wrong with using it in this way, indeed doing so is common in healthcare ethics (see Harris, 1985, p. 195; Dworkin, 1988, p. 108; Levy, 2014, p. 298; O'Neill, 2002, p. 23). But having the same word mean two different things, both of which are important, opens the door to considerable misunderstanding if we are not careful. For this reason I will generally only use the term 'autonomy' to refer to a person's capacity to affect the way their life goes. When talking about sovereignty accounts of autonomy I will use 'authority' or 'sovereignty' instead.

If chronic illness compromises a person's personal autonomy, it can also have a negative effect on his well-being (Kelleher, 2014, p. 27). As such, there are two ways of thinking about what healthcare professionals are, or should be, trying to do when treating their patients. We can, as outlined earlier, think of them as aiming to benefit their patients (Cullity, 2007, p. 19; Beauchamp and Childress, 2009, pp. 206–207). Alternatively, we can think of them as aiming to counteract the way illness impairs their patients' autonomy (see Richman, 2004; and for a related view about the aims of public health policy see Owens and Cribb, 2013, p. 269). The two are clearly linked. As David Molyneux points out,

> the benefit that medicine brings often operates through an increase in autonomy—for example, the benefits of a hip replacement come from not just the cessation of pain, but the mobility that allows patients to start controlling their lives again.
> (Molyneux, 2009, p. 246)

Treatment for chronic illness does not cure the patient, but it does enable him to get on with his life. Perhaps not to the extent that he could if he were not ill, but at least to a greater extent than he could if he were not treated. It is at least in part because treatment enables people to do this that we think of it as a benefit. Because of this it would perhaps be a mistake to characterise the conflict outlined at the start of the previous paragraph as being solely between respect for autonomy and beneficence (particularly if we take the requirement to respect autonomy to include a requirement to promote or enable it). Instead it may be more illuminating to conceptualise the problem as a conflict between enabling the patient to be more autonomous in the long term, and respecting his autonomy in the short term. How this conflict should be handled has received little attention (but see Levy, 2014). The main exception to this is work on pre-commitment devices in the treatment of those with certain types of mental illness (see, for example, Elster, 2003; Robertson, 2003; Andreou, 2008; Brock, 2003; Dresser, 1982; Davis, 2008; Spellecy, 2003; Walker, 2012a). While the problems here are different, drawing on that literature can perhaps provide a way into resolving them.

In addressing these problems we also have to think about where, if at all, healthcare professionals' responsibilities end. Where the patient is actively involved in managing and treating his own condition he is not merely a patient. He is also an agent. Treatment will only succeed if both he and the healthcare professionals treating him do their part. As such, we might reasonably ask whether those healthcare professionals have a continuing obligation to help him where he persistently fails to do so. Suggesting they might not, is likely to be controversial—shouldn't healthcare professionals do everything they can to help their patients? But we need to guard against two things here: 1. setting up an unrealistic ideal, and 2. ignoring the patient's agency. With autonomy comes responsibility. If people are governing their own lives, deciding what to do in the light of what is important to them, this cannot be avoided. That does not necessarily mean that they should be blamed or held to account when things go wrong. Instead it means that they cannot rely entirely on others. Where a patient is having surgery it may be reasonable to think that it is the responsibility of the surgeon and her team to ensure the treatment is performed successfully. In contrast, where treatment is co-operative it would be odd to place responsibility entirely on the shoulders of one of those involved. Indeed, to do so risks perpetuating a hierarchical relationship between healthcare professional and patient. It is reasonable to expect the parents of a young child to help him again and again despite the fact he continually fails to do what he has agreed to do. It is much less clear that competent adults can reasonably expect other people to do likewise when they similarly fail to stick to their part of the agreement.[16] Raising this topic takes us onto contentious ground. But it cannot be avoided. As we will see in chapter six how we deal with it depends in large part on how we conceptualise the role of both healthcare professionals and patients when it comes to treating chronic illnesses.

In that chapter I will argue that it is a mistake to think of these roles in isolation from each other. It is easy to think of healthcare professionals and patients purely as individuals, each of whom is pursuing their own aim (to help their patient and to get appropriate treatment respectively).

But when thinking about the treatment of chronic illness it is more useful to think of them as working together to achieve a common aim (captured in the patient's treatment plan). Doing so has several advantages. To begin with, it highlights the fact that in cases of chronic illness the patient is typically an integral, and essential, part of the treatment team. How extensive his role is will, of course, vary from case to case—depending both on what is required and on what he can do. But in many cases treatment will simply be impossible without his active input. The patient must therefore be treated as a member of the team, and accorded the respect owed to him as such. That means he needs to be recognised as an agent, rather than thought of simply as a patient. Doing this may be particularly important where the patient is an older adult (as many of those with chronic illness are). Given the existence in most countries of widespread negative attitudes about the capabilities of older people (World Health Organization, 2015, pp. 10–11), attitudes that conceptualise the old as incapable, there is a significant risk that their role in managing their own illness will be missed. That can result in a failure to treat them with the respect they are owed. Of course, some of those in this age group have severe cognitive and/or physical impairments that significantly restrict what they can do. The impact of that on healthcare professionals' obligations when treating patients with chronic illness will be considered throughout the coming chapters. But most of those with chronic illness, including most older patients with chronic illness, do not fall into this category. They either have no such impairment or have an impairment that does not render them completely incapable of playing an active role in their own treatment.

Conceptualising treatment of chronic illness as a shared activity also affects what we say about healthcare professionals' responsibilities in cases of patient non-adherence. If we focus solely on the individual actions of healthcare professionals and patients, interventions to improve patient adherence are likely to appear unacceptably paternalistic. They will look like cases in which a healthcare professional attempts to bring it about that her patient does what she (the healthcare professional) thinks is best for him (the patient), and in which she does so because she thinks that that is what is best for him. Furthermore, any failure to adhere will appear to be the patient's sole responsibility. That in turn might be thought to affect what he is owed if, as is likely, his non-adherence negatively affects his future health. In particular, it might be argued that he should receive lower priority for treatment than those who are not responsible for their condition.

Drawing on work in the philosophy of joint action (Bratman, 1993, 2014; Gilbert, 2014; Searle, 1990; Velleman, 2000) I will argue that there is a way to respond to both these concerns. The fact that patients are working with the healthcare professionals treating them to achieve a common aim both places obligations on those involved, and changes the dynamic of their relationship. The problem caused by non-adherence ceases to be that the non-adherent patient is not being benefitted (a framing that presents it as a problem for the healthcare professionals involved, and one that they need to solve). Instead the problem is that non-adherence gets in the way of healthcare professionals and patients achieving their shared aim. That, in turn, affects how we conceptualise interventions aimed at improving adherence. These are no longer cases where a healthcare professional is intervening to achieve her own aims, but rather ones where she acts with the intention of bringing the shared activity back on track. I argue in chapter six that this means such interventions are not problematically paternalistic. That healthcare professionals and patients are engaged in a shared activity also affects what the latter are owed where they do not adhere. It would be incompatible with the obligations entailed by that shared activity to respond to such non-adherence by withdrawing future help. That would guarantee its aims are not achieved. That in turn, or so I will argue in chapter six, affects what we should say about patient responsibility and the allocation of healthcare resources.

Taking this approach also reveals that in many cases the people who are acting together to manage a patient's illness, or to deliver treatment, are not just the patient and the various healthcare professionals involved in his care. Family members are also frequently important members of this team. That is most obvious where the patient is either a young child or an adult with significant mental or physical impairments (as will be the case with some older patients with chronic illness), though it is not restricted to such cases. Like patients, these other people can fail to adhere, and like patients they can do so either intentionally or non-intentionally. Determining what healthcare professionals should do when this happens requires paying close attention to the role of the family (or other volunteer carers) in the delivery of treatment—something that is particularly important in the treatment of chronic illness given the nature of that treatment and the demographics of those who need it. That will, in turn, lead us into considerations of when information about the patient can permissibly be shared with those non-professionals involved in their care—something that needs to be done if they are to help the patient. Because medical information is typically either confidential or private, there is a general presumption against sharing it. But that presumption does not apply in all cases, and can get in the way of providing high quality care. Navigating these issues requires detailed consideration of why, and when, sharing medical information is wrong. These two topics (carer non-adherence, and confidentiality/privacy) will form the substance of chapter seven.

So far in this section the focus has been on what happens when an agreed treatment plan is not working as well as expected. But healthcare professionals also need to take account of the possibility that the plan needs to be changed to reflect changing circumstances. Examples of where they might need to do this include:

- There is a change in the patient's ability to treat himself. This could be due to features of the treatment (as a result of treatment the patient can now do things he previously could not). It could be due to the patient's illness (despite treatment the patient's condition has continued to decline and is now interfering with his ability to treat himself, or his illness has caused other health problems that in turn interfere with these abilities). Or it could be due to things that are independent of both the illness being treated and the treatment for it (for example, the patient's mental capacities have declined due to the onset of dementia).
- There is a change in external conditions that mean the treatment needs to be adjusted (for example, pollen levels rising in the case of a patient with severe asthma).
- The patient develops a new condition that potentially interacts with either his existing one or the treatment for his existing one. This is not unusual among older patients, who frequently develop more than one chronic illness (known as multimorbidity). In Germany, for example, it is estimated that 24% of those between 70 and 85 have five or more diseases at the same time (World Health Organization, 2015, p. 26).
- The patient has been assisted in caring for himself by someone who is not a healthcare professional and that assistance is no longer available (his care-giver has become too ill to continue, or has moved away, or has died).
- A new treatment has been developed for the patient's condition. While the treatment he is currently on was the best available, this may no longer be the case. However, given that treatments have different effects on different patients, it is unclear whether the new treatment really would be better for him all things considered.

Whether the treatment needs to be altered, and if so how, requires a decision. It thus returns us to the problems outlined in section 1.4 above. In doing so, however, it also introduces new questions. For example, healthcare professionals may need to decide whether it really is the case that the treatment needs to be changed, or whether it would be better to deal with (or help the patient deal with) those factors that may interfere with its effectiveness. That in turn raises questions about the scope of healthcare professionals' obligations—ones that we will not be able to answer until we have clarified what healthcare professionals should be aiming to do when treating those with chronic illnesses.

In contrast to the voluminous work on ethics and consent, the topic of assisting patients to treat themselves has been substantially ignored by

28 *The Problem*

ethicists. That is not because it raises no important or challenging questions. As we have seen it does. To address these questions we need to get clearer about what healthcare professionals' obligations are. We will also need to pay close attention to the temporal aspects of illness and its treatment. For example, we will need to consider how the long term effects of short term interventions affect what healthcare professionals should do. Finally, we will need to consider the ways in which treatment is provided. Assistance can be given in ways that are supportive and respectful, or in ways that are intrusive, heavy handed, and dominating. This matters ethically. Addressing all these issues will be the task of chapters six, seven, and eight.

1.7 Advising and Preventing

Healthcare professionals give treatment to their patients and help those patients treat themselves. But that is not all they do. They also tell their patients, among other things, how to identify the early signs of illness (for example, how to carry out self-diagnoses for breast or testicular cancer); how to reduce their chances of becoming ill or their illnesses becoming worse (by making changes to their diet or by doing more exercise); and how activities (such as smoking) they are either engaging in, or may start to engage in, could affect their health. This type of work is important in managing, controlling, and preventing chronic illness. At first sight there is nothing morally problematic about any of it. But is there a positive obligation to provide some, or all, of this information? If there is, what explains that and how much information do healthcare professionals have an obligation to provide?[17] We will answer these questions in chapter eight.

As we have already seen, existing work on healthcare professionals' obligations to disclose information to patients has focused on two things: what is required for informed consent; and the connection between withholding information and failing to respect autonomy. The former is not relevant here, and it is doubtful that the latter covers everything that matters. There is a difference between saying 'Mary withheld information from Joe' and saying 'Mary did not give information to Joe'. The former, unlike the latter, implies that Mary chose not to give Joe the information. It is that choice, and the reasons behind it, that mean withholding information is sometimes incompatible with respecting autonomy. As such, that healthcare professionals should not withhold information from their patients, does not reveal much about what they have a positive obligation to tell them (see Gert, Culver, and Clousen, 2006, p. 37).

In uncovering those positive obligations we might start by turning to the idea that healthcare professionals ought to enable their patients to be more autonomous. As a general rule the more relevant information a person has, the more autonomous (the more able to effectively shape

The Problem   29

their life according to their plans, values, and commitments) they are (Harris, 1985, p. 198; Beauchamp, 2005, p. 316). If this is right and if healthcare professionals have an obligation to enable their patients to be more autonomous, the former would have an obligation to tell the latter anything that they (the healthcare professionals) know that might be relevant for their (the patients) future choices. But that is not all. Healthcare professionals would also have an obligation to disclose information (such as that about a terminal diagnosis) that might indicate a change in the patient's circumstances, and thus that the patient may need to rethink what he is going to do.

While such an approach may initially look promising it faces two problems. First, it is potentially very demanding. Healthcare professionals would have an obligation to tell their patients everything that might be relevant to a patient's future decisions, and that could be anything at all. Second, in some situations it is strongly counterintuitive. When we are focused on treatment we tend to think that healthcare professionals should tell their patients about both the risks and benefits of different options. But when we are focused on prevention we tend to think something different. Perhaps healthcare professionals should tell their patients about the risks of drinking heavily, but they have no obligation to tell their patients about the pleasure some people get from drinking heavily. That is, in this context people generally see nothing wrong with healthcare professionals providing a partial, and one sided, picture. However, if the reason patients should be told relevant information is that this promotes their autonomy, it *is* wrong—healthcare professionals are not providing, and may be deliberately withholding, information that would enable their patients to be more autonomous. If in some contexts (treatment decisions) healthcare professionals have an obligation to ensure their patients know about both the risks and benefits of things they might choose to do, why is it that in other contexts (preventative medicine) there is no such obligation? At first sight it is not clear how an account based on an obligation to enable patients to be more autonomous can answer this question. Doing so is important, however, particularly in the context of treating chronic illness—because in that context treatment sometimes is prevention.

The above might suggest that respect for autonomy is not the operative value here, and I will argue in chapter eight that it is not. Perhaps, instead, what is important is that providing information to patients is a way to benefit them. That would seem to capture many people's intuitions about the heavy drinking case. However, it is not clear that it can explain their different responses to the treatment and prevention cases. It also involves a judgment about what is best for, or what would benefit, the patient all things considered. To say that healthcare professionals should disclose information that would benefit their patients, or would help the patient to choose the option that would be best for him, is to presume that healthcare professionals can identify this information. But, as we saw in section 1.4 above, it is not clear that healthcare professionals are in a suitable epistemic position to make such judgments. That a patient's long term health might be improved if he avoids certain activities, does not necessarily mean that he would be better off all things considered if he avoids them. That depends on details of his life—details that the healthcare professionals treating him are unlikely to have.

Untangling these issues is the topic of chapter eight. There I will argue that while healthcare professionals have an obligation to tell their patients how to protect their future health, this is not because they have an obligation to enable their patients to be more autonomous. It is instead for a combination of two reasons. First, healthcare professionals (like everyone else) have a duty to warn. They should tell their patients about the risks associated both with the patient's current behaviour, and with things they have reason to think the patient may do. This obligation falls on them because they have this information and it is likely that the patient does not. Second, where healthcare professionals and patients are acting together, as described above, sharing information is sometimes necessary if they are to achieve their common goal. Where a healthcare professional has such information, she will thus have good reason to pass it on to her patient. It is a combination of these two reasons that explains why healthcare professionals have obligations to give their patients the kinds of information listed above. But those obligations are limited, and there is consequently a limit on what information front line healthcare professionals should be required to give their patients.

1.8 Conclusion

The aim of this chapter has been to show that the treatment of those with chronic illnesses requires sustained ethical attention. It is not possible simply to extend what has been said about the treatment of other kinds of condition—acute or terminal illnesses—to these cases. Doing so would miss much that is ethically important. This is not to say that that other work is not useful. It is. But it needs to be adapted and supplemented if it is to give us a complete account of what healthcare professionals should do. Having identified the need for this, we now need to make a start at meeting that need. We do so by first looking at the important issue of choice.

Notes

1 In doing so the focus will be on individual healthcare professionals in the world as it is. For that reason I will not be addressing questions about what resources should be made available for treating patients with chronic illness. While that is a significant question, individual healthcare professionals must work with what they have. It is what their obligations are in that situation that is the concern here.

2 This account might appear to incorporate disabilities as chronic illnesses, and much has been written in the healthcare ethics literature about disabilities. It will only do so, however, if disabilities are illnesses. I do not intend to enter that debate here. Suffice it to say the focus of this book is not on disabilities, it is on diseases like diabetes, Parkinson's disease, asthma, cancer, and arthritis.

3 In this section I will be providing a brief overview of five chronic illnesses: asthma, diabetes, Parkinson's disease, osteoarthritis, and rheumatoid arthritis. Information about these, their symptoms, and the available treatments is provided in summary form by both the National Health Service in the United Kingdom (www.nhs.uk/conditions/) and the Centers for Disease Control and Prevention in the United States (www.cdc.gov/DiseasesConditions/). The available treatments will in practice vary from country to country.

4 Talk of the functions of the body, and even more so of parts of it, raises its own questions (something explored in depth by Tim Lewens; see Lewens, 2015). Here I am using the term in a non-technical sense.

5 Characterising chronic diseases in this way is to adopt a value neutral approach. As such, it has strong affinities with naturalistic accounts of 'health' and 'disease', such as those proposed by Christopher Boorse (Boorse, 1977, 1997). On Boorse's account a 'disease', or more recently a 'pathology', is an impairment of normal biological function (relative to an individual of the same gender and age), and 'health' is the absence of disease (Boorse, 1997, pp. 7–8). I do so because this is the account that is prevalent in medical practice (Venkatapuram, 2011, pp. 44–48)—indeed Boorse's aim in developing his account has been to understand and clarify the concepts implicit in that practice (Boorse, 2011; see also Lewens, 2015, p. 181). Characterising chronic illness in this purely descriptive way means that more work is needed to show that it is normatively significant (Lewens, 2015, pp. 175–202). In what follows I do this by arguing that alleviating and preventing the symptoms of chronic illness benefits the patient, and that healthcare professionals have an obligation to benefit their patients. It might, however, be thought that characterising chronic illness in this way is a mistake. In everyday usage terms like 'health', 'disease', and 'illness' are not normatively neutral—health is good, and disease and illness are both bad. To capture that idea a different kind of account is needed, one that builds values into the meaning of these terms. For this reason, among others, naturalistic accounts like Boorse's have been challenged. The alternative is to adopt a normative account. Whilst naturalistic accounts characterise disease in terms of biological impairment or malfunction, normative accounts do so in terms of welfare or 'badness' (see Lewens, 2015, p. 176). And while naturalistic accounts characterise health as the absence of disease, normative accounts do not limit it in that way. According to Nordenfelt, for example, "A is in health if, and only if, A has the ability, given standard circumstances, to realize his vital goals, i.e. the set of goals that are necessary and together sufficient for his minimal happiness" (Nordenfelt, 1987, p. 97). On this kind of normative account we would need to characterise chronic illness in a different way—for example, by saying that it compromises the patient's health by making it harder for him in normal circumstances to realise his vital goals (though this will not distinguish chronic illnesses from things like poverty). I do not intend to enter this debate about how best to characterise 'health', 'disease', or 'illness'. As we will see (in chapter six) what follows for healthcare professionals' obligations is in practice remarkably similar whichever route we take.

6 In this book I will be focusing on situations involving two people: a healthcare professional and a patient. Talking about such situations is clearer if the

32   *The Problem*

people involved are of different genders. For that reason in this chapter, and in all odd numbered chapters, the healthcare professionals will be female, and the patients male. In chapter two, and all even numbered chapters, things will be reversed so that the healthcare professionals are male and the patients female.

7 The term 'informed consent' is also used is to refer to an autonomous authorisation. That is closer to the way I am using 'consent'—it is something that makes an act morally permissible. But in that case it is unclear what the word 'informed' adds. By definition all consent makes an act permissible, not just consent that is informed. It may be that only acts that are informed can be cases of consent—but in that case the 'informed' is telling us something about what is needed for consent, not telling us something about the type of consent that is needed.

8 This means that steps that make consenting harder (as in more stringent institutional consent procedures) not only place restrictions on what healthcare professionals may do, they also make it harder for patients to get the treatment they want. Whether it is justifiable to do this is sometimes missed in discussions of consent because the focus is on the healthcare professional not the patient.

9 This example comes from Keith Frankish.

10 Given the account of chronic illness developed here, some cancers count as chronic illnesses.

11 The family member might in fact be a healthcare professional—as when a nurse is looking after her sick son—but in these cases they are not acting in the role of healthcare professional.

12 Whether respecting autonomy has this positive aspect may be doubted. I will argue in chapter eight that it does not.

13 In medical practice there has been a shift to thinking in terms of shared decision making (see, for example, Coulter and Collins, 2011; Cribbs and Donetto, 2013; Edwards and Elwyn, 2009; Elwyn, Tilburt, and Montori, 2013; Godolphin, 2009; Friesen-Storms et al., 2015). While what this means in practice is not always clear, in general it picks out a middle way between two contending positions: that healthcare professionals alone should make decisions, and that patients should get the treatment they want. It does so by drawing on, and combining, the values of benefitting patients and respecting their autonomy. The approach taken here thus addresses, albeit indirectly, the reasons for thinking that decision making should be shared. Furthermore, as we will see, it reaches the same conclusion (with some exceptions). But that can only be the conclusion of the argument, it cannot be the starting point. Given our concerns there are three reasons we need to start from the specific obligations of healthcare professionals. First, it keeps attention squarely on what matters for our purposes—what should the healthcare professional *qua* healthcare professional do. Second, it enables us to clarify what it means to say that decision making should be shared, where it should, in a way that is grounded in healthcare professionals' obligations. Third, it enables us to see where and when shared decision making is important, and where it is not.

14 Alternatively if he is a child she could seek his parents' agreement that either they or he will do what is required.

15 In English both of these could be described as consenting, but to avoid confusion I will only use this term to refer to the latter

16 Where moral theorists have addressed what is required of us where someone else is not doing their part, they have normally been concerned with failures to help third parties (see, for example Singer, 1972; Unger, 1996). In

particular they have investigated situations where the cost to each of us will be low if we all do our part to help those in need, but would be very high if the entire cost fell on a few people. The situation I am concerned with here is different. It is a case, to adapt one of Singer's examples, where walking past a pond I see you drowning. I throw you a life belt and pull you to the shore. I explain to you where to get buoyancy aids that will prevent this happening again (I even give you them). The next day as I walk past I see you drowning again, you have left the buoyancy aids at home. I pull you out, and explain how to avoid this happening again (I give you some more buoyancy aids). Next week I walk past I see you in trouble again (yet again you have not taken the buoyancy aids with you). I pull you out, I explain how to avoid this. And so on, week after week. Am I obliged to keep doing this indefinitely? Or does there come a point where I am no longer required to do so?

17 Healthcare professionals may have contractual obligations to provide some or all of this information to their patients, but that is not my focus here.

2 Working Out What Will Benefit Patients

2.1 Introduction: The Epistemic Argument

Healthcare professionals' obligations are often expressed in highly abstract terms—for example, that they should benefit, and should not harm, their patients (see Beauchamp and Childress, 2009; Gillon, 2003). To fulfil these obligations a healthcare professional must first work out, for each of his patients, what in practice this requires (Kelleher, 2014, p. 32). As we saw earlier doing this is difficult. It requires him to assess both what other people (including his patient) will do in the future, and how different treatments will affect his patient as a person (rather than simply as an organism). He can only do that with any degree of accuracy if he knows how the patient is likely to behave and what matters to her (her goals, her values, her commitments). In practice he is unlikely to know this in the required level of detail. How, then, should he proceed?

Here I want to investigate an answer to this question that has two parts. First, there are several ways healthcare professionals could try to work out what to do, not all of which will be available on every occasion and not all of which will be appropriate in every context (they may, for example, vary depending on the local culture). These include working it out by themselves, consulting with colleagues, asking the patient, asking the patient's family, and tossing a coin. Some of these methods are more likely than others to lead to actions that will benefit and not harm the patient. The first part of the answer is thus that when healthcare professionals are attempting to work out what will benefit or harm their patients they should use the most reliable method of doing so available to them. This will not guarantee that they always do what will benefit their patients, nor does it guarantee that they will never harm them. No method will get the right answer on every occasion. But it does mean that they have the highest chance of doing so. Using the most reliable method also protects the healthcare professional if things go wrong. A healthcare professional who decides what to do by tossing a coin is open to criticism in a way that one who attempts to work out what is best for his patient using a more reliable method is not.

Second, where the patient is a competent adult the most reliable method of working out what will benefit, or harm, her is to tell her what the different treatments involve (including any benefits or side effects) and let her decide. According to John Stuart Mill each competent person has a better understanding of how different options will affect them (how they will interfere with or promote their goals, projects, or values) than anyone else (Mill, 1859/1974, p. 143). A patient thus has at least some of the information the healthcare professionals treating her lack. She also has considerable experience in making decisions about what to do in the light of her situation and the things that are important to her. As such, she is (at least once she has been informed about the different treatments available) in a better position to make the required assessment than those healthcare professionals, and so is more likely than them to choose the treatment that is best for her (Coggon and Miola, 2011, p. 544). Indeed if we adopt an informed preference satisfaction account of well-being, what she would choose in these circumstances is what is best for her as a person (Richman, 2004, pp. 109–110; Higgs, 2006, p. 615).

This does not cover all cases. A young child, for example, is unlikely to be a good judge of what is in her own best interests. However, in general her parents will be good judges of this (see Archard, 2007, pp. 312, 317). They understand their child and what is her interests in a way that the healthcare professionals treating her do not. As such, providing them with relevant information and letting them choose is likely to be a reliable way of determining what is best for her. Parents can play that role because they know their child well and care about her wellbeing. The same is frequently true of those caring for adults who cannot make decisions for themselves—as some patients with chronic illness cannot. They also know the person they are caring for well and have her best interests at heart. By parity of reasoning, therefore, where an adult patient is unable to make decisions for herself, healthcare professionals should provide information about available treatments to those caring for her and find out what treatment they think best. This gives them evidence about what will benefit or harm their patient they would otherwise lack.[1] This is not to ignore the fact that some carers of adult patients are not motivated solely by the patient's wellbeing. But we should not overstate this problem. The same is true of some parents and that is not taken to undermine the idea that parents should generally both be told about treatments available for their children and have a say in what treatment their children receive.[2]

If we put all this together we end up with the following argument:

1. Healthcare professionals should both benefit and avoid harming their patients.[3]

2. Where there is more than one way to work out what will benefit, or harm, a patient, healthcare professionals should use the most reliable available method.
3. The most reliable method for determining what will benefit, or harm, a patient is (a) where she is a competent adult to give her information about possible treatments (e.g. what each involves, their benefits and costs, and any risks involved) and let her choose or (b) where she is not a competent adult to give those caring for her that information and let them choose.
4. Therefore, healthcare professionals should provide information about possible treatments to (a) the patient where she is a competent adult, or (b) to her carers if she is not. They should then do what she, or they, choose on the basis of this information.

This is the epistemic argument for giving information to patients or their family members, and letting them choose what treatment to have. Your reaction to it is likely to depend (at least in part) on which examples come most easily to mind. If you focus on difficult cases—for example, whether or not a cancer patient should have chemotherapy—it may seem plausible. On the other hand, if you focus on cases where a patient wants treatment that will not benefit her—for example, where she asks for antibiotics to treat a viral infection despite having been told these will not help—it will not. Faced with these different reactions the temptation is to argue that one of them is mistaken. For instance, we might, following Ronald Dworkin, argue that cases like the latter give good reason to reject the claim made in premise three of the argument above (see Dworkin, 2006, pp. 359–360). This temptation should be resisted. I am going to argue that both reactions are correct. We should not expect the best approach to making decisions to be the same irrespective of the circumstances of the decision (including the setting in which the decision is being made).

Developing this argument will take some time and requires us to look at the scope as well as the content of each premise of the epistemic argument. In this chapter I will focus on the normative and epistemic claims made in premises one and two of the argument above, leaving the empirical claims made in premise three to chapter three. Before getting into the details of the argument, however, I want to make two points that are important for what follows. First, we should not think of making choices or decisions as a purely cognitive process. Making a choice, or coming to a decision, sometimes requires acting as well as thinking. For example, as we saw earlier, working out what is best for a patient might involve trying a certain treatment and seeing how it goes, or adopting a 'wait and see' approach. As such, particularly in cases of chronic illness, it is not always possible to draw a sharp line between working out what treatment will benefit a patient and delivering treatment to that patient. In making choices, or coming to decisions, it is also not unusual to involve other people. When faced with an important decision an individual might consult with those close to her, or those she thinks have relevant expertise. She might even defer to someone she thinks knows more about the issues than she does. These possibilities are at the heart of the above argument. It is important to bear in mind that they are open to patients as well as healthcare professionals.

Second, patients may sometimes think that one of the healthcare professionals treating them is better placed to make the right choice than they are, and so seek to make their decision by asking him what he would do, or what he would recommend. This need not mean that the patient wants no involvement in deciding what to do. She may still want the opportunity to choose, even if she does not want to make that choice on her own—for example, where she values choice for symbolic reasons (to be discussed in chapter four) rather than instrumental ones. Standardly discussions about patients who do not want to choose have focused on consent (see, for example, Beauchamp and Childress, 2009, pp. 131–132). Because our concern in this chapter is with choice (not consent) the issues are different.[4] If the argument above succeeds these patients are simply wrong about who is best placed to make decisions about their treatment. In trusting a healthcare professional to decide (and deferring to him) they are trusting someone with less expertise and less relevant knowledge than they have themselves. To the extent that institutional informed consent regulations undermine this trust, according to the argument we are considering here this should not be seen as a problem—contrary to what Onora O'Neill argues (see O'Neill, 2002). Rather it should be welcomed.

With these preliminaries out of the way it is now time to return to the epistemic argument for giving information to patients with chronic illness, or their carers, and letting them choose what treatment to have.

2.2 What Is It Exactly That the Healthcare Professional Is Attempting to Determine?

The idea that healthcare professionals should not harm their patients is well established—going back at least as far as the Hippocratic Oath (see Beauchamp and Childress, 2009; Gert, Culver, and Clouser, 2006). Similarly, it is relatively uncontroversial that healthcare professionals should benefit their patients (though as we saw in chapter one this is not the only way to conceptualise the role of medicine). There is, as Tom Beauchamp and James Childress put it,

> an implicit assumption of beneficence in all medical and health care professions and their institutional contexts. Promoting the welfare of patients—not merely avoiding harm—embodies medicine's goal, rationale, and justification.
>
> (Beauchamp and Childress, 2009, p. 205)

Or, as Garrett Cullity puts it,

> The relationship between health care professionals and their patients is governed by a mutual understanding that the role of the former is to use their medical expertise for the benefit of the latter.
>
> (Cullity, 2007, p. 22)

To fulfil these obligations healthcare professionals need to work out what will benefit, or harm, their patients. Does it also mean they need to work out is best for their patients all things considered? Both Paul Kelleher (2014, p. 45) and Robert Veatch (2006) have argued that it does not. In this section I will argue that it does (subject to certain constraints to be explained later). In doing this I will also be arguing that the obligation to benefit and the obligation not to harm should (at least in this context) be combined—as is the case in some older accounts in bioethics, such as the Belmont Report (see discussion in Beauchamp, 2010c).

It will be useful to start by focusing on healthcare professionals' obligations to benefit their patients. In contrast to their obligations of non-maleficence, these cannot be satisfied by doing nothing. They require the healthcare professional to act, and there are potentially many different ways he could act. Here context matters. People seek out (or are taken to) healthcare professionals when they are ill, or think they are ill. They do not seek them out when they have other types of problem—for example, if they are short of money or want a divorce—except where these other problems are also making them ill. Equally people seek out different healthcare professionals depending on the particular problem they have. They go to the dentist when they have toothache, for example, but not when they have stomach ache. That is because healthcare professionals have particular medical (but not financial or legal) expertise, and access to resources for treating illnesses (but not other problems). Both their expertise and the resources available to them will vary depending on their situation, and where in the world they are working. There is also, as we have just seen, a mutual understanding between healthcare professional and patient that the healthcare professional's role is to use his *medical* expertise to help the patient.[5] Given that role, healthcare professionals only have an obligation, *qua* healthcare professionals, to help their patients deal with problems where those problems are ones that can be dealt with using that expertise and those resources.

As this account makes clear there are only certain types of problem, and certain ways of addressing those problems, that fall within the remit of the healthcare professional's obligations *qua* healthcare professional. What they have an obligation to do is further restricted by the available resources (something that may vary considerably from place to place), and the limits placed on what they can do with those resources. As Emily Jackson points out, even if exercise is beneficial to health the health service is not required to provide running shoes to patients (Jackson, 2012, pp. 17–18), and the same is true of healthcare professionals. They have neither access to special resources to pay for such shoes, nor an obligation to pay for them out of their own pockets. Equally, financial assistance may benefit patients but this does not mean healthcare professionals should provide that assistance, even if they should provide medications of comparable value (Kelleher, 2014, p. 45). Neither state funded healthcare systems nor medical insurance provide money for healthcare professionals to give out in this way, and it would a misuse of funds were a healthcare professional to do so.

Taking all this into account we can characterise a healthcare professional's obligation of beneficence this way: he should help his patients where, given his expertise and the available resources, he can do so. He can only do this once he knows what their problem is. Finding that out might take a bit of work, and in some cases will require obtaining his patient's consent either to perform an examination or to carry out tests (we will look at what that, in turn, requires in chapter five). But once he has done this he will often find there are several things he could do for his patient. He thus needs to make a decision. His role is to use his medical expertise and the resources available to him to tackle and, if possible, to alleviate his patient's problem, but as it turns out there are several ways of doing that (Kelleher, 2014).[6]

In any given situation the different options open to a healthcare professional are unlikely to benefit his patient equally. Given this, and that the reason he has for doing any of them is that it will benefit his patient, the obvious way to resolve his epistemic problem is to compare the benefits provided by each treatment, and choose the one that produces the most benefit. Suppose, for example, that a doctor has identified two treatments—A and B—that would benefit his patient. The only difference between them is that A would provide more benefit than B. In this situation if the doctor were to give his patient treatment B, he would rightly be criticised. This could be because doing so is irrational—he has reason to do B (it would benefit his patient) but more reason to do A (it will provide more benefit to his patient). Or, it could be because he has not benefitted her to the extent that he could have—there is more that he could have done to benefit her and no reason not to do so. If this is right, then healthcare professionals ought to do what is best for their patients, not simply what will benefit those patients.

However, some caution is needed here. The world of healthcare is frequently not as simple as suggested by this example. In practice treatments work differently in different patients, and often come with side effects. Suppose some patients who get treatment A suffer harmful side effects that reduce its overall benefit. Those patients may (depending on the details) have been better off getting treatment B, whereas those who do not experience the side effects are better off getting treatment A. It can even be uncertain before giving a treatment whether it will benefit the patient all things considered—it may produce considerable benefit for most patients, but leave a small minority worse off than they were before. In that case before giving the treatment a healthcare professional will not know if it will benefit or harm his patient.

To work out what to do in these cases the healthcare professional concerned must take into account both the potential benefits and the potential harms of each option (remembering that no treatment is always an option). He has two ways of doing this. He could attempt to work out what he has most reason to do. He has a reason to give his patient treatment A—it might benefit her and he ought to do what will benefit her. He also has a reason not to give his patient that treatment—it might harm her and he ought not to harm her. By weighing these reasons (along with his reasons for and against giving his patient treatment B) he can work out whether he has more reason to give her A than to give her B.[7] Alternatively, he could attempt to work out whether giving his patient A has a higher expected utility than giving her B—taking account both of the size of the potential harms and benefits involved, and of the probability of these occurring. Whichever option he takes he will, in effect, be working out what is (all things considered) best for his patient. Doing this is the only way he has of knowing what his obligations of beneficence and non-maleficence require of him in the situation he is in. That is, in practice healthcare professionals should work out what is best for their patient, and then do that.

Saying that healthcare professionals should do what is 'best' for their patients here does not mean that they should do what will in fact provide those patients with the largest benefit—what Michael Zimmerman describes as the 'objective' account (Zimmerman, 2008, pp. 2–5 and 17–33). It means that they should do what has the best prospect from the epistemic position at the time the decision is made—what Zimmerman calls the prospective account (Zimmerman, 2008, pp. 6–7 and 33–56). What is prospectively best for a patient need not be what is objectively best for him. To see this, suppose that in our earlier example treatment A has a 99% chance of completely curing the patient (call this a utility of 100) and a 1% chance of leaving her very badly off (with a utility of 1). In contrast, treatment B is guaranteed to produce only a partial cure (with a utility of 70). The patient's doctor gives her treatment A and unfortunately she ends up with a utility of 1. The doctor in this example has done what is prospectively best for his patient but has not done what is objectively best for her.

There are good reasons for preferring the prospective account. As already described, in many situations it will be impossible to determine in advance what is objectively best for a patient, but it may nevertheless be possible to determine what is prospectively best for her. To work out what is objectively best a healthcare professional would need to know how different treatments will in fact affect his patient, and the underlying uncertainty means this is not always possible. He may be able to reduce this uncertainty—for example, by trying out a treatment and seeing how it affects the patient. Doing so provides new information, changing the epistemic situation, and so potentially changing what is prospectively best for the patient. Where complete certainty is obtained, if it ever is, what is prospectively best for the patient will be the same as what is objectively best for her. As such, what is prospectively best can be determined in a broader range of cases than what is objectively best, and agrees with what is objectively best in those cases where the latter can be determined. It is therefore more useful when we are concerned, as we are here, with practical reasoning and decision making.

A second reason for preferring the prospective account is that sometimes a healthcare professional should do something he knows is not objectively best for his patient, even if his sole concern is to benefit her. To see this, consider the following example developed by Frank Jackson (Jackson, 1991, pp. 462–463—this example is extensively discussed in Zimmerman, 2008, ch.1). There are three drugs available for treating a patient: A, B, and C. If treatment is not given now the patient's condition will be incurable. One of these drugs will completely cure the patient, one will kill her, and one will provide a partial cure. The doctor knows that drug A will provide the partial cure, but does not know which of B or C will completely cure, and which will kill, the patient. Assuming there is no way to determine which option is which, Jackson argues that the doctor should give the patient treatment A. Intuitively this is correct. But if it is correct then we are denying that the doctor ought to do what is objectively best for his patient. Instead we think that he should do what is prospectively best for her.

It is important to see that saying healthcare professionals should do what is prospectively best for their patients is not the same as saying they should do what they believe is best for their patients. Saying the latter would be to adopt what Zimmerman calls a 'subjective' account (Zimmerman, 2008, p. 5), and there are good reasons not to do that. To determine what has the best prospect requires investigative work and at least some attempt to acquire relevant information. In contrast, the subjective account places no such requirement on healthcare professionals. If a healthcare professional believes that a certain treatment is best for his patient, even if this is just the result of a guess, on that account he should give it to her. On the other hand, if he has no beliefs about what is best for his patient, according to the subjective account there is nothing he ought to do (for a related point when it comes to subjective accounts of what is morally required see Zimmerman, 2008, p. 14). He ought to do what he believes is best for his patient, but he has no beliefs about what is best for his patient. That looks clearly wrong—he should do something, even if this is only to seek out relevant information. For these reasons the subjective account should be rejected.

It will be useful to pause here and summarise where we have got to. I have been arguing that to fulfil their obligations to benefit and not harm their patients, healthcare professionals should do two things. First, they should work out what, given their expertise and the resources available to them, they can do that might benefit their patients. Second, they should work out which of those things would be prospectively best for those patients, and do that. While the resulting position might be captured by saying that healthcare professionals should do what is best for their patient, doing so could be confusing. In part this is because of the point we have just been discussing—'best' needs to be interpreted as 'prospectively best' not 'objectively best'. But it is also because the position I have been arguing for has a narrower scope than might be suggested by that wording. On the account developed here healthcare professionals only have an obligation to do what, of the things they can do given their medical expertise and the resources available to them, is best for their patients.

Narrowing the scope in this way is important because it enables us to respond to two challenges Robert Veatch has made to earlier versions of the argument outlined in section 2.1 (Veatch, 2006). Veatch argues, first (p. 643), that giving a patient information about available treatments and letting her choose cannot ensure that those treating her do what is best for her. At most it can tell them which of the options they offer is best for her. But what is all things considered best might not be one of those options. Veatch is right about this, but it is not an objection to the position I have been arguing for. As I have set it out a healthcare professional's reason for trying to work out what is best for his patient is practical, not theoretical. It is a way to determine what he needs to do to fulfil his obligations to benefit, and not to harm, her. As such, the only options he needs to consider are ones he could in fact take given his medical expertise and the resources available to him as a healthcare professional. It is no part of my argument that doing so will guarantee that he does what is objectively best for his patient. Indeed, as I have been stressing, the problem healthcare professionals face is that nothing can guarantee that.[8]

Veatch's second criticism is that some things that might benefit a patient are ones healthcare professionals should not do for other reasons (Veatch, 2006, p. 643). This usefully highlights the point that doing what is prospectively best for their patients is not the only obligation healthcare professionals have. It does not, however, challenge the argument here. Just as practical considerations limit the range of options healthcare professionals need consider, so too do normative considerations. Effectively those things a healthcare professional should not do even if they were what was best for the patient are in the same category as those things he cannot do because he lacks the necessary resources to do them—they are not among the list of open and available options he is trying to decide between.

Working Out What Will Benefit Patients 43

That, however, might look too fast. Introducing a normative constraint on what counts as an available option might seem to create problems of its own. An example will help to show why. Suppose that a healthcare professional works out that there are two ways to benefit his patient (A and B), and that A is prospectively better for the patient than B. He now seeks his patient's consent and finds that she will not consent to A, but would consent to B. This is not a situation where the benefit of doing A is so large that it would justify acting without the patient's consent. What should he do? The obvious answer is that he should do B. But B is not what is prospectively best for his patient, and so on the account developed here there is no obligation to do it. He should do what is prospectively best for his patient, and B is not what is prospectively best for his patient. It will not do, in response, to say that when working out what to do he should only consider those things that are morally permissible. At the time he is trying to decide what to do neither A nor B is morally permissible because, at that time, he has consent for neither.

The appearance of a problem here stems from an overly static picture of how people make decisions. Working out what is prospectively best for a patient takes work. Something that might at first sight appear to benefit her may after further investigation look less promising. For example, a doctor might judge that a particular course of medication would benefit his patient. But if she will not take the medication, prescribing it will provide no benefit at all. As such, to work out what is prospectively best for his patient he needs to investigate whether or not she will take the medication if he prescribes it. Doing so will normally require talking to her (or those around her). Patient involvement in decision making is here an important part of determining what is prospectively best for the patient—not because she is the best judge of what will benefit her, but because her doctor needs to know what she will do in the future.

Just as working out how much different treatments are likely to benefit a patient requires investigation, so too does working out whether they would be morally permissible. If the argument we are investigating in this chapter succeeds, the two may seem to go together. The most commonly discussed reason for thinking that giving treatment would be impermissible without consent is that doing so would fail to respect the patient's autonomy. But according to the argument we are considering, healthcare professionals should work out what is prospectively best for their patients by telling them what the treatment involves and letting them choose (or, if they are not competent, by telling their carers what it involves and letting the carers choose). They should then give the patient the treatment that she (or her carers) have chosen. At first sight that does not look as if it involves any failure to respect autonomy. However, appearances here are deceptive. Acting in this situation would only avoid the wrong of failing to respect autonomy if choice and consent were the same, and as I have stressed they are not. That the patient has chosen a treatment does not mean she has consented to it (nor does it mean she will consent to it). So giving her the treatment she chose could still fail to respect her autonomy.

So imagine the following is the case. A healthcare professional has worked out both that there are several things he could do that would benefit his patient, and that what is prospectively best would be wrong if done without her consent. He thus has conflicting obligations—the treatment he should give to satisfy his obligation of beneficence, he should not give due to his obligation to respect autonomy. The way to proceed here is not, as suggested by some authors (for example, Beauchamp and Childress, 2009, pp. 16–24), to balance or specify these conflicting demands. It is to try to dissolve the conflict by obtaining his patient's consent. This is part of working out what he should do. If his patient refuses, there is still more work to do. He should try to find out why she refuses—perhaps, for example, her refusal stems from a misunderstanding that can be overcome. It is only when he has exhausted these options that he needs to consider whether giving what he thinks is the best treatment would be permissible despite the lack of consent. In doing that he needs to do more than just balance two conflicting moral principles. If the law states that no competent person shall be given medical treatment without his consent, and this is a competent patient, then that matters too. Indeed, it may turn out to be decisive (one of the problems with using a framework of four *prima facie* principles as popularised by Gillon [2003] and Beauchamp and Childress [2009] is that considerations of this type can be hard to see). It is only at this point that the treatment comes off the table. If the patient will not consent and it would be all things considered wrong to give the treatment without consent, then that treatment is not really available. What the healthcare professional should provide in that case is the treatment, out of those that remain, that is prospectively best for his patient. In the example used to set up this problem that is B, and so that is what he should do.

The purpose of this section has been to investigate premise one of the argument we started with—'healthcare professionals should both benefit and avoid harming their patients'. We have seen that in its original form it does not adequately capture healthcare professionals' obligations, but that it can be reformulated to do so. The revised version states that 'healthcare professionals should do what, of the things they can do given their expertise and available resources, is prospectively best for their patients'. Although this is not the same, the epistemic challenges it creates *are* the same. Healthcare professionals need to assess which option, albeit from a narrower range of options, is prospectively best for their patients. That, in turn, means they need to assess how each available treatment will affect the patient as a person, and it was this that created the epistemic challenge. The argument we are investigating here is a response to that challenge—it argues that there are ways for healthcare professionals to make the required assessment by outsourcing it to those who have the relevant expertise. For all that has been said so far it can still do so.

2.3 Should Healthcare Professionals Always Use the Most Reliable Methods?

Having considered the first premise of our original argument in some detail it is now time to turn to premise two: 'where there is more than one way to work out what will benefit, or harm, a patient, healthcare professionals should use the most reliable available method'. While this claim is not discussed in the existing literature, something like it is needed to link the claims that do appear (patients are the best judges of their own interests, and healthcare professionals should do what is best for their patients). At first sight it might appear uncontroversial. As we have seen, healthcare professionals could work out what to do using a variety of methods, and some of these are more likely than others to select the option that is prospectively best for their patients. Tossing a coin to decide what to do, for example, would be irresponsible because it takes unnecessary risks with patients' wellbeing. Those risks can be avoided if healthcare professionals use a more reliable method to make their decision. However, saying that this is what they should do runs into two problems: 1. it ignores the fact that different ways of working out what is best for a patient come with different costs, and 2. it cannot deal with what I will call transitional cases (which turn out to be particularly important in chronic illness). Let us consider these in turn.

My initial formulation of premise two focuses on only one way in which methods for working out what is best for patients can vary—their reliability. However, those methods will also vary in other ways, some of which matter when working out what healthcare professionals should do. One of these is their costs. Suppose, for example, that a healthcare professional could use either method C or method D to work out what is prospectively best for a patient. Method C is more reliable than method D, but using it takes a lot more time and effort. Using method C thus has considerable opportunity costs—the additional time and effort it requires means the healthcare professional has less time available to actually treat patients. Given these costs it is pertinent to ask whether he would be justified in using method D instead. If C is only slightly more reliable than D, it seems that he would—that very small benefit would not be worth the costs of obtaining it. However, we might think differently if this is a life or death decision. Given the stakes involved healthcare professionals should take the additional time to ensure that the right choice is made. Things might again look different if there is only a small difference in the costs of C and D. In that case even if the increased benefit of using C is small it may still be worth the additional cost.

It appears from this that whether it is justifiable to use a cheaper but less reliable method to work out what is prospectively best for a patient depends on three things:

1. The difference in cost—the larger the difference in cost the more justifiable it would be to use the cheaper method all else being equal.
2. The difference in reliability—the greater the difference in reliability the less justifiable it would be to use the cheaper method all else being equal.
3. What the stakes are if the wrong choice is made—the higher the stakes the less justifiable it would be to use the cheaper method all else being equal.

As such, saying that healthcare professionals should always use the most reliable method (as I did earlier) is wrong. Sometimes they should, but at other times they should not.

This matters for two reasons. The first stems from the fact that much work in both medical ethics and healthcare ethics has focused on cases where the stakes are high—that really are matters of life and death. As we have just seen, in these cases healthcare professionals should use the most reliable method available to work out what is best for their patients. If telling patients about the available options and letting them choose is the most reliable method (and we have yet to assess that claim), it follows that in these cases healthcare professionals should do what informed consent procedures say they should do (where this is for purely epistemic reasons). But that may be a consequence of the fact that the stakes are high. Where the stakes are lower things might be different. For example, on the account developed here patients with moderately severe polyfocal ventricular arrhythmia—to use an example from Veatch (Veatch, 2006, pp. 640–641)—would not need to be told about the whole range of different medications available, all of which vary only slightly in their efficacy and possible side effects.

The second is that it affects how much information patients should be given. The argument we are considering in this chapter relies on the idea that an informed patient is a better judge of what is best for her than an uninformed patient. Were this not the case there would be no epistemic reason to tell patients anything about the available treatments. Of course this does not mean that patients are in one of two states: informed or uninformed. In practice they could be at any point on a scale from understanding nothing about the available treatments to understanding all that there is to know about them. Providing information to the patient is a way to move her along this scale towards greater understanding (though beyond a certain point it may no longer do so[9]). Doing this takes time, and the more information provided the more time it takes. There are likely to be diminishing returns when carrying out this process. Learning something about the available treatments from a starting point of knowing nothing will make a big difference to how well a patient can assess what is best for her, but after a certain point providing more information is unlikely to make any difference to her ability to do so.[10] The costs, in terms of time, of obtaining additional information are also likely to go up the more the healthcare professional has already divulged. There is a core of information that is readily available, other information is something he will need to search for. For these reasons, even if it is true that the more information a patient has the better a judge of what option would be best for her she is, it will not follow that healthcare professionals should tell her everything about the options available to her. How much they should tell her will vary from case to case (in part dependent on the stakes involved).

Methods of working out what is best for a patient differ in both their costs and their reliability. But they may differ in other ways too—for example on occasion there may be independent reasons for thinking that a particular method would involve doing something morally wrong. From the fact that a person ought to do X and doing Y will enable them to do X it does not always follow that they ought to do Y (see Raz, 2011, pp. 149–157). To see why this matters consider the case of an adult patient who is unable to make decisions for herself. In setting out the argument at the start of this chapter I said that in this case the most reliable method to determine what is best for the patient is to give those caring for her relevant information and let them decide. However, that information (which is likely to include information about the patient's past medical history and the nature of her illness) is frequently confidential or private. As such, passing it on to the carer of an adult patient— particularly where that patient was competent in the past—is likely to be wrong either because it breaches the duty of confidentiality or because it violates the patient's privacy.[11] Where this is the case healthcare professionals will have a reason, in many cases an overriding reason, not to share the information. Alternative methods of working out what is best for patients would not be ruled out in the same way. So even if providing information to carers and finding out what they prefer would be the most reliable way to work out what is prospectively best for a patient, there will be times when that method should not be used.

As with the points made earlier this reveals that the requirement to use the most reliable available method to work out what is best for patients is at best a *pro tanto* obligation. Whether or not the most reliable method should be used will vary depending on the details of the case—taking account both of the healthcare professional's other moral obligations, and the costs involved in finding and providing additional information.

There is however a second problem with my initial formulation of premise two, one that is potentially more significant. That argument made two empirical claims. First, that where the patient is a competent adult she is a better judge of what is best for her than anyone else (including the healthcare professionals treating her). Second, that where the patient is not a competent adult, her carers are better judges of what is best for her than anyone else (including both healthcare professionals and the patient herself). Because whether or not a patient is competent changes over time, this implies that who is the best judge of a patient's best interests also changes over time. For example, it implies that as an adult's competence declines due to the onset of dementia there comes a point at which she is no longer the best judge of her own interests; and that as a child grows up there comes a point at which she becomes the best judge of her own interests.[12] These changes do not happen overnight. Instead they take place over an extended period of time. During that transitional period it will sometimes be unclear who is the best judge of what is best for the patient. This creates a problem for the argument we are investigating. It says that healthcare professionals should use the most reliable method to work out what is prospectively best for their patients, but during this period it is unclear what method is most reliable.

There is a fairly obvious way for healthcare professionals to proceed in cases like this—where considerations of privacy and confidentiality allow, tell both the patient and those caring for her about the available options. If they agree on what should be done, the healthcare professional involved will have good evidence that that is what is prospectively best for his patient. Difficulties will only arise if they disagree, and that is likely to be rare. While work in ethics tends to focus on cases of disagreement, that is because such cases are particularly challenging, not because they are common. Of course, sometimes those involved will disagree. The healthcare professional then has more work to do to find out why, and to figure out how to proceed. Reasonable as this response is, accommodating it requires fairly substantial changes to the above argument.

To see why, we need to start by looking more closely at the different kinds of reason healthcare professionals have in these cases. Our starting point in this chapter was that a competent adult has expertise in making decisions about what will benefit or harm her that healthcare professionals lack. She also has relevant information they lack. As such, when trying to work out what to do a healthcare professional has reason to tell his patient about the available treatments and find out which one she prefers. Doing so tells him something he does not know, and cannot find out in any other way. He also has reason to think that the treatment she chooses is prospectively better for her than the alternatives. Indeed, if she is a better judge of this than anyone else (including him), he will have decisive reason to think this. Any reason he has for thinking differently will be outweighed by that provided by her informed (and voluntary) choice. Finally, given that he ought to do what is prospectively best for her, he has reason to do what she chooses. That is, he ought to show her choice what Suzanne Uniacke calls compliance respect (Uniacke, 2013).

The situation we are now considering is one in which the patient's informed (and voluntary) choice does not give the healthcare professional decisive reason to think that the treatment she chose is better for her than the alternatives. He potentially has a stronger reason for thinking that it is not (provided by her carer's informed and voluntary choice)—though whether or not that is stronger will depend on the details of the case. However, he still lacks relevant information and expertise that she has, and so still has reason to tell her about the available treatments and find out which she prefers. It is not, in this case, that doing so is the only way to find out how they will affect her as a person. Telling relevant family members about those treatments and finding out which they prefer will also do so. It is that doing so is a relatively easy way to find out something relevant he does not know, something that he cannot find out *more reliably* in any other way. What is important in this case is that he has no reason to think that one of the options he has—telling his patient and finding out what she prefers, or telling her carers and finding out what they prefer—is more reliable than the other. Things would be different if his patient's carers were better placed to work out what is best for her than she is herself—as will be the case, for example, when she is very young child. In that case the healthcare professional will always have more reason to think that what her carers choose is best for her, than to think that what she chooses is best for her (assuming they are different). As such, he has no epistemic reason to tell her about the different options and seek her choice about what to do (though that does not mean he has no reason of any kind to do so). Doing so would take time and would produce no benefit.

What this case shows is that sometimes healthcare professionals should, for epistemic reasons, tell their patients about available treatments and find out what they prefer, even where they have no good grounds to think that the patient is the best judge of what is best for her. In doing this it also challenges the idea that healthcare professionals should always show their patients' choices compliance respect. In the situation just described the patient's choice gives her doctor some reason to think that the treatment she has chosen is better for her than the alternatives offered, but that reason is not conclusive. Her doctor must also take account of any other evidence he has about what is best for her—particularly if it points in a different direction—and work out on the basis of this what he has most reason to do. That is, in this case he should show his patient's (and his patients' carer's) choices what Uniacke calls consideration respect—he should take them into account and give them due weight when deciding what to do, but need not necessarily comply with them (Uniacke, 2013).

2.4 Interim Conclusion

We have now looked at the first two premises of the epistemic argument for telling patients (or their carers) about available treatments and letting them choose. It should be apparent that that initial argument was both incomplete and potentially misleading. It ran into trouble dealing with transitional cases (young people in the process of becoming adults, and adults in the process of losing competence). It was also overly simple, in that it ignored both some of the uncertainties and some of the practicalities (such as limited time) that exist in healthcare.

We have also seen that, while it identified two different scenarios healthcare professionals need to deal with (competent adult and child/incompetent adult) there are in fact three—exemplified in the argument above by the competent adult, older child/patient losing competence, and young child/incompetent adult. The essential features of these can be characterised as follows (starting with those identified in the original argument):

1. Cases where the patient's informed choice will provide better evidence about what is prospectively best for her than any other source of evidence that might be available to the healthcare professional. In these cases the healthcare professional should tell his patient about the available options, let her choose which to take, and show her choice compliance respect.
2. Cases where the evidence about what is prospectively best provided by the patient's informed choice would not be as good as other evidence the healthcare professional has or could obtain. In cases of this type the healthcare professional has no epistemic reason to tell his patient about the available treatments and let her choose which to have.
3. Cases where a patient's informed choice would provide valuable evidence about what is prospectively best for her, but other sources of evidence would also be useful and may outweigh it. Transitional cases like the ones we have just been looking at fall into this category. In these cases the healthcare professional should tell his patient about the available treatments, let her choose which she thinks is best, and show her choice consideration respect.

The existence of this third category is important for reasons other than the transitional cases we have focused on so far. It reveals that the epistemic argument for thinking that healthcare professionals should provide relevant information to their patients and let them choose what treatment to have does not rely on the idea that the patient is a better judge of what is best for her than anyone else. As such, our original argument as set out in section 2.1 above included (as premise three) an empirical claim that was too strong. We can rewrite that argument to take account of this, as well as all the other points made in this chapter as follows:

1. Healthcare professionals should do what, of the things they can do given their expertise and available resources, is prospectively best for their patients.

2. If one of the available methods for working out what is prospectively best for their patients is more reliable than any of the others, healthcare professionals should all else being equal use that method.
3. In some situations (a) the most reliable method of working out what is prospectively best for a patient is to tell her about the available treatments (e.g. what each involves, their benefits and costs, and any risks involved) and let her choose. In others (b) it is to tell her carers about those treatments and let them choose.
4. Therefore, if the situation is as in (a) healthcare professionals should provide information about possible treatments to the patient and let her choose which to have. If the situation is as in (b) they should provide that information to her carers and let them choose which she should have. They should then do what she, or her carers, choose on the basis of this information.
5. Where none of the available methods is more reliable than each of the others, healthcare professionals should use a mixture of methods to determine what is prospectively best for their patients.
6. In this situation, if providing information to the patient (or her carers) would provide valuable evidence about what is prospectively best for her, then all else being equal healthcare professionals should provide that information to her (or them), and find out what treatment she (or they) prefers. Healthcare professionals should show the resulting choice consideration respect.

There are two things about this argument that I want to highlight. First, it is weaker than the argument we started with—hedged about with qualifications and exceptions (the 'all else being equal' clauses). As such, it would not support introducing institutional informed consent regulations on the grounds of promoting patient well-being, in the way that (as we saw in chapter one) is advocated by some writers (for example, James Stacey Taylor; see Taylor, 2005a). Second, it includes two distinct empirical claims—in premises three and six. Rejecting one need not involve rejecting the other. We thus need to investigate both. This will the topic of the next chapter. I will argue there that even for competent adult patients in some situations we should reject both claims. However, in others we should accept one or the other of them. The details matter, and what is required of healthcare professionals epistemically will differ depending on the details of the case.

Notes

1 It would not constitute consent—and nothing said here implies that it would make giving the treatment morally or legally permissible.
2 The cases where a patient is a young child and those where she is an incompetent adult are not exactly parallel. Concerns about confidentiality and

52 *Working Out What Will Benefit Patients*

    privacy arise in the latter, in a way that they do not in the former. We will return to these later in this chapter, and in chapter seven.
3. This is only a *pro tanto* requirement because the obligation to do what is best for the patient can in some circumstances be overridden—for example by the need to respect autonomy.
4. Because consent is distinct from choice, consent in these cases might not be needed—as will be the case where the doctor's response when asked what he would do is, 'I wouldn't do anything for the time being and see if it develops into something worse'.
5. The reason for this is, at least in part, contractual—he is employed to do just this. But healthcare professionals may also have voluntarily taken on a moral obligation to benefit their patients in this way at the time they became a healthcare professional.
6. In doing this he must choose between the options that are actually available to him, and so should ignore any treatments he cannot access—for example those that are not funded by the healthcare system for which he works. What treatments are accessible in this way is likely to vary considerably from place to place. As such, what healthcare professionals have an obligation to do will also vary. It might be thought that if a treatment benefits patients then it should be made available to them. Whatever the rights or wrongs of this, it is irrelevant here. Healthcare professionals have to deal with the patients in front of them, and for all practical purposes if they cannot get a medication they cannot give it to those patients.
7. This process will be familiar to many readers because, while I have expressed it in terms of weighing reasons, it is similar to that of balancing conflicting *prima facie* principles (for a discussion of what this involves see Beauchamp and Childress, 2009, pp. 19–24).
8. That healthcare professionals should benefit and not harm their patients may also mean they have other obligations—such as to conscientiously and diligently investigate what they could do to benefit their patients. What Veatch's criticism points to is that this might not be adequately done.
9. For example, because she comes to her limits of taking in information, and so pays no attention to anything else she is told.
10. This is not to deny that in some cases it might. But healthcare professionals cannot know this in advance. The only way to ensure this does not happen would be to tell the patient anything that might be relevant (which could be anything). In practice this is simply impractical.
11. Whether and when it would be wrong on these grounds will be considered in detail in chapter seven.
12. Much of the discussion of this latter transition in the healthcare ethics literature focuses on whether or not teenagers are autonomous (see, for example, Dickenson, 1994; Parekh, 2007; Manson, 2015; Walker, 2016). In contrast my focus here is on whether or not they are a better judge than their parents of what is prospectively best for them.

3 Is an Informed Patient's Choice Good Evidence That the Option Chosen Is What Is Best for Him?

3.1 Introduction

Healthcare professionals ought to benefit, and ought not to harm, their patients. In chapter two I argued that working out what exactly these obligations require is difficult—particularly when patients are treating themselves (as they frequently are in cases of chronic illness). Faced with a specific patient a healthcare professional must assess what is wrong with him, what (if anything) she can do to help him, what other people (including the patient) will do in the future, and how each of the available treatments will affect him as a person (rather than simply as a biological organism). In that chapter I also suggested a way of responding to this challenge. That suggestion, as we have seen, relies on two empirical claims—telling patients (or their carers) about the available treatments and letting them choose is either 1. the most reliable way of working out what is prospectively best for the patient, or 2. a way to obtain valuable evidence about what is prospectively best for him that cannot be more reliably obtained in some other way. It is now time to assess these claims. At first sight they look problematic. Over the last few decades considerable evidence of systematic bias in reasoning has been uncovered (for an overview see Kahneman, 2011; or Thaler, 2015). This evidence, along with evidence showing patients' sometimes limited understanding, has been used to question the adequacy of informed consent procedures (on bias in reasoning see: Beauchamp, 2011; Levy, 2014; Felson and Reiner, 2011, and on misunderstanding see: Corrigan, 2003; Dawson, 2004; Iltis, 2006; Hoffman and Del Mar, 2015). Our concern in this chapter is not with informed consent. But the same evidence might suggest that it does not follow from the fact that a patient (even an informed patient) chose a treatment, that that treatment is best for him. If that is right, then it will also show that the choices of informed carers (including parents) may not be good evidence about what is best for those they are caring for. Family members and other carers are as prone to misunderstanding and reasoning biases as anyone else.

However, assessing the implications of this evidence requires care. Evidence about biases in reasoning casts doubt on the idea that patients will always choose the treatment that is best for themselves. It also shows that patients are more likely to make some kinds of mistake when reasoning than others. But it does more than that. It shows that healthcare professionals make the same kinds of mistake as their patients. Consider the following example. There are two treatments for lung cancer: surgery and radiation. Five-year survival rates favour surgery, but it carries a greater risk in the short term. That risk can be expressed in two ways: 1. the one month survival rate is 90%, or 2. the mortality rate in the first month is 10%. How the risk is expressed affects the choices people make—told that the one month survival rate for surgery is 90%, 84% of participants chose surgery; but told the one month mortality rate for surgery is 10%, only 50% chose surgery (McNichol et al., 1982). The participants in this experiment were physicians, not patients. According to Daniel Kahneman this shows that "physicians are just as susceptible to the framing effect as medically unsophisticated people" (Kahneman, 2011, p. 367). Other experimental work shows that physicians, like patients, are also subject to other reasoning biases—for example, base rate neglect (see Gigerenzer, 2008). Biased reasoning cannot be avoided simply by changing who is doing the reasoning. Similarly, while patients (or their carers) might not understand, or might misunderstand, relevant information, this is also a problem for healthcare professionals. Indeed, that the latter's understanding is limited is what created the epistemic problem in the first place.

Because both patients and healthcare professionals experience reasoning biases and lack full understanding when making decisions, it would be problematic to focus only on how these affect patients. Working out what the evidence shows about the relative reliability of decisions made by healthcare professionals, patients, or patients' carers would also be difficult—particularly if we consider the full range of situations where these decisions need to be made. Fortunately doing so is not necessary. An alternative is to structure the argument around the three different scenarios identified at the end of chapter two (and exemplified there by the situations of the young child/incompetent adult, the older child/adult losing competence, and the competent adult). This is the approach I will adopt here, taking account of the empirical evidence where this is relevant. I will argue that sometimes there is no epistemic reason for healthcare professionals to provide information about different options to anyone (even competent patients), sometimes they should provide that information to patients (or their carers) and show the resulting decision consideration respect, and sometimes they should provide that information to patients (or their carers) and show the resulting decision compliance respect. This is undoubtedly more complex than some other accounts. However, this complexity is needed to adequately deal with the range of situations healthcare professionals find themselves in when treating patients with chronic illness.

3.2 Where Patient Involvement Is Not Needed to Determine What Is Best for the Patient

The problem we are investigating here is that healthcare professionals lack any special expertise in working out what will be best for their patients as individuals. However, we should not overstate the extent of this problem. Some decisions require no such expertise. Deciding what diagnostic tests to carry out, for example, does not normally require any assessment of how different tests would affect the patient's wellbeing—simply because the tests themselves are unlikely to affect it. Healthcare professionals will also normally be much better placed than their patients to make these decisions. As such, there is no epistemic reason to seek the patient's input when making decisions of this type (though their consent may well be needed). Having said that, healthcare professionals often do need to make decisions requiring an assessment of how different courses of action might affect their patient as a person—decisions about treatment, for example, or decisions about where care will be delivered (at home, in hospital, or in a care home). Even when we restrict our attention to these decisions there are situations where the epistemic argument fails to get off the ground. These fall into two categories: 1. where no special expertise is needed to make the decision; and 2. where there are good reasons to think healthcare professionals have more expertise than their patients (or their patients' carers). We will take these in turn. In doing so it will sometimes be clearer to use examples concerning treatment for acute conditions. Where this is the case, that is what I will do. An account of what healthcare professionals should do needs to be able to cover all the situations in which they find themselves.

In both medical ethics and healthcare ethics it is normal to focus on the difficult cases. They present the most pressing ethical issues, and require the most sustained ethical reflection. But not all cases are difficult. Some, indeed many, medical decisions are remarkably straightforward. Here are two examples. One, a patient goes to his doctor with a bacterial infection, one that can be cleared up with a widely used antibiotic that has, at worst, minor side effects. Given that he has gone to his doctor for help (and it should not be forgotten that this might mean he has had to take time off work and trek across town for his appointment) it takes no great expertise to work out that prescribing those antibiotics is best for the patient. The doctor can do this herself. Indeed, from the patient's perspective if she cannot—if she needs his input to work out whether a course of antibiotics is best for him given he has a bacterial infection—she is not much use as a doctor. Two, a patient goes to his doctor with a potentially fatal condition for which there is a relatively safe and straightforward treatment—think of something like a ruptured appendix. As in the first case, working out that giving the treatment—for example removing the appendix—is what is best for the patient requires no special expertise. The stakes may be high here but the choice is not hard. In cases like those just described there is no reason to think that healthcare professionals lack the expertise to work out what is prospectively best for their patients.

It might be objected that this moves too fast. There could be special circumstances that mean, for a particular patient, things are not as straightforward as they appear. Perhaps, though more detail would be needed to make this convincing. Suppose however that there are, what of it? If the patient is conscious, competent, and understands that these special circumstances apply this will become clear fairly quickly. He will not take the antibiotics (and will likely tell his doctor this when she starts to write out the prescription), or he will not consent to the appendectomy (and again will likely tell her this as soon as she proposes it). Patients are not passive. They can and do bring up information they think is relevant without waiting to be asked. Indeed, if they are autonomous this is precisely what we should expect them to do. On the other hand, if the patient is not conscious or does not recognise there are these special considerations, the healthcare professional has no way of taking account of them whatever she does—even telling her patient about the available treatments and seeking his choice would not do so. Either way, the mere possibility that there are special, and very unusual, cases does not mean that healthcare professionals should always tell their patients about the available options and seek their input about what would be best for them. Doing so has costs of its own—it takes time that could be more effectively used elsewhere, and could undermine the patient's trust in his doctor.

The cases we have just been looking at are straightforward. They are not ones where the epistemic argument gives any reason to tell patients about available options and seek their choice, simply because they are not ones where the problem that argument is designed to solve exists. There are other, less straightforward, cases where that problem does not exist either. These are ones where working out what is prospectively best for a patient involves assessing the impact on his life of a significant change that he has not, but others have, experienced—for example, where one of the available options (treatment or no treatment) will leave the patient blind, render him impotent, or alleviate his current chronic pain. In these cases it turns out that those who have experienced that change are a better source of evidence about how it will affect the patient's life than his own choices about what to do.[1]

When assessing how a major change will affect their life, people have two options: simulation or surrogation (for an overview see Gilbert, 2006, pp. 225–226). When using the former they imagine what their life would be like after the change—what it would be like if they were blind, say, or if their pain had gone. In contrast, when using the latter they take the experiences of those who have experienced that change—who have become blind, or pain free—as a surrogate for what life would be like for them were they to experience it. That is, they take the surrogates' level of well-being as the basis for determining what their own level of well-being would be were they in the surrogates' situation. While the former takes close account of the specifics of a person's life, the latter does not. As such, there is no reason to think that the individual him or herself will do it better than anyone else (such as their doctor).

The available evidence suggests that surrogation is in general more accurate than simulation (for an overview of this evidence see Gilbert, 2006, pp. 224–228). There are two reasons for this. First, when people imagine themselves in a different situation they do not imagine it in all its details. If they imagine being blind, for example, their focus will be on what is most salient about being blind—they would no longer be able to see. Other things that contribute to their well-being (such as playing with their grandchildren, eating good food, or listening to music) and that they could still do if they lost their sight are not as salient, and so are apt to be forgotten. As such, people tend to underestimate how well their own life would go (or how well other people's lives would go) were they to become blind or suffer some other loss (Gilbert, 2006, p. 104). Conversely, when imagining what life would be like without their current chronic pain people are likely to overestimate how well it would go—they imagine the pain gone but do not take account of all the other pains and frustrations that would remain (such as their stressful job, or their annoying neighbours). Second, people tend to underestimate how resilient they are and how quickly they will adapt to their new situation. Studies of those who have experienced a major change in their lives— either positive or negative—show that while there is a short term effect on their well-being (as assessed by them), this effect does not last (Taylor, 1983). This is not something that people always anticipate when these sorts of change happen to them (see Wilson and Gilbert, 2003; Gilbert and Wilson, 2009).

Taken together this all suggests that simulating—imagining what it would be like—systematically leads people to overestimate how well their life would go if some positive change (such as their pain going) occurs, and to underestimate how well it would go if some negative change (such as losing their sight) occurs. So far, however, it does not show that surrogation would be any better. Other experiments, albeit not directly related to healthcare, point to the possibility that it would (see Gilbert et al., 2009; Walsh and Ayton, 2009). Those who have already experienced some change are not affected by the biases that come with using simulation—they do not need to imagine what it would be like to be blind or without chronic pain, they just have to report on how well their lives are currently going.

But there might seem to be an obvious problem with using a surrogate to assess how well a person's life will go after some change. The surrogate is different from that person, and so how a particular change—such as going blind—will affect the latter, will also be different. Perhaps it will. But we need to remember that while there are undoubtedly lots of ways in which people differ, there are also lots of ways in which they do not. These similarities can be overlooked because we are usually more concerned with what makes people different from others than with what makes them alike. As a result we can exaggerate those differences—as Daniel Gilbert puts it,

> Because we spend so much time searching for, attending to, thinking about and remembering these differences, we tend to over-estimate their magnitude and frequency, and thus end up thinking of people as more varied than they actually are.
>
> (Gilbert, 2006, pp. 231–232)

It is this that explains why participants in the experiments referred to above were better at assessing how they would feel in some future situation if they did not try to work this out by using their imaginations, but instead relied on the experience of others. Importantly for our purpose here one of the things people have in common is the ability to adapt their lives to take account of new circumstances.

In saying this I am not saying people are all exactly the same, with no important differences between them. As such, who is used as a surrogate matters. An athlete may argue that how losing a limb affected the well-being of non-athletes is not likely to reflect how it would affect him. But if it turns out that other athletes who have lost a limb adapted well and were not noticeably worse off in the long run, this may be good evidence that he will do the same. Of course, he may not—in which case losing a limb may make him much worse off. Using surrogates to assess how well someone's life would go is not infallible. But then neither is using our imagination to simulate what life would be like after a major change. The claim here is simply that if a person wants to assess how a major change he has never experienced would affect his well-being, he would be better off relying on the experiences of those who have lived through that change than on his own imagination.

What are the implications of this for the argument that healthcare professionals should provide information to patients (or their carers) for epistemic reasons? In many cases none. Much of the time patients do not need to work out what life will be like in some situation they have never experienced to judge which treatment (including having no treatment) would be best for them. Treatment, if they get it, frequently restores patients to a condition they have been in before. For example, where they have a chronic condition they will often have received that very treatment before, and so know how it affects their life. Furthermore, in some cases no usable or useful information from surrogates will be available—either because it has never been gathered, or because it does not provide a clear picture. Think, for example, of a situation where those who have received a certain treatment strongly disagree about its effect on their wellbeing. Faced with this situation, looking at how the lives of others have gone will give no guidance about what would be best for a given patient. Falling back on using experience and imagination, with all their flaws, is then the only option.

Having acknowledged all that, however, sometimes healthcare professionals do have information about how significant changes most people have never experienced (such as losing a limb, or going blind) affected the well-being of previous patients. Where this is the case, they could either use this to work out what will be best for their current patients (using surrogation), or pass it on to those patients to let them decide what treatment (if any) would be best for them. The evidence suggests the former is likely to be better than the latter. If patients are told about different options, including how those options affected the lives of previous patients, they are likely to try to figure out what is best for themselves using simulation (Walsh and Ayton, 2009). And that, as we have seen, can get in the way of making a good decision. Suppose, however, that they do not, and instead use surrogation. In that case they would be replicating something the healthcare professional could do just as well herself. Either way there is little reason to think the patient (even when suitably informed) will be a better judge of what option would be best for him than the healthcare professionals treating him.

Thus, at least in cases of this type a healthcare professional will have no epistemic reason to provide information to her patients and find out what treatment they prefer. It must be stressed that this does not mean there is no obligation to provide information to patients in these cases. Doing so may be necessary for other reasons, for example to obtain valid consent. Nothing said here affects that (though as we saw earlier consent is not always needed before enacting decisions about what to do). Given that some decisions about the treatment of children or incompetent adults also require an assessment of what life would be like for them if one course of action, rather than another, were taken, similar considerations will apply there. This will, for example, be the case where decisions are being made about what would be best for a patient if he loses the capacity to choose for himself. Similarly, if the best evidence concerning how well a child's life will go after a certain treatment is how well other children's lives went after they had that treatment, healthcare professionals can work this out for themselves. As such, there is no epistemic reason to provide information to the child's parents when trying to determine what would be best for him—at least in cases of this type. Something similar will be true with regard to the carers of adult patients who lack competence. People do not lose their reasoning biases just because they are thinking about someone else's wellbeing.

3.3 How Are Patients Making Decisions When Asked to Make Them?

As we have just seen, sometimes there are no epistemic reasons to tell patients (or their carers) about available treatments, and let them choose what treatment is best for them (or the person they are caring for). Cases of this type fall into one of three categories: 1. where the patient is not a competent adult there is no need to tell him about the available treatments and find out what he prefers (from chapter two); 2. where the decision about what is best for the patient is straightforward; and 3. where the decision hinges on an assessment of how well the patient's life would go after some change he has not experienced but others have. While some healthcare decisions fall into one or other of these categories, many do not (including many decisions about the treatment of chronic illness). We now need to turn to these other cases. In doing so it will be useful to start by making explicit two assumptions the epistemic argument makes: 1. when making decisions patients[2] are trying to work out what is best for themselves (and nothing else); 2. when making decisions patients take account of all the relevant information they have. There are at least some cases where these assumptions can be challenged (though that they can be challenged in some cases does not mean they can be challenged in all). If those challenges succeed, this will limit the range of cases where the epistemic argument gives good reasons for healthcare professionals to provide information to patients and let them choose what treatment to have.

When investigating this, it is useful to begin by recognising the different tasks healthcare professionals and patients face. Healthcare professionals, as we have seen, have to work out which of the available options is prospectively best for their patients. Patients, on the other hand, have to work out what option to take. The idea that their choice reveals something about what is best for them assumes that in doing this they take their task to be the same as that of the healthcare professionals treating them. If they do not, there is no reason to think that the options they choose are better for them than any others. But the assumption that this is what patients are doing can be challenged. Rather than trying to work out what is best for them, they could be satisficing—that is, choosing an option they judge is good enough without attempting to work out whether it is the best available option (for an account of what satisficing involves see Simon, 1997, pp. 118–120). Alternatively they could be taking account of things other than their own well-being when making their decision—either the interests of other people (see Molyneux, 2009, p. 247), or their own moral judgements (see Veatch, 2006, pp. 641–642). Taking account of other people when making treatment decisions may be uncommon, but could happen—though it may be more likely in medical research where the choice to participate may be based on a desire to

An Informed Patient's Choice 61

benefit others in the same position. For an example of how a patient's moral judgment might affect her choice consider a woman who judges that having an abortion would be best for her but that it would be wrong to have one and so refuses it (Veatch, 2006, p. 642). While these cases do not involve chronic illness, if they show there is a flaw in the epistemic argument, that would cast doubt on whether there are ever epistemic reasons to think healthcare professionals should disclose relevant information to their patients. We therefore need to consider them here.

A defender of the epistemic argument might respond to the idea that people are sometimes motivated by things other than their own interests by denying that this ever happens. Since at least the 17th century people have argued that apparently altruistic or moral behaviour is really motivated by self-interest (for an early example see Hobbes, 1650, p. 12). For example, they may argue that the woman in our earlier example does not want to do what she thinks is morally wrong because she will feel guilty if she does. She also expects sanctions, from both her community and God, if she has an abortion—sanctions she is keen to avoid. Similarly, it may be argued that the apparently altruistic research participant is really motivated by the praise she believes she will receive for taking part in the research. Those who argue in this way are usually advocates of psychological egoism, one of the most influential theories of human motivation. Psychological egoism holds that people are only ever motivated by self-interest. According to C. Daniel Batson its advocates have been in a majority in Western philosophy and psychology (see Batson, 1991). It has been both influential and persistent in classical economics (for a discussion see Sen, 1979, p. 87).[3] And, arguably, it is the theory of motivation that forms the background to many of our most successful social and political theories (see Flanagan, 1991, p. 108; Blackburn, 1998, p. 134). Given all this it would be unsurprising if any appeal the epistemic argument has relies on a (usually unspoken) assumption that psychological egoism is correct.[4]

However, this response, challenging the idea that people are ever motivated by things other than self-interest, is not the way I intend to proceed. Doing so would require defending psychological egoism, and while that theory has been very influential it has also faced a barrage of criticism (see, for example, Butler, 1726; Broad, 1950; Feinberg, 1965; Nagel, 1970; Sen, 1979; Rachels, 1999; Batson, 1991; Flanagan, 1991; and Sober and Wilson, 1998). Given my aims there is an easier way to defend the argument introduced in chapter two (one that has the additional advantage of dealing with cases where the patient is satisficing). This is to argue that even if patients are sometimes motivated by things other than their own interests this does not pose a problem for that argument. To see why, think back to the woman who refuses an abortion because she thinks it is wrong (and assume for the moment she is a competent adult). For reasons we looked at in chapter two her moral objections effectively mean abortion is not an option her doctor needs to consider when trying to work out what is prospectively best for her. She will not consent to having an abortion, and if she will not consent it will not happen. Whether or not it would be best for her is strictly speaking irrelevant—it is not in practice an available option.

Where a patient's choice is partly determined by her moral objections, the situation is thus as follows. Her choice indicates that the treatment chosen is, of those she considers morally permissible, best for her. Those treatments she would reject on moral grounds are not (despite appearances to the contrary) actually available. If consent would be needed for those treatments, as in the abortion example, she will not consent and so giving the treatment would be wrong. Even if consent would not be needed (or it would in the circumstances be all things considered permissible to act without consent), in practice the treatment is still not available. Delivering that treatment effectively will require the patient's co-operation—she must take the prescribed medicine, or follow the treatment plan—and given her moral objections this co-operation is not likely to be forthcoming. Those treatments rejected on moral grounds are not, therefore, options healthcare professionals need to consider when working out which of the available options is prospectively best for their patient—which as we saw in chapter two is what they need to do.

Where the patient chooses treatment she does not think is best for her because she takes account of its effects on others, healthcare professionals face a different problem. The treatment she has chosen will be one they judge would benefit her—if it was not, it should not have been offered. The patient now knows that that treatment is available. Knowing that, she is unlikely to agree to, or co-operate with, any of the alternatives offered. Because the patient's co-operation is needed for most treatments to be effective, in practice this means that none of the other options are available as a way to treat her. That is, just as in the case where a patient's choice is influenced by her moral objections, where a patient's choice is not entirely based on self-interest this has the effect of narrowing down the list of options that need to be considered when working out what to do.[5]

The possibility that patients' choices are not based entirely on their own interests does not, therefore, challenge the argument we are considering here—that for epistemic reasons healthcare professionals should both tell their patients about the available treatments, and find out which one the patient thinks is best.[6] It is true that in these circumstances, contrary to what the epistemic argument assumes, a patient's choice may not tell us much about what is best for her. Instead it reveals that some treatments that might have looked attractive are not really live options (at least for this patient). That is, it clarifies the range of treatments the healthcare professional must choose between if she is to fulfil her obligations to benefit, and not harm, her patient. She must do what, of the available options, is prospectively best for that patient and the epistemic argument tells her how to work this out. Finding out which options are in fact available is just as important when doing this, as finding out which of the available options would be best for the patient.

The problem we have just been considering is that when choosing what treatment to have patients may not be focusing solely on their own well-being. We have seen that this does not challenge the epistemic argument for telling patients about different treatments and letting them choose. There are, however, two further potential problems for that argument looming nearby. The epistemic argument not only assumes that patients are solely focused on themselves, it also assumes they approach decision making in a certain way—taking all the information they have about possible treatments (including what they involve, and what the benefits and side effects of each are) and using it to calculate which one would be best. The problem is that patients may not be doing that. First, patients, like healthcare professionals, have more than one way to make a decision. They could, as just explained, work out what to do for themselves taking account of all the available and pertinent information. Alternatively, they could ask for advice from others and incorporate that into their decision, they could ask others what they would recommend (or do) and choose that (effectively using the other person as a proxy decision maker), or they could toss a coin. Which method they use will vary depending on the details of the case—for example, they may be happy deciding for themselves in simple and relatively straightforward cases, but want to include others (such as family members) if the decision is more complex or has weightier consequences. Because social norms about how decisions should be made vary from place to place, which method they use is also likely to be affected by their cultural context. Second, patients may not reason in the relatively systematic way suggested by the epistemic argument. We will look at these in turn.

We can begin by thinking about how, and why, patients might involve others in their decisions. While some healthcare decisions are relatively straightforward (do I take these antibiotics?), others are not (do I start chemotherapy?). People only need to make these decisions when they are ill. That is not a time they are likely to be at their informed best—they may be tired, anxious, and in pain. These are not ideal conditions for making important decisions (Levy, 2014, p. 297; Manson and O'Neill, 2007, pp. 5–6). It would not be surprising, therefore, if people wanted some help—particularly where their condition is serious or their options are difficult to assess. Indeed, there would be something odd if they did not consult their spouse or partner, if they have one, in these circumstances. This is in part because they may need their spouse's help and co-operation to carry out any decision made—where, for example, treatment requires adjustment to their diet, or would significantly affect some area of their shared life. But it is not just that. Sharing important decisions is part of what it is to be in a close relationship of this type. Within a close relationship the image of the independent decision maker is no ideal—though whether the patient acts as an independent decision maker should not affect how he is treated (for a related point see May, 2005).

To some extent the issues here shade into those we have just been considering. When making a decision about what to do patients are likely to take account of how different options might affect their family, as well as how those options might affect themselves (see Hardwig, 1990, p. 6). However, things are a bit more complicated than that. How a treatment would affect a patient's partner may affect his judgment about what is best for him—if it is bad for them, it is also bad for him given their importance to him. How exactly it does this is something the healthcare professional will not know, adding to the difficulty of working out what is best for her patient. And, as such, reinforcing the need to make use of the patient's expertise when working out what is best for him. The problem for the epistemic argument arises when the balance in decision making shifts, so that effectively the patient's partner is making the decision. For example, suppose that after talking it over with his wife a patient tells her that he does not know what to do, and asks for her advice. She says she thinks he should take treatment A (rather than B), and on that basis he tells his doctor he will have A. In this case it is not at all clear that giving the patient information and letting him choose has made use of his expertise in determining how different options will affect his wellbeing. But according to the epistemic argument the reason for providing that information is precisely to take advantage of that expertise.

None of this is to say that his wife's decision is a bad one. In this situation she may be about as good a judge of what is best for her husband as he is. Rather it is to point out that even if a patient has chosen a particular treatment this does not necessarily mean that he has worked out, taking account of the information he has been given, that that treatment is best for him. As such, it would be problematic for his doctor to assume, on the basis that the patient is the best judge of his own interests, that she has conclusive reason to think that the treatment he chose is better for him than the alternatives. She should of course still respect her patient's choice. But the relevant sense of 'respect' here is consideration respect, not compliance respect.

Further grounds for thinking that consideration respect is all that is required (at least for epistemic reasons) comes when we turn to the second problem mentioned above—the way patients make decisions even when they make them themselves. As we saw in chapter one, informed patients do not always make informed choices. One reason for this is that patients do not approach medical decision making knowing nothing—particularly where there are ongoing meetings between patient and healthcare professional as will frequently occur in the treatment of chronic illness. As such, any information the healthcare professional provides is adding to, or correcting, information the patient already has. To see the problem this can create imagine the following scenario. A patient has been diagnosed, and a meeting is now scheduled to decide what treatment he is to have. He arrives at this meeting having already made up his mind. Perhaps he has investigated options on-line, or perhaps he knows people with his condition and has seen what they do. His doctor now provides him with fuller information about his options, including (let us suppose) information about potentially serious side effects of that treatment of which he was unaware, or information about a newly available treatment. What will he do? Rationally, perhaps, he should reconsider his choice in the light of this new information. It is pertinent to that choice, and potentially shows he has made a mistake. But that does not mean he will reconsider his choice. People do not always open up their decisions for reconsideration just because new information has become available, even when they should. Sometimes they just stick with their original choice. Even if he does reconsider what to do, his earlier choice may well bias his reasoning—what in the literature is known as confirmation bias (see Nickerson, 1998; Kahneman, 2011, pp. 80–81; Levy, 2014, pp. 295–297). Having already decided on one option, A, he may treat information that supports A as more relevant or more authoritative than information that suggests A is not the best choice.[7]

That the patient has already made up his mind is not the only reason he might not take account of relevant information when making decisions (Walker, 2017). To see this, think about how you would decide what to do when you are uncertain about what will happen, and the alternatives you face carry both risks and benefits—something that is not unusual in healthcare. The available evidence suggests that in this situation you are unlikely to proceed by rationally weighing up the risks and benefits of each option, even if you think you should (Goldman, 2009, pp. 1–5). Instead you are likely to use shortcuts, heuristics, or rules of thumb (see Gigerenzer, 2000; Gigerenzer and Selton, 2001; Gigerenzer, 2015). As Gigerenzer has argued there need be nothing irrational about this. What heuristic is used will vary from person to person and from situation to situation. But the essence of them all is that they do not make use of all the information available—instead focusing in on only one or two key factors. Another, related, feature of decision making is that frequently some information is more salient for a decision maker—it grabs their attention more—than other information they have. As a result, the latter can be overlooked, and the former given more weight than it really deserves. This may be a particular issue in medical decision making because of the presence of visceral factors, such as pain, that focus attention on them (Loewenstein, 1996). When a person is in pain, especially if it is severe, this can so grab their attention that all they really care about is getting rid of it. Other factors may then get little look in when making decisions about what to do. Similarly, when anxious or tired (as may well be the case with patients facing decisions about their illness) people may become more risk averse in ways that affect what they choose to do. Taken together this all means that, as Neil Manson and Onora O'Neill put it, patients can "mistakenly dismiss important information as routine or trivial, or react to routine information with misplaced or disproportionate dread or fear" (Manson and O'Neill, 2007, p. 5).

These features of everyday decision making matter. The epistemic argument outlined in chapter two relies on the idea that an informed patient is a better judge of what is best for him than an uninformed patient. That is why it does not simply say that the patient should make the choice, but that the patient should be told about the available alternatives (what they involve, their benefits, any side effects they might have, etc.) and then make that choice. That idea, in turn, relies on the assumption that informed patients will use the information they have been given. If they do not, their decision is no more likely to be accurate than that of an uninformed patient. The problem we are now considering is that that assumption might be (at least partially) wrong, suggesting in turn that the epistemic argument incorporates an over-idealised view of how patients go about making decisions. That it might be wrong, however, does not mean there is no epistemic reason for healthcare professionals to tell their patients about the available treatments and seek their choice. By doing so they obtain useful evidence about how different options will affect their patient as a person—evidence they cannot obtain more reliably in any other way. Nor does it mean there is no reason for them to respect that choice (to show it appropriate consideration). However, it does cast doubt on the idea that the patient's choice is an informed choice, and so for epistemic reasons should be shown compliance respect. Providing patients with relevant information and seeking their choice about what to do will tell healthcare professionals something about what will benefit the patient, and may tell them something about what is important to him. But that choice may not be as informed as might have been thought (despite the patient both having and understanding relevant information).

In saying this it is important not to overstate the case. That patients sometimes act in the ways described above does not mean they always act in those ways. Sometimes they really will take the time to work out what is best for themselves, and do so carefully and systematically. This may be particularly likely where either the patient has considerable experience of living with his illness (as will be the case with treatment for many chronic conditions) or where the decision is not straightforward but is weighty (as in many of the cases standardly discussed in the ethics literature). Where this is the case, nothing said in this section challenges the idea that healthcare professionals should show compliance respect for their patients' choices for epistemic reasons. The arguments here sound a note of caution about doing so, they do not show that this is never required.

3.4 The Problem of Risk and Uncertainty

I argued in chapter two that for healthcare professionals to fulfil their obligations to benefit, and not harm, their patients they must work out what is prospectively best for those patients, and then do that. Working this out requires assessing the ways different treatments could affect the patient as a person. But it requires more than that. What is prospectively best is also affected by the chances of different possible outcomes occurring. As such, working out what is prospectively best for a patient requires combining how different treatments might affect their well-being with the likelihood that each of those effects will occur. How people do this is influenced by their attitude to risk. We have touched briefly on how risks are incorporated into decision making, but so far have said nothing about how attitudes to risk might matter when deciding what treatment to have (or what treatment to give). It is to this that I now want to turn.

When acting involves taking a risk, we need to assess whether this is a risk worth taking—are the potential benefits large enough to be worth the risk?[8] Those working in decision theory have developed tools to help make this kind of assessment—typically making use of expected utilities (for a good introduction to this topic see Gilboa, 2010). At its most basic, working out the expected utility of an action requires four things: 1. identifying all the things that might happen if you act that way; 2. for each of those calculating both their utility (or disutility) and the probability that they will occur; 3. combining these by multiplying the utility by the probability; and 4. adding together the results from each possible outcome to give the overall expected utility. This can then be compared with the expected utility of the other available options. This process builds in attitudes to risk. It also normally requires using subjective probabilities—the decision maker's best estimate of how likely something is to happen—because this is all that is available.[9] Expected utility theory is a complex and highly technical subject. Fortunately there is no need for us to go into it here. It is highly unlikely that either healthcare professionals or patients go through this process when making treatment decisions (though it may in some contexts be possible to model their choices as if they were). Indeed, it may be doubted that doing so would be rational given that they frequently lack both time and relevant information (see Gigerenzer, 2015). Instead of reaching for the tools provided by decision theory healthcare professionals and patients alike are more likely to use heuristics and past experience when deciding what to do. For this reason in what follows I will not be using the terminology of expected utility. I will instead describe the problem in more general terms—is the risk (in a colloquial sense) worth taking given the alternatives, the potential benefits, and the size of the risk (taking account of both its likelihood and its impact on well-being)? Working out whether a treatment is prospectively better for a patient than the alternatives requires that we somehow answer this question—indeed, they are effectively the same question.

Incorporating risk into decision making creates a problem—people have different attitudes to risk. This is in part because some people are more risk averse than others. But it is also because their attitudes to risk can vary depending on who is running the risk. For example, they may be more sanguine about risks when someone else is facing them, or alternatively want to shield others (such as their children or elderly parents) from risks they would happily take themselves. So, whose attitude to risk should we incorporate in decisions about what is prospectively best for a patient? Equally, while all those involved may agree that certain things would benefit (or harm) a patient, they may reasonably disagree about the relative size of the benefit or harm. That is, their characterisation of how good or bad a particular outcome is may differ, even if they agree that the outcome is either good or bad (Gert, Culver, and Clouser, 2006, pp. 12–13). So whose weighting of the benefit or harm should be used in working out what is prospectively best for a patient? In line with the argument we are considering, we could attempt to answer these questions by assessing who is likely to be the best judge of whether a risk is worth taking. But to do that we would need to know what the right attitude to risk is, and we do not (indeed it may be doubted whether there is a 'right' attitude). An alternative is to think about who might be the appropriate judge of whether a risk is worth taking. Someone might be the appropriate judge because they are the best judge—the one most likely to get the right answer. That is what we have been focusing on. But where there are risks involved something else matters too—who runs the risk. In the cases we are concerned with—the treatment of a particular patient—the risk will be run by the patient. If the treatment is given, he is the one who may suffer harm. If the treatment is not given, he is the one who must forego a benefit. As such, it seems reasonable to think that (assuming he understands the benefits and risks involved, and can make decisions using this information) he is the appropriate person to decide whether this is a risk worth taking.

While this conclusion comes out of our investigation into the epistemic problem healthcare professionals face, it does not rely on the idea that patients are the best judges of their own interests. It also does not obviate the need for healthcare professionals to work out what is best for their patients. There is an asymmetry in how we should think about patients and risk. If a patient judges a treatment is not worth the risk given the alternatives available to him (again assuming he understands all the relevant facts), it would be inappropriate to force him to take that risk simply because his doctor thinks differently. In contrast, the mere fact that he thinks something is a risk worth taking does not mean that healthcare professionals ought to give it to him. Their obligation to benefit, and not harm, him may mean they should not do so. They should, however, take his views seriously, particularly if this is a treatment other patients are given. Healthcare professionals (and carers) may at times be too risk averse when making decisions—particularly where their patients are older adults, as many patients with chronic illness are. Indeed Atul Gawande has argued that, "our most cruel failure in how we treat the sick and aged is the failure to recognize that they have priorities beyond merely being safe and living longer" (Gawande, 2014, p. 243). That is, while healthcare professionals should show compliance respect for a choice not to have a treatment because it is too risky, or the potential benefits are not sufficiently high given the possible side effects, they need only show consideration respect for choices to have that treatment. This only applies where the patient himself is in a position to make the choice. While the carers of a patient can certainly disagree with healthcare professionals about whether a treatment is, or is not, too risky given the alternatives, they themselves would not be running the risk. As such, nothing said here suggests that healthcare professionals should show compliance respect for a carer's refusal of treatment for the person he or she is caring for, or a parent's refusal of treatment for his or her child, on the grounds that the risks outweigh the benefits.

The argument just outlined is restricted in two ways. First, it only applies to those patients who can understand relevant information and use it to make a decision about what to do—that is, it is limited to those patients who are competent. Second, it relies on the idea that patients not only have the ability to understand but do in fact understand that information. The extent to which patients understand what they are told, however, has been challenged, and this challenge has been particularly sharp when it comes to their understanding of risks. Those making that challenge have typically focused on its implications for consent (see, for example, Corrigan, 2003; Dawson, 2004; Iltis, 2006; Hoffman and Del Mar, 2015). It is not hard to see why. If, as the standard picture claims, it is wrong to give a competent patient treatment without his informed consent, and informed consent requires substantial understanding, then patients who do not understand have not consented. While our concern at this point is not with consent, we need to consider this challenge here because it appears to undermine the usefulness of what I have just said.

Empirical work on misunderstanding by patients has focused on information about the likelihood of harms or benefits occurring as the result of an intervention. Following a systematic review of the available evidence, Hoffman and Del Mar concluded that "the majority of patients overestimated intervention benefits and underestimated harm" (Hoffman and Del Mar, 2015, p. 274). The extent of the misunderstanding varied considerably across the studies included in Hoffman and Del Mar's review—both in terms of the proportion of patients who misunderstood and in terms of how much they misunderstood. For example, the proportion of participants who overestimated the benefit of an intervention varied between 7% and 94% depending on the study, and there were also cases where participants underestimated the benefit (Hoffman and Del Mar, 2015, p. 278).

In the face of this evidence there are different ways we might proceed. One is to argue that it undermines the position being considered in this chapter. Given the extent of patient misunderstanding there is little reason to think that telling patients about different treatments will help healthcare professionals work out what is best for those patients. Nor is there reason to think patients ought to be the ones to decide if the risks associated with certain treatments are worth taking. The problem with this response is that it both leaves healthcare professionals with fewer resources for making choices about what treatment to give, and ignores the extent to which they themselves lack understanding. This problem could be avoided by adopting an alternative response—one that says that the argument we have been looking at is incomplete. Merely providing patients with information is not enough, it might be argued, healthcare professionals should also take steps to ensure that that information is understood (as is sometimes argued in relation to the consent process). However, this response in turn faces a problem. Ensuring that a patient has understood the information given to him takes time and energy. That is, it has a cost, and as I argued in section 2.3 the benefits obtained from using a more expensive method to work out what is best for a patient may not justify the costs of doing so. For example, time spent checking the understanding of one patient is time not spent treating patients, and given the necessary trade-offs it is unclear that doing so is the best use of a healthcare professional's time.[10] Furthermore, introducing such a requirement creates a hurdle patients need to jump in order to get treatment, and it is not clear that placing such hurdles in patients' way is justifiable.

What we should conclude from all this depends on the details of the case. Sometimes, as with some decisions about cancer treatment, the seriousness of the underlying condition combined with the potential harms attending the treatment mean the healthcare professional may have considerable doubt about what would be best for her patient. In such cases the patient's input plays a particularly important epistemic role. These are also cases where it is reasonable to think the patient is the appropriate judge of whether the potential benefits are worth having given the possible side effects. Moreover, these are not cases where treatment is usually given straight away, and they are cases where there is normally ongoing discussion between healthcare professional and patient. As such, there will usually be time to ensure both that patients are well informed and that they understand the information they have been given. In these circumstances the idea that healthcare professionals should provide information and take steps to ensure that it is understood before concluding that a particular treatment is best for their patient is not unreasonable.

These are precisely the cases that have been at the centre of debate in healthcare ethics. However, what is true of them is not necessarily true of other cases healthcare professionals confront. It is the significance of what is at stake, that is the very features that make them serious, that is the determining factor here.

3.5 Conclusion

Back in chapter two we started with a fairly simple argument—healthcare professionals should provide information to patients and let them choose what treatment to have because this is the most reliable way to work out what is needed to fulfil their obligations to benefit, and not harm, their patients. As we have seen, in this simple form it faces significant problems. In some cases (those that are straightforward, or where the decision rests on how well the patient's life will go after a change he has not, but others have, experienced) there turns out to be no epistemic reason to tell patients anything about the different treatments—except what is needed to determine whether they would follow the treatment plan. In others, the argument shows that healthcare professionals should provide information to patients, and seek their choice, but should treat this as only one relevant source of information. The patient's choice should thus be shown consideration respect, but need not be shown compliance respect. In yet other cases the original argument seems to work, and may even be strengthened to include a requirement that healthcare professionals ensure the information provided is understood. In these cases they should show their patients' choices compliance respect—where this is purely on the basis that this is what is prospectively best for the patient. Finally, we also saw that where there is a risk involved in giving treatment patients are often the appropriate judges of whether the risk is worth taking.

The kinds of case where the original argument works best are those where the stakes are high, there is disagreement about the effects of different options, and there is time to engage at length with the patient. These are the kinds of case that have been the focus of much of the work in both medical ethics and healthcare ethics. Drawing conclusions from a relatively narrow set of examples like this is, however, problematic, giving a distorted picture of healthcare professionals' obligations. That is particularly the case when we move to consider the treatment of chronic illness. What healthcare professionals should do there will vary with the details of the case. There is in practice no way to argue on epistemic grounds that there is always a reason for healthcare professionals to provide information (or particular types of information) to their patients and let their patients chose what to do. There is also no way to argue on the basis of selected examples that healthcare professionals' obligations to benefit, and not harm, their patients do not give them an obligation to tell their patients about different treatments and do what the patient chooses. As we have seen the situation is far messier, and more complex, than that. Before attempting to impose some order on this situation, it is worth looking at other arguments for thinking that healthcare professionals should provide information to patients and then do what the patient chooses—those based on the need to respect autonomy. These will be the focus of the next chapter.

Notes

1. It is worth noting that while the idea that we are in general the best judges of our own interests is often attributed to J.S. Mill, in his *Principles of Political Economy* Mill himself acknowledged that in cases like this where people lack relevant experience they are not good judges of what is best for them (see Young, 2008, p. 219 fn.18).
2. In this section I will omit explicit references to carers for the most part. This is simply for clarity, and does not mean that the argument here does not apply equally to them.
3. Sen, like Batson, is an opponent of psychological egoism, and sets out in this paper to challenge it.
4. Psychological egoism can appear cynical. But whether it is depends on how we characterise what counts as a benefit. For example, on preference satisfaction accounts of well-being, getting what we prefer benefits us. To incorporate moral judgments, while retaining the idea that people are solely motivated by their own interests, this account characterises moral judgments as preferences—rather than side constraints (see Hausman, 2012, p. 35). So, the woman who refuses an abortion because she judges it is morally wrong, prefers not doing what is morally wrong to the benefits she foresees from having an abortion. Because this is what she prefers, contrary to appearances not having the abortion is better for her than having it. We can say something similar about the apparently altruistic research participant. He prefers taking part in the research and advancing knowledge to any benefits he might receive from not participating. So, taking part satisfies his informed preferences, and thus is what is best for him.
5. Discovering that they are not available may, as we saw in chapter two, only become apparent as a result of telling the patient about them.
6. Theoretically there is one exception to this—where a healthcare professional knows for certain that her patient would refuse a possible treatment on moral grounds. Given the argument here she would have no reason to tell her patient about that option. She knows that it is not a live option, so whether or not it would be best for him is irrelevant. Such cases are likely to be extremely rare, if they exist at all. It is much more likely that the patient's moral objections only become apparent while telling him about the treatments available.
7. It should be remembered that healthcare professionals (like all humans) are also subject to confirmation biases. Thus their judgment may sometimes be faulty for the same reasons that the patient's may be faulty.
8. The term 'risk' is being used here in its everyday sense and so incorporates both risks and uncertainties.
9. Even if we know that one out of every hundred people who get a certain treatment experiences a given side effect, it does not follow that there is a 1% chance that a particular patient will experience it (though this may be a reasonable starting point in estimating the subjective probability). Population

level figures average over differences in the population that affect how likely something is to affect individual members of that population.

10 It might be objected here that when dealing with a patient the well-being of that patient should be a healthcare professional's sole concern. However, this claim is ambivalent between two readings. On the one hand, it could mean that the decision about which treatment to give should be determined solely by what will benefit that patient (other factors such as the cost of the treatment or the length of waiting lists should play no role). On the other, it could mean that in dealing with a patient considerations about things other than the well-being of that patient should play no role in how the patient is dealt with (including how much time to devote to him). The possible objection here relies on the second reading. That second reading is, however, implausibly strong. It would rule out any form of triage, and require a healthcare professional to continue to deal with a patient with a minor condition even if an emergency life-threatening case comes in.

4 'It should be up to the patient what happens to her'

4.1 Introduction

The argument of the last two chapters characterised choosing as the healthcare professional's responsibility. Out of all the things he could do for his patient, he must choose the one that is prospectively best for her. Only in that way can he fulfil his obligation to benefit, and not harm, her. But this whole approach may look mistaken. Isn't it up to the patient what treatment (if any) she receives? Isn't is also up to her whether she goes home to receive care, or receives it in an institutional setting? The impetus behind these questions is that what happens should be up to the patient, not the healthcare professional. She should be the one to choose. This is not because her choosing is sometimes a way to help other people determine what is best for her (as discussed in chapters two and three). It is because it is her choice to make. This line of thought is rooted in another obligation that healthcare professionals are standardly thought to have—the obligation to respect their patients' autonomy (Dworkin, 1988; Gillon, 2003; Stoljar, 2007; Beauchamp and Childress, 2009, pp. 99–148). The requirement to respect autonomy was largely ignored in the previous chapters. It is to it that that we now turn. In doing so our focus needs to narrow—what we say will only apply to patients who are autonomous (in a sense to be described below), and not everyone with chronic illness is.

When working out what respect for autonomy requires, it is useful to start by asking a more basic question—what normative restrictions (or requirements) are placed on healthcare professionals by the fact that many of their patients are autonomous? There are two ways someone might answer that question. First, the fact that a patient is autonomous means that things, including treatment, should not be imposed on her. Her freedom, what Isaiah Berlin called her negative liberty (Berlin, 1969, pp. 122–131), should not be infringed precisely because she is autonomous. Treatment that a patient has voluntarily agreed to is not imposed on her. So, according to this way of answering our question, to avoid acting wrongly healthcare professionals need to obtain their patient's consent before acting. Second, the fact that a patient is autonomous means that other people (such as healthcare professionals) should not make decisions about things like treatment (or where to receive care) on her behalf—where to decide is not just a cognitive act but affects what happens. This answer also concerns the patient's freedom, but here it relates to what Berlin called her positive liberty (Berlin, 1969, pp. 131–134). As such, what it says healthcare professionals need to do if they are to adequately respect their patients' autonomy is different—they should, for example, allow their patients to choose what treatment to have. These answers locate the wrong of failing to respect autonomy, if it occurs, at different places. The first locates it at the time treatment is given (the treatment is imposed on the patient without her consent); the second locates it at the point decisions about what treatment to give are taken (the healthcare professional decides this for his patient). This in turn means that according to the second answer, but not the first, a healthcare professional who gives no treatment could still fail to respect his patient's autonomy (for example, by deciding that no treatment will be given, rather than allowing her to make that choice). That is, the second answer, unlike the first, places positive obligations on others (a point made explicitly by Feinberg in relation to the sovereignty account of autonomy; Feinberg, 1986, p. 53).

While these two ways of thinking about what respect for autonomy requires are not in competition with each other, they are very different. The first focuses on consent—what is needed to respect autonomy is that the patient makes the proposed act permissible. The second focuses on choice—what is needed to respect autonomy is that the patient gets to choose what treatment (if any) she has (or that she gets to make some other choice such as whether she will be treated at home or somewhere else). Because of this they raise different issues, and may place restrictions on healthcare professionals in different areas of practice. As such, they need to be looked at separately. This chapter will focus on choice, leaving consent to chapter five. In making this split I am breaking apart issues that are frequently conflated in the existing literature. For that reason these two chapters need to be read together. On its own neither gives a full account of what respect for autonomy requires of healthcare professionals, nor covers all the topics that would standardly be dealt with under that heading.[1]

To assess whether respect for autonomy really does mean patients should be the ones to choose, we first need to get clearer about what is meant by both 'respect' and 'autonomy'. Let us start with 'autonomy'. As is well known this word has been used to capture many different ideas, all related to self-governance (Dworkin, 1988, pp. 3–6; Arpaly, 2003, pp. 117–148; Taylor, 2005b; Stoljar, 2007). Not all these are relevant for our purposes. However, even if we restrict ourselves to the ways 'autonomy' is used in healthcare ethics we find it referring both to features of choices, and to features of individuals (Wilson, 2007, pp. 353–356). In both this chapter and the next my focus will be on the latter. What the relevant feature of individuals is, has also been a matter of some disagreement. According to some accounts it is a capacity that people have; according to others it is a standing or authority (such as sovereignty) they possess. There is, however, no reason to think that we need to choose between these. My interest here is not in working out what the right way to interpret 'autonomy' is (if that task even makes sense). It is with the obligations of healthcare professionals. And, as we will see, both the fact that some patients have a certain capacity (as on capacity accounts of autonomy) and the fact that they have a certain standing (as on sovereignty accounts of autonomy) matter when doing that. In this chapter my focus will be on autonomy as a capacity, while in chapter five (when we look at consent) the focus will be on autonomy as standing or sovereignty. Referring to both of these features as 'autonomy' would, however, create confusion. So, as far as possible in what follows I will avoid using that term.

If autonomy is a feature of individuals, we need to reconsider what we mean by 'respect'. In chapters two and three I made use of Suzanne Uniacke's distinction between consideration respect and compliance respect (Uniacke, 2013). Because both of these concern how we should respond to choices people have made, however, neither can capture what it is to respect autonomy as a feature of individuals. Taking the term 'respect' to have its standard meaning in English we could interpret the idea that healthcare professionals should respect autonomy (taken as a feature of individuals) in one of two ways. First, we could interpret it as referring to what Stephen Darwall calls 'recognition respect'—that a person has the feature of being autonomous means healthcare professionals should respect them in virtue of the fact they have it (however well or badly they use it) (Darwall, 1977). Alternatively, we could interpret it as referring to what he calls 'appraisal respect'—to the extent that someone uses their autonomy to live an autonomous life they should be respected, and the more autonomous their life the more highly healthcare professionals should respect them. It is the former that is most relevant for the arguments being considered here.

With those terminological points out of the way we are almost ready to begin. Arguments relating to autonomy and patient choice normally take it that autonomy is a capacity people have (though for an exception see Feinberg, 1986, pp. 52–97). For example, according to an influential line of argument, autonomy is the capacity people use to shape their lives and it is this that means patients should be the ones to determine what happens to them, including what treatment (if any) they receive. In this chapter I will start by looking in more detail at what autonomy as a capacity is, before (in section 4.3) rejecting this argument. There is, however, another way to argue that because patients are autonomous they should be the ones to choose, one that is more successful. This is that whether healthcare professionals choose for someone or allow her to choose for herself, communicates something about how they see her—that she is or is not competent, or that she is or is not a moral agent they need to treat as an equal. This argument, based on the idea that choice has what Tom Scanlon calls 'symbolic value', will be introduced and defended in section 4.4.

Before getting into these arguments, however, I want to explain briefly why I am not looking directly at the idea that healthcare professionals should respect their patients' autonomous choices despite the prevalence of such accounts in the literature. There are two reasons for this. First, there is no real controversy over whether healthcare professionals should show consideration respect for patients' autonomous choices—indeed, there is no real reason to restrict this requirement to those choices that are autonomous. Doing so only requires healthcare professionals to give due weight to their patients' choices when deciding what to do (something everyone should do in the face of other people's requests or expressed preferences anyway; see Raz, 1986, pp. 36–37; Owens, 2012, pp. 85–87). In contrast the idea that they should show compliance respect for patients' choices is much more contentious. Such a requirement would mean healthcare professionals should do what their patients' autonomously choose, whatever that is. If we adopt a very minimal account of what makes a choice autonomous, this is implausible (Manson and O'Neill, 2007, pp. 19–21). Even if we characterise an autonomous choice, as Tom Beauchamp does, as a choice that is intentional, voluntary, and informed (Beauchamp, 2005, pp. 314–316), it still needs some defence. As a general rule the mere fact that someone who has relevant understanding has voluntarily and intentionally chosen that I do something, does not mean I am required to do it. There may be exceptions to this, but if there are these will need to refer to things other than the fact that the choice is autonomous. For example, that a patient is autonomous may mean that their autonomous choices should be complied with. Whether or not they should, is, in part, the focus of this chapter.

Second, focusing on respect for autonomous choice would miss things that are important for both consent and choice. The idea that healthcare professionals should respect a patient's autonomous choice tells us what is required in the light of that choice—what they should do, or not do, given that the patient has chosen as she has.[2] It places no restrictions on what they may do if the patient has not made a choice, simply because in that situation there is no choice to respect. However, the idea that it is wrong to give a competent patient treatment unless she has consented does place restrictions on what healthcare professionals may do where a patient has made no choice. Think about a competent patient who has not been told anything about a proposed treatment, and so has neither chosen it nor consented to it. Giving her the treatment would be wrong, but this cannot be because it would fail to respect her autonomous choice—she has not made an autonomous choice. Equally, the idea that it should be up to patients what treatment (if any) they receive is not reducible to the claim that healthcare professionals should show compliance respect for their patients' autonomous choices. If it is correct, it means healthcare professionals should allow their patients to choose and not act until they have chosen. As with consent, this places restrictions on what is done before the patient chooses, and so cannot be fully captured by the need to respect autonomous choice.

4.2 The Capacity to Choose and the Value of Choice

Those who think of autonomy as a capacity, think of it as the capacity to govern oneself. What is required to have that capacity is captured in the following two accounts: one from Raanan Gillon, the other from Gerald Dworkin. According to Gillon, autonomy is "the ability and tendency to think for oneself, to make decisions for oneself about the way one wishes to lead one's life based on that thinking, and then to enact those decisions . . ." (Gillon, 2003, p. 310). According to Dworkin,

> Autonomy is a second-order capacity to reflect critically upon one's first order preferences and desires, and the ability either to identify with these or to change them in light of higher-order preferences and values. . . . Autonomy is not simply a reflective capacity but also includes some ability to alter one's preferences and to make them effective in action.
>
> (Dworkin, 1988, p. 108)

There are important differences between these accounts but here I want to focus on what they have in common. Both take it that autonomy includes a cognitive capacity—a capacity, that is, to stand back from your immediate desires and think about which you will act on, or what you will do, in the light of your goals, your values, and your other commitments. But it includes more than that. Autonomy also requires the capacity to enact your chosen desires, and to put your plan into action. It is the combination of these two capacities—to reflect and to act—that enables you to make your life your own.

Both of these capacities come in degrees—people can be more or less autonomous, and this can vary over time. The extent to which they can exercise these capacities also varies. They may, for example, have the capacity to understand their situation, to reflect on what they want to do, and to make choices on the basis of that reflection (they are, that is, competent), but be unable to exercise those capacities well because they are in pain, tired, distracted, intoxicated, or in the grip of strong emotion. Equally, while someone may be able to plan their life, their ability to do so effectively can be compromised by lack of information (for example, about what might follow from their actions) or by the kinds of cognitive biases briefly discussed in chapter three (Levy, 2014). Limits are even more evident when it comes to a person's capacity either to enact their decisions (Gillon, 2003, p. 310), or to make them effective in action (Dworkin, 1988, p. 108). Sometimes their ability to do this is restricted by an internal compulsion or addiction (see, for example, Frankfurt, 1988; Levy, 2006). Far more frequently it is limited by external features of the world in which they live. Many of the things people value or want can only be obtained with the co-operation and assistance of others—co-operation and assistance that may not be forthcoming. This is particularly the case when they are ill. People visit their doctor, for example, because they cannot get rid of their pain, or manage their illness, without his assistance. They need both his expertise and the resources he can get for them. Even if he advises them to take an over the counter medicine, they are still reliant on others—to manufacture the medicine, to deliver it to a local shop, and to sell it to them.

Of course, when exercising their capacity for autonomy—that is, when reflecting on what to choose, and what to do—people generally take account of what is possible. It would be irrational not to. What help they are likely to get in enacting their choices is affected by what someone in their position can reasonably expect other people to do. If it should be up to them as patients what treatment they receive, they could reasonably expect to be able to enact their choice to have a certain treatment. But if what treatment they receive is not up to them, they could not. As such, it would seem that people only have the capacity required for autonomy (in the sense spelt out by Gillon or Dworkin) if it is already the case that what treatment they receive should be up to them. But if that is right, we cannot argue that patients should be the ones to choose on the basis that they have that capacity.

This problem can be avoided by adopting a narrower account of what it is to be autonomous—one that refers only to things the individual has (the ability to reflect, to plan, and to decide) and things he lacks (compulsions or addictions). The capacity to enact our choices would then not be part of autonomy, but something separate—such as freedom or liberty (for a related split see Coggon and Miola, 2011, pp. 525–526). Doing this would bring the account of autonomy into line with that adopted by at least some other writers. For example, Tom Beauchamp and James Childress argue that "Law, medicine, and, to some extent, philosophy, presume a context in which the characteristics of a competent person are also the properties possessed by the autonomous person" (Beauchamp and Childress, 2009, p. 113). The characteristics of a competent person, in turn, are described as the ability to "understand a therapeutic or research procedure, deliberate regarding its major risks and benefits, and make a decision in the light of this deliberation" (Beauchamp and

Childress, 2009, p. 114). Taken together these imply that autonomy is a purely cognitive capacity and does not include the capacity to enact one's decision.[3]

On this revised account a person is autonomous if they have the ability to decide what to do, or what they want to happen, in the light of their own values, aims, and commitments. They have the capacity, that is, to choose what treatment (if any) to have. But that they have this capacity is not in itself sufficient to show that they should be the one to choose. After all, there are many other equally autonomous people who also have the capacity to do so (including those treating them and members of their family). What we need is an explanation of why the fact that a patient has this capacity means that the choice should be hers, not theirs, to make. As we have seen, different possible explanations are available—all relating in some way to the value of being the one to choose. Making that choice could be valuable to the patient for instrumental reasons—it is the best way to ensure that his own well-being is promoted (Mill, 1859/1974; Dworkin, 1988, pp. 111–112; Scanlon, 1998, pp. 251–252; Owens, 2012, pp. 166–167). We looked at this idea in some detail in chapters two and three so will not repeat it here. But choice is not only valuable for instrumental reasons (Dworkin, 1988, p. 112; Scanlon, 1986, 1998, pp. 251–256). It can also be important for 'symbolic reasons' (Scanlon, 1998, p. 253), or because as Dworkin puts it, "The exercise of the capacity of autonomy is what makes my life *mine*" (Dworkin, 1988, p. 111). Whether either of these gives good grounds for thinking that what treatment a patient receives should be up to her is something we now need to investigate.

4.3 Choice and the Autonomous Life

The capacity to make choices for themselves, and to enact those choices, is important to people (where it is) because it is only by exercising this capacity that they can make their lives their own. As Neil Levy puts it,

> The autonomous agent must actually rule, or be capable of ruling, herself. That is, she must be capable of shaping her life as she wants: in accordance with her values, her projects and her conception of the good.
>
> (Levy, 2014, p. 298)

Or, as Gerald Dworkin argues, it is by choosing for ourselves and enacting those choices that we "define our nature, give meaning to our lives, and take responsibility for the kind of person we are" (Dworkin, 1988, p. 108). Having only the more limited capacity outlined in the previous section is not enough—though it may be necessary—to ensure that someone's life is autonomous in this way (see Berofsky, 1995, p. 28).

They also need to both exercise that capacity, and affect the way their life goes by doing so. To see why, imagine two people with similar capacities to plan, to reason, and to choose (neither of whom suffers from a compulsion that would prevent them from acting on their choices). The first uses these capacities to think about what she wants to do, to make plans for her life (and figure out how to achieve them). She also reflects on the values that are important to her and adjusts them in the light of that reflection. The second does none of this as far as she can—she does what she is told, always defers unthinkingly to those in authority, and holds fast to the values she acquired in childhood without ever reflecting on them. Though they have the same capacity for autonomy, the first person lives a more autonomous life than the second. She alone has made her life her own.

To the extent that living autonomously in this way is valuable (and for the sake of argument I will assume that it is) it requires that people take control of their lives. It is not enough that what happens is what they would have chosen, it must happen because they chose it. We want, as Peter Bieri puts it, "to determine our lives ourselves . . . to be able to decide for ourselves what we do and what we do not do" (Bieri, 2017, p. 6). Isaiah Berlin captures the basic idea well when (talking about positive liberty) he says,

> I wish my life and decision to depend on myself, not on external forces of whatever kind. I wish to be the instrument of my own, not of other men's acts of will. I wish to be a subject, not an object; to be moved by reasons, by conscious purposes, which are my own, not by causes which affect me, as it were, from outside. I wish to be somebody, not anybody; a doer—deciding not being decided for, self-directed and not acted upon by external nature or by other men. . . . I wish, above all, to be conscious of myself as a thinking, willing, active being, bearing responsibility for his choices and able to explain them by reference to his own ideas and purposes.
> (Berlin, 1969, p. 131—according to Gerald Dworkin this passage captures the flavour of his conception of autonomy; Dworkin, 1988, p. 107)

This idea has considerable resonance for many people—particularly when it comes to major areas of their lives. People generally want the decision about what work they do, who they live with, if they marry (and if so to whom), and whether they have children to be their own. Were someone else to decide these things for them they would not be in control of their own life, they would be being governed by other people not by themselves.

Decisions about what medical treatment to have appear important in the same way. Just as it should be up to the individual herself if she marries (and if so to whom), it seems it should be up to her what medical treatment (if any) she receives. If someone else makes that decision, they are effectively governing her life—she is, in Berlin's terms, being decided for, not deciding. By deciding for her, that is, the other person compromises her ability to live as autonomously as she might. If living a more autonomous life is valuable, this is something they ought not to do. As such, healthcare professionals should not make choices for their patients (where those patients have the capacity to decide for themselves). This is, in outline, the argument I want to consider in this section. It grounds patient choice in the value of living an autonomous life (the kind of life only those with the capacity for autonomy can live). I will argue that it does not work. In doing so I will not challenge the idea that living more autonomously in the sense just described is valuable, at least for many people. That account does not characterise the autonomous life as one that is self-sufficient, as is sometimes assumed by critics of the role of autonomy in bioethics (see discussion in May, 2005). It only requires that others do not make important choices about how a person's life goes on her behalf. Instead I will argue that even if living more autonomously (in this sense) is valuable, it does not mean that what treatment a patient receives should be up to her. The idea that it should, implies both that 1. if she chooses it, it should be done, and 2. that if she does not choose it, it should not be done. The latter, however, also follows from the idea that treatment should not be imposed on patients without their agreement or permission. As such, to avoid intuitions about consent getting in the way of our assessment of the argument, in what follows I will generally use examples where the patient chooses treatment (rather than ones where she refuses it).

Arguments based on autonomy risk giving the impression that, were it not for the healthcare professional's interference, patients would be able to enact their decisions and in doing so determine the way their lives go. But of course they cannot. As we have already seen, lots of things can get in the way of a person being able to enact his choices. While these might all interfere with his autonomy, they do not all wrong him. It is easiest to see this by using a non-medical example. If Joe's plan to marry Jean is frustrated because she dies in an accident this is unfortunate, but if it is frustrated because Jean's father prevents the marriage both Joe and Jean have been wronged (her father has not respected their autonomy). Jean's death does not alter the fact that it is Joe who is governing his life, but her father's intervention does. The morally important difference between these cases is not simply that in the latter Joe's choice is frustrated by the actions of another person. Suppose that Jean refuses to marry Joe. Her actions prevent him from enacting his choices (just as much as those of her father in the first example). But she cannot be said to have acted wrongly by setting back, or failing to respect, his autonomy. In making her decision Jean is deciding what she is going to do—will she marry Joe or not—and as an autonomous individual this is a choice she is entitled to make. If Joe were to attempt to force her to marry him, or to make this decision for her, he would be wronging her in exactly the same way as her father would wrong him were he to prevent the marriage.

This example illustrates two points that will be important in what follows. First, some of our choices, including some of our most important choices, affect other people in ways that would be wrong without their agreement or co-operation. Joe's choice to marry Jean can only be enacted in a way that is not morally wrong if Jean voluntarily agrees to marry him. That is, at least morally a person's autonomy is limited by the autonomy of others. Second, where we cannot enact a choice on our own, there are two ways in which other people can prevent us doing or getting what we choose. On the one hand those whose co-operation is needed can do so by refusing to co-operate (as when Jean refuses to marry Joe). On the other, third parties can intervene to prevent the people involved from co-operating with each other (as when Jean's father prevents the marriage). These differ morally, and raise different questions. Because this book is about the obligations of healthcare professionals I will have nothing to say about third party interventions. In healthcare these usually occur when the state prevents patients from accessing services that at least some healthcare professionals would (in the absence of that prohibition) be willing to provide—examples that have been extensively discussed in the literature include abortion and euthanasia. The question of whether, and if so when, such interventions are morally justified is a significant one. However, to engage with it would take us too far from our concerns here.

How does all this relate to choices about treatment for chronic illness? For a patient to enact a choice to have treatment she usually needs the co-operation of others—typically some combination of healthcare professionals, family members, and volunteer caregivers.[4] Suppose, therefore, that a patient wants a certain treatment, and approaches her doctor to get it. Just as Jean in our earlier example must decide whether she will marry Joe, so the healthcare professional in this situation must decide whether he will give his patient that treatment. Suppose he decides not to. His decision means she does not get it, but this is not necessarily a case of his governing her or making a decision on her behalf. He is, like Jean, making a decision on his own behalf about what he will do, and does so in the light of his own goals, values, and commitments (including those that he accepts as part of his role as a healthcare professional). As an autonomous agent it is not clear why that would be wrong. It is precisely what is required for him to act autonomously, and the starting point of the argument we are considering here is that acting autonomously is valuable.[5]

That might look too fast. To see why consider the following example: Paula wants a hip replacement operation but her doctor refuses to perform it. He might do so for different reasons. Perhaps there is a regulation in place that means women with her condition should not receive this operation, and he is unwilling to break the regulations to help her. In that case when refusing he is not making a decision on her behalf, and hence this is not a case of him governing her. But what if his reason for refusing is that he thinks the operation would be bad for her—that she is making a bad choice, one she is likely to regret? In that case it does look as if he is making a decision on her behalf. Such a refusal looks paternalistic, and paternalism is generally taken to be a failure to respect autonomy.

However, some care is needed when assessing this example. We have already seen that choice can be valuable for more than one reason. As will become apparent later, the symbolic value of choice means that if other patients are allowed to choose whether to have this operation it would be wrong to deny Paula the same opportunity. Considerations of this type may affect our intuitions about the case, and we need to put them aside for the time being. For our present purposes the key question is whether in refusing to perform the operation Paula's doctor is preventing her from governing her own life. It is not clear that he is. The point of the marriage example was to show that there are moral limits on self-governance. In making choices about what to do or how we want our future to go, we must take account of the fact that other people are also autonomous. In choosing to have an operation Paula is not only choosing what she wants, she is inevitably making a choice about what she wants other people to do—in this case that she wants her doctor to replace her hip. Her autonomy, her ability to govern herself, does not extend to governing others (they must have the same ability to govern themselves). As such, her doctor's refusal to perform the operation is not really a wrongful interference with her autonomy at all. His decision may frustrate Paula's plans, but this in itself does not make it wrong on the grounds of failing to respect her autonomy (any more than Jean's refusal to marry Joe would be wrong on those grounds). That this is the case is even clearer when we move away from examples involving surgery. Suppose, for example, that Jill, a seventy-year-old woman, chooses to receive treatment at home so she can be cared for by her son, rather than staying in a care home. If her son is happy with this decision then there is no problem. But what if he is not? The value of living autonomously does not mean that Jill alone should be the one to make that choice. Acting on her choice would frustrate her son's ability to live autonomously. The problem being highlighted here is that although we usually describe a patient's choice as being about what will happen to her, it can often equally accurately be described in other ways: as a choice about what other people will do (e.g. what treatment they will give her) or a choice about which people will help her (e.g. her son or the care home staff). These other people also have the capacity for autonomy. If living autonomously is valuable (which is a starting assumption of this argument), it must be valuable for them in just the same way that it is for her.

If this is right, the mere fact that the patient has the capacity for autonomy (and that living autonomously is valuable) places no obligations on healthcare professionals to give their patients the treatment they choose. Furthermore, were a patient to insist on a healthcare professional providing her with the treatment she wants (or anything else for that matter), she would be wronging him by failing to respect his autonomy. This does not mean that healthcare professionals never have an obligation to help patients achieve their goals, or allow patients to decide what to do. It is the more limited claim that there is no requirement to do any of this simply because the patient has a particular capacity (the capacity for autonomy). If it should be up to patients what treatment (if any) they get, we need to look elsewhere for the reason.

Two objections are likely to be raised at this point. The first is that the analogy to marriage that I relied on earlier is inappropriate because there is something distinctive about healthcare. Even if respect for autonomy does not impose a general obligation to let other people choose what will happen, it might be argued that it does impose such an obligation on healthcare professionals. For this objection to work some reason for thinking that things are different in healthcare is needed, and that reason must relate to the idea of enabling people to live more autonomously. That is not an easy task, and I am not aware of any such reasons.[6] In saying this I am not denying that healthcare professionals have obligations to assist their patients, or to do things that will help make their patients more autonomous, that other people may not have. If, as I argued in chapter two, healthcare professionals have an obligation to do what is prospectively best for their patients, this will ground just such an obligation. Where a patient is ill and seeks help to overcome that illness, her doctor will have an obligation to help her—and in doing so will normally enable her to be more autonomous. This obligation, however, is rooted in the obligation to benefit, not the obligation to respect autonomy. We will also see in the next section that healthcare professionals have obligations, within limits, to let patients choose and do what the patient has chosen. But the argument that they have those obligations will not in any way rest on the value of individuals shaping their lives in accordance with their values, goals, and commitments. Finally, in some cases healthcare professionals will have contractual obligations to let patients make certain choices, and then to do what the patient chooses. In such cases the reason they should enact the patient's choice is because they have voluntarily agreed to do so when signing the contract—again it does not stem directly from the need to respect patient autonomy.

The second objection likely to be raised here is that my choice of examples obscures the fact that sometimes healthcare professionals really can act in ways that govern their patients' lives. Suppose that rather than refusing a hip replacement operation Paula wants, her doctor performs a hip replacement she does not want. Isn't this a case where he denies her the chance to govern her own life, and isn't that wrong? It is undoubtedly the case that Paula's doctor in this scenario has acted wrongly. But, the reason it is wrong is not that he has denied Paula a choice she ought to have, and thus prevented her from making her life her own. This is in part for the reason we have just seen—to say that the choice should be hers is to say both that if she has not chosen something her doctor should not do it, **and** that if she has chosen something he should do it—and saying the latter is problematic.[7] But it is also because such an account has problems explaining why actions of this type are always wrong. To see why, consider the following two examples (neither of which involves a chronic illness). In both examples the patient has agreed to an operation while unaware that it will make him sterile.[8] Robert is in his mid-sixties. Several years ago he committed to living a celibate life as part of a religious order. He never wavers in this commitment. In performing the procedure that sterilises Robert his doctor does not decide for him that he will not have children, and impose that choice on him. Robert has already made that choice for himself—albeit the method he has adopted is different. Because of this, in acting as she does Robert's doctor neither intervenes in a way that shapes his life, nor sets back his ability to choose and enact the choices that matter for him. While she does take away Robert's ability to change his mind and enact that change, it is far from clear that taking away a possibility he neither wants nor values wrongs him. In contrast to Robert, Tim is a young sexually active man at the time the procedure is performed. However, unknown to both Tim and his doctor he is unable to have children. As such, the procedure does not in fact affect his ability to shape his life as he chooses. He could not choose to have children and enact that decision before the procedure, and he cannot do so after the procedure. In these two examples the doctors involved are not really governing the life of their patients. They do not, by their actions, prevent their patient making his life his own. As such, if their actions are wrong—and they are—the reason for this cannot be that they have set back their patient's ability to govern his life, or his chance to shape it in the way he chooses. To see why it is wrong we need to look elsewhere—either to the symbolic value of choice (to be considered below), or to the importance of consent (to be considered in chapter five).

In looking at these examples my focus has been on the consequences of acting—how it affects (or in the cases of Robert and Tim does not affect) the way a person's life goes. This focus is in turn a consequence of the account we are considering here, with its conceptualisation of choice as a way people shape their lives. To the extent that choosing what treatment (if any) to have does that, it does so in virtue of the way it affects their future. People generally do not choose treatment for its own sake, they choose it as a way to achieve some end or goal—to cure their illness,

'It should be up to the patient'   87

to alleviate their pain, to enable them to continue to live independently, etc. However, it might be argued that this focus on consequences misses something important. Medical interventions frequently involve actions that are wrong independent of their consequences. Carrying out an operation, for example, involves doing something to the patient's body, and morally that seems to matter. Doesn't the fact that it is her body mean that it should be up to her whether or not it is done? I will argue in the next chapter that it does. But we cannot argue that acting in this way is always wrong on the grounds that denying patients the chance to make this choice undermines their ability to shape the way their life goes. The reason that doing something to a patient's body without her consent is morally wrong is that it would violate her bodily integrity. It is not wrong because it sets back her opportunity to shape her life in the way that she chooses, or to make her life her own. To see this we only need to look at interventions that violate a person's bodily integrity but have no effect on how her life goes. Suppose, for example, that you were to take a mouth swab from a sleeping patient without her knowledge (Archard, 2008). This would be a violation of the patient's bodily integrity, and wrong on that basis, even though it does not affect how the patient's life goes and does not interfere with her ability to make her life her own. It is even possible, as David Owens has argued, to seriously violate a person's bodily integrity by raping them without them ever becoming aware of the rape (Owens, 2011, p. 416), and so without it affecting the way the victim's life goes. That would not affect the fact that the rape was wrong. This is not to deny that violations of bodily integrity sometimes have serious adverse consequences. But as Owens argues, where they do, this is, at least in part, because the person concerned knows that the violation has occurred, and thus that they have been seriously wronged (Owens, 2011, p. 416). In explaining why such violations are wrong we need to turn, as we will in chapter five, to a different type of account—one that focuses explicitly on consent, not choice.

The argument of this section has been that the capacity to live autonomously does not support the idea that what treatment (if any) a patient receives should be up to her, even if we accept that living autonomously is valuable.[9] While the focus has been on autonomy as a capacity (and as a value), it should not be difficult to see that accounts which conceptualise autonomy as sovereignty will face similar problems. Medical treatments (at least those that are our concern here) require people other than the patient to act (or refrain from acting). Whatever the limits of an individual's sovereignty (and we will look at this in more detail later) it cannot give them authority over what other people do. If it did, those others would not be sovereign. But healthcare professionals are as autonomous as their patients. That is, a patient's sovereignty cannot extend to her having the authority to require her doctor or other healthcare professionals to act in the way that she chooses (whether that be to have a treatment

88 'It should be up to the patient'

or not to have it) if they are also to be autonomous. In this the sovereign individual is like the sovereign state—on which the idea of autonomy as sovereignty is based (see Feinberg, 1986, pp. 47–51). Of course, sovereignty does require that others cannot do things to us (to invade our territory). But as we will see in chapter five this is best captured by the idea that what the patient has authority over (if he is sovereign) is what it is permissible to do to him, rather than what is done to him (as Feinberg argues; see Feinberg, 1986, pp. 47–51). And here again we are in the realm of consent rather than choice.

4.4 The Symbolic Value of Choice

As we have just seen the idea that what happens, or what treatment is given, should be up to the patient cannot be defended by focusing on autonomy as a way people shape their lives. However, this does not mean it cannot be defended. Doing so requires moving to a different account of the value of choice. The argument in the previous section took it that choosing is valuable because it is by choosing that people make their life their own. This is the, frequently unstated, starting point of those writers who stress autonomy as a capacity. But as we have seen choice can also be valuable for other reasons, ones that have not been extensively explored to date in the healthcare ethics literature. The most important of these for our purposes is that who gets to choose matters symbolically (Scanlon, 1998, pp. 253–256). It is to this account that I now want to turn.

Scanlon develops his ideas about the value of choice as part of his general account of what people owe others (Scanlon, 1998). On that account choosing is valuable for three reasons. One of these is that being allowed to choose, and even more being prevented from choosing, sends a message about how others view the person concerned. As Scanlon puts it,

> In a situation in which people are normally expected to make choices of a certain sort for themselves, individuals have reason to value the opportunity to make these choices because not having or not exercising this opportunity would be seen as reflecting a judgment (their own or someone else's) that they are not competent or do not have the standing normally accorded an adult member of the society.
> (Scanlon, 1998, p. 253)

These are judgments people want to avoid. As such, having the opportunity to choose, or being allowed to choose, is valuable to them because "it is an important form of recognition as competent independent agents" (Scanlon, 1998, p. 256). Being denied that opportunity is potentially "demeaning" (Scanlon, 1998, p. 253), and "would stigmatize those who are interfered with by labelling them as immature or incompetent"

(Scanlon, 1998, p. 254). While Scanlon's concern is not with healthcare, encounters with doctors and other healthcare professionals are ones in which people are normally expected to make certain types of decision for themselves. Furthermore, situations where the symbolic value of choice comes into play are not limited to those where people are *expected* to make choices, they also include situations where people are generally *allowed* to make choices. As David Owens points out,

> If I live in a society in which most people are allowed the choice of whether to wear a crash helmet whilst cycling, the fact that I (and people like me) are deprived of this choice will be demeaning. It carries the message that they are competent to decide this matter but I am not.
>
> (Owens, 2011, p. 409)

It is undoubtedly the case that in contemporary medicine adults are generally allowed to make choices about what treatment (if any) they will receive.

Because of this, healthcare professionals who deny their patients a choice about what treatment to have, wrong those patients. They do so by acting in a way that demeans the patient, and fails to recognise her as a competent agent. Their actions, we might say, belittle their patient and that is incompatible with treating her in the way she deserves to be treated. There is a clear link here to the idea of respecting patients who are autonomous (in the sense of having a certain capacity as outlined in section 4.2 above). Only patients who are autonomous (in that sense) can be wronged in this way by denying them a choice. It is not demeaning to be treated as lacking competence if one does lack competence. As such, we could reasonably express this point by saying that to respect the autonomy of competent patients healthcare professionals should allow those patients to choose what treatment (if any) to have. However, doing so might be misleading. The idea that choice is important for symbolic reasons, and that this is why patients should be able to choose what treatment to have, is substantially different from the dominant accounts of respect for autonomy in the literature. As we will see these differences have important implications for what healthcare professionals ought to do.

In uncovering these implications it will be useful to start by contrasting the idea that choice is valuable for symbolic reasons with the idea that it is valuable for instrumental reasons. While the latter is committed to the idea that the patient is the best judge of her own interests, the former is not. When it comes to the symbolic value of choice what matters is simply that the patient has the opportunity to choose. She can make her choice using whatever method works best for her. She might, for example, weigh up the costs and benefits herself, or consult with others (her family, friends, doctor, religious advisor), or defer to someone else whose judgment she trusts. Which method she uses is irrelevant as far as the symbolic value of choice is concerned. All that matters is that she gets to make the choice—it is not imposed on her. Forcing, manipulating, or deceiving the patient into making a particular choice is not consistent with recognising that she is competent to make that choice herself. That is, on this account as long as the patient has made a voluntary choice to have (or not have) a particular treatment she has not been wronged. Things are different if the reason the patient should have a choice is that she is the best judge of her own interests. As we saw in chapter two, on any such account some ways of deciding what treatment to have will be ruled out. For example, it would make no sense, on that account, for her to defer to someone else when deciding what treatment to have. This restriction on how the patient makes her choice causes problems for instrumental accounts—as we saw in chapter three. Accounts based on the symbolic value of choice avoid these problems. They also better capture our intuitions in cases where a patient who has been given no choice nevertheless receives the treatment she would have chosen had she had one. If the value of choice is instrumental it does not look as if this patient can reasonably complain that her doctor has acted wrongly—choice is valuable because it is a way to ensure she gets what is best for her, and she would not be better off if she had been given a choice. On the other hand, if the value of choice is symbolic this patient does have a reasonable complaint. Her doctor has treated her in a way that is belittling and that fails to recognise her as a competent person.

These differences affect what a healthcare professional should do in at least some cases. Suppose, for example, that a patient is not sure what to do and asks her doctor what he advises or what he thinks the next step should be. If his concern is with the instrumental value of choice, the patient's doctor should resist answering this question. But if it is with the symbolic value of choice he need not. On that account there is no reason not to tell his patient what he thinks would be best for her. Indeed, if (as I argued in chapter two) healthcare professionals should do what is prospectively best for their patients, there are good reasons to think he should. Doing so is a way to bring it about that he both avoids demeaning his patient by denying her a choice and does what is prospectively best for her. The requirement that patients be the ones to choose precludes their doctor choosing for them. It does not preclude their doctor either providing advice about what he thinks is best, or attempting to persuade them to take the option that he believes is best (something that would be ruled out according to instrumental accounts of the value of choice).

Grounding the idea that patients should be the ones to choose on the symbolic value of choice also differs in practice from accounts that ground it on the value of making one's life one's own—particularly when it comes to the kinds of choices patients should be allowed to make, and which patients should be allowed to make them. Denying a person a choice is not always demeaning, and does not always express any judgment about their competence. For example, while regulations restricting the number of hours a person can work restrict choice (they remove the option to work more hours) they do not necessarily treat anyone as incompetent—rather they protect people from being forced to make certain choices (Scanlon, 1998, p. 254). The same will be true for some public health regulations that restrict choice. It is also the case that some choices—such as whether or not to have treatment that would be ineffective given the patient's condition—are not ones that anyone is allowed or expected to make. As such, denying a patient this choice would not carry the message that others are competent to choose but she is not. Denying patients the option of choosing a treatment that is not funded by the local health authority, or the relevant insurance provider, carries no such message either. Because of this, to avoid sending a demeaning message, healthcare professionals only need to allow their patients to choose between those locally available treatments they judge would benefit their patients. That is, if choice is valuable for symbolic reasons, patients should be allowed to choose between those treatments her healthcare provider makes available for people with her condition—what Sven Ove Hansson calls, in a different context, those "therapeutic options proposed by medical professionals" (Hansson, 2013, p. 120). This account provides no support for the idea that patients should be able to demand services that would not generally be provided in similar circumstances to other patients.

While this section has concentrated on choices about treatment, its argument has wider implications. Some of the choices made in healthcare settings are about other things—for example, choices about when to eat or bathe, when to get up or go to bed, what to eat, and what to do to fill one's time when in a hospital or care home. Just as it is possible to wrong patients by denying them a choice about what treatment to have, it is also possible to wrong them by denying them choices about these other things too. Denying such choices is not always wrong—the message sent by denying someone a choice is always context dependent. But where doing so would send a message that a competent patient is not competent, denying her the opportunity to choose is wrong in exactly the same way as denying someone a choice about what treatment to have would be wrong. This may be particularly important when it comes to long term care for older patients. Giving these patients choices over the details of their lives is a way of recognising that they are "competent independent agents" (Scanlon, 1998, p. 256) and still have the standing "normally accorded an adult member of the society" (Scanlon, 1998, p. 253).

Given the way they are sometimes treated older patients, including those with declining cognitive capacities, may be particularly sensitive to the messages sent by being denied choices. That is particularly important in the context of treating patients with chronic illness for two reasons.

First, older adults, as we saw in chapter one, are more likely to experience chronic illness than those who are younger. Second, widespread ageism means that such patients may be treated as if they are unable to decide for themselves even where they are. Decisions may be made for them, which would not be made for younger patients whose situation is otherwise similar. As such, these patients may reasonably chafe against attempts by others to choose for them, in part as a way to resist attempts to treat them as if they are no longer competent. Older children with chronic illnesses may also be particularly sensitive to the symbolic value of choice. They might well be denied a choice—technically they are still children—but may also very much value the recognition that comes with being allowed to make that choice. Looking in a bit more detail at people in these groups will enable us to tease out the account being developed here in a bit more detail, and also allow us to address a potential problem for it.

Many, indeed most, older adults and older children can make choices—they can understand information, deliberate about what to do, and choose on the basis of that deliberation. How well they do this will vary, but there is no reason to think they will all fall below the threshold of competence used for the rest of the adult population. This raises a question—on the account being developed here, is the threshold for being allowed to choose the same as the threshold for counting as having the capacity for autonomy (that is, for being competent)? To answer that question we need to focus on whether denying certain individuals a choice would demean or belittle them, not on whether those individuals are autonomous. Doing so is complicated because it will vary depending on the nature of the choice. It may be belittling to deny a person choices over what to eat, but not to deny her choices over what medical treatment to have. In this it is no different from any other account—for example if we treat 'autonomous' and 'competent' as having the same threshold we would need to recognise (as is standardly the case) that whether someone passes this threshold is task specific (see discussion in Beauchamp and Childress, 2009, pp. 112–114) or that there are spheres in which a person is autonomous and others in which she is not (Berofsky, 1995, p. 31).

Suppose that for the moment we restrict our attention to choices about whether or not to have treatment. It might appear that someone competent to make this choice should be allowed to do so because to deny her that opportunity would be to treat her as incompetent (which she is not). However, this creates a potential problem. It is easiest to see this where the patient is an older child (as some patients with chronic illness are). The problem is not that such children might choose to have a treatment that is bad for them. As we have seen, the options patients should be allowed to choose between are only those that would generally be made available to someone with the patient's condition. The problem is that they might choose not to have treatment that would be very beneficial for them. This is sometimes captured in the literature as an asymmetry between being able to consent to and being able to refuse treatment (for discussion of this kind of case see Walker, 2016).[10]

There are two ways we might attempt to respond to this problem. The first focuses on the relevant contrast class. According to the account being developed here the problem with not giving patients an opportunity to choose is that it treats them differently than others (who would be given that opportunity). To apply this account we need to have some idea who the relevant 'others' are. Suppose we say that in the case of children the relevant contrast class is other children. In that case the problem with older children could be avoided. They are children and children are not generally expected or allowed to make choices over what treatment they will have. Such an approach is unlikely to succeed. As I have stressed when it comes to the symbolic value of choice what matters is whether denying choice sends a message that is demeaning or belittling to the person concerned. In part that depends on whether they are competent to make a choice (and some older children are). It also depends on social norms and common practice. Common practice in healthcare can be characterised either as allowing those who are competent to make choices over what medical treatment they receive, or as allowing competent adults to make choices over what medical treatment they receive. The latter is more restrictive, but the limitation to adults (that is a restriction based solely on age) seems arbitrary—were we to deny all those over sixty choices about what treatment they receive this would not avoid the problem that denying such choices would be demeaning (indeed it would exacerbate the existing ageism such patients face). We might more reasonably think that the restriction to adults is based on the idea that denying choice to adults is demeaning or belittling, in a way that denying choice to children is not.

The alternative is to argue that while all those who are competent should be allowed to choose, it is nevertheless sometimes acceptable to override those choices. As patients people might value having the opportunity to choose, and for that choice to affect what happens (it ensures they are recognised as competent agents). But they also value other things, like avoiding harm. Because they are not infallible judges, and sometimes make poor choices, things they value can come into conflict—as when they choose something that is harmful, or refrain from choosing something that would be beneficial. Healthcare professionals ought both to avoid imposing treatments on their patients and do what is best for them. Where a patient refuses treatment that would significantly benefit her they cannot do both. As such, a decision about what is most important will need to be made. As we have seen, this situation is familiar (perhaps particularly for those who adopt a four principles approach). It is relatively straightforward to see how the problematic cases involving older children can be dealt with on this approach (see Walker, 2016). Where healthcare professionals have good reason to think that acting on the patient's choice would be very harmful to her, so that the value of avoiding that harm outweighs the value of having her choice enacted, there is no need for them to act on that choice. In practice such cases are likely to be rare. That the choice may be overridden does not mean the patient has not been offered a genuine opportunity to choose. There is no reason for the healthcare professional to even consider whether a particular choice (such as to have no treatment) would be overridden until it actually happens. And even where the patient chooses something harmful, overriding that choice is not the first thing he should do—explaining the possible harms, and ensuring his patient has not misunderstood relevant information comes first. It may also not be possible in practice for him to override her choice (particularly where that is a choice not to have treatment) or overriding it may be unjustified for other reasons. That is, at the time the patient makes her choice there is no reason to think that she will get the treatment whatever she says, and hence no reason to think she does not really have a choice.

On this account the problem is not with how older children should be treated, it with how competent adults should be treated. In practice competent adults are frequently treated as having a right to refuse treatment, a right that is sometimes enshrined in local laws. For example, according to Margaret Brazier and Emma Cave in the United Kingdom, "The right of the patient who is sufficiently rational and mature to agree to that treatment is a basic human right" (Brazier and Cave, 2007, p. 99). Such an absolute prohibition cannot be defended on an account that starts from the symbolic value of choice. To support it we would need to move to an account on which competent patients have absolute authority over either what treatment they receive or what treatment it is permissible to give them (for an example see Feinberg, 1986, pp. 47–97). That is, we would need to move to a specific account of consent. We will consider such accounts in the next chapter.

Finally, the argument we have been looking at in this section appears to give good grounds for introducing regulations that stipulate competent patients must be given a choice about what (if any) treatment to have—such regulations would help to guard against actions that wrong the patient by treating them in a demeaning or belittling way. But it does not support the idea that healthcare professionals should not act until their patients have made an informed choice (in the sense usually spelt out in informed consent regulations). What matters on this account is that the patient gets to choose what treatment (of those that are standardly offered to patients in his position or with his condition) she receives. Suppose that a patient chooses to have a certain treatment without taking any notice of (or perhaps without even being told about) the potential risks involved. She has made a voluntary choice, and as such would not be belittled or demeaned if she is given that treatment. We may think it would be unwise for her to choose without more information, but this does not mean she has not voluntarily chosen. For this reason the idea that the choice should be the patient's does not impose any obligation to tell her about the different treatment options available, beyond what is required for her to be able to make a choice (though as we have seen this needs to be done in a way that neither coerces nor deceives her). How much information that is is likely to vary from patient to patient. While some patients may be happy to make a choice without knowing much, and perhaps preferring not to know much, about possible consequences or the risks involved, others will want a lot more information before they choose. While everyone can make a choice without knowing much about the available options, not everyone is willing to do so. They may phrase this unwillingness by saying they cannot choose unless they have more information, but we should not be misled by the literal meaning of what is said here. This distinction between what is needed for a person to be able to choose and what is needed for him to be willing to choose is also important when it comes to consent. For that reason we will come back to it in the next chapter.

4.5 Conclusion

In this chapter we have been investigating whether it should be up to patients what treatment (if any) they have. I have argued that there is a sense in which it should. If other people are allowed, or expected, to make certain choices, then they should be allowed to make those choices too. In practice this means that healthcare professionals should allow competent patients to choose between the available and effective options (remembering that no treatment is always an option). The reason for this has nothing to do with the value of living autonomously. It is because denying choice in this situation would treat the patient in a demeaning or belittling way. To some, perhaps most, readers this account will seem inadequate. It says that the patient should be allowed to choose, but does not require that her choice be informed. It requires consistency, but does not say why it would be wrong to deny everyone a choice. It could not, for example, explain why it would be wrong to impose treatment on others in a situation where no-one is expected or allowed to make decisions about their own treatment. Finally, it does not require that healthcare professionals do what the patient chooses if they believe that doing so would harm the patient.

That it does not capture everything that matters, however, should not be surprising. At the start of this chapter I distinguished two ways in which healthcare professionals can wrong their patients: 1. imposing treatment on the patient without her consent, and 2. choosing for the patient what treatment she will have. In this chapter we have only been concerned with the latter. The idea that it is wrong to impose treatment on a person without her consent has yet to be addressed. Similarly, we have not yet looked at what is required for consent (that is, what is required for an act to make permissible what would otherwise have been wrong). For example, we have not looked at whether only those who are suitably informed about a treatment (what it involves, its benefits and side effects) can consent to it being given. It is to these questions that we now need to turn. They are not questions about choice, but about the morality of giving treatment. As such, when looking at them we will focus only on consent (making permissible) and leave questions of patient choice to one side. While in both healthcare ethics and medical ethics it is usual to combine consent and choice, as I have been stressing the two are importantly different both conceptually and in practice. The wrong, where it is a wrong, of denying patients a choice over their treatment, is different from the wrong of imposing treatment on them without their consent. While it is possible to wrong a patient in both ways (and such cases have played a prominent role in the literature), they do not necessarily go together.

Before moving on, however, it is worth briefly explaining how the arguments we have just been looking at relate to those in chapters two and three. While the starting point for this chapter was healthcare professionals' obligation to respect autonomy, those earlier chapters started from their obligations to benefit and not harm their patients. One difference that our starting point makes is fairly clear. Obligations to benefit and not harm can, as we saw in chapters two and three, mean that the carers of incompetent patients (including the parents of a child) should have a say in what treatment is given. In contrast, obligations to respect autonomy do not. When we turn to competent patients the picture turns out to be much messier—reflecting the realities of healthcare practice. To capture it we need to focus on three distinct categories:

1. **Cases in which healthcare professionals should seek their patient's informed choice and show that choice compliance respect for epistemic reasons.** These, as we saw in chapters two and three, fall into two distinct categories: 1. cases where it is reasonable to judge that the patient (or her carer) is the best judge of what is best for her, 2. cases where the patient is the appropriate judge of whether a risk is worth taking in light of the potential benefits of taking it. In these cases, healthcare professionals have an obligation to provide relevant information to patients (or their carers) and in at least some cases take steps to ensure that that information is understood. If healthcare professionals do all this, as required by the epistemic argument looked at in chapters two and three, they will also have done everything required to ensure that they do not demean their patients. They will have given their patients a choice about what treatment to have (where the relevant choice is between those treatments (or other options) that are both available locally and therapeutically beneficial).

'It should be up to the patient' 97

2. **Cases in which the epistemic argument fails to provide any reason to seek input from the patient.** In these cases there will often still be a requirement, arising from the argument in this chapter, to give the patient a choice about what treatment to have. That argument does not require that that the patient make an informed choice, as that is usually understood in healthcare ethics. As such, in contrast with cases in the first category, there is much less of an onus on healthcare professionals to provide information to (or to ensure the understanding of) their patients. Problems could occur if the patient does not choose the option that the healthcare professional judges is best for her. However, such problems are likely to be rare—for cases in this category what is best for the patient is frequently clear cut. Where they arise further work is needed to find out what has been missed or misunderstood either by the patient or the healthcare professional. Where this does not resolve the issue a choice still has to be made. That will require balancing the requirement not to demean the patient with the requirement to do what is prospectively best for her.
3. **Cases, perhaps the majority, in which the epistemic argument requires healthcare professionals to seek their patient's (or the patient's carer's) informed choice, and to show that choice consideration respect.** In these cases the healthcare professional has two independent reasons to show her patient's choice consideration respect—doing so is needed both to work out what is best for her, and to avoid acting in a way that demeans her. As with cases in category one, the first of these also gives her reason to provide relevant information to the patient. Because the obligation here is only to show consideration respect, sometimes a healthcare professional should not do what her patient has chosen (though in practice such cases may be rare). These will be times where, having taken account of the patient's choices, she judges both that (a) something else is better for her and (b) what she has chosen is sufficiently worse for her that all things considered he has greater reason to do what she has not chosen (the additional benefit) than what she has (the benefit that option will provide *plus* the need to avoid demeaning her).

For cases falling into either 2 or 3 above there may be disagreement between patient and healthcare professional. Deciding what to do in such cases requires weighing up all the reasons for and against the different options. If a patient has not chosen a particular treatment there will normally be several reasons not to give it to her. In addition to those mentioned above these can include the practical difficulties of doing so, and that the patient has not consented to the treatment (where consent is needed to avoid wrongdoing). Where this is the case these all need to go into the calculation about what to do.

Notes

1. It is worth noting here a difference between treatment and research. Respect for autonomy in research will typically only require consent. The researcher is the one who chooses what is being investigated and who would be a suitable participant. He then needs those individuals to consent to being included in the research. Given the strong connections between research ethics and medical ethics this might explain why choice is often conflated with consent. Indeed, Tom Beauchamp has stated that in setting out early guidelines for research ethics it was argued that respect for persons applied to informed consent (with no mention of anything else) (see Beauchamp, 2010c, p. 9).
2. In saying this I am taking 'respect' to have its standard English meaning. Some authors, as we have seen, give it an extended meaning, so that it covers things like enabling a person to make an autonomous choice (see Beauchamp and Childress, 2009, p. 104; Beauchamp, 2010b, p. 37; Levy, 2014). I will argue in chapter eight that doing so is a mistake.
3. Because competence is standardly taken to be task specific (see, for example, Beauchamp and Childress, 2009, p. 112), they also imply that autonomy is task specific.
4. Those cases where she can treat herself without anyone's help are not ones we need consider here, given our concern is with the moral obligations of healthcare professionals.
5. Of course, a doctor's situation is not exactly like Joe's. He may have contractual obligations that mean he must give his patient the treatment she requests. For the purposes of the argument here I am putting any such obligations to one side. What they consist in will vary considerably from place to place.
6. We will investigate the idea that healthcare professionals should enable their patients to be more autonomous in chapter eight below. However, even if they do (and as we will see I am sceptical about that) it does not follow that they should always do what their patients choose. Some further argument would be needed to support that conclusion.
7. It may not appear problematic because our intuitions can be misled by cases where it looks as if the choice really is the patient's to make. Suppose, for example, that Paula's doctor has decided that a hip replacement would be prospectively best for Paula, but he will not perform it unless she consents. In that case if Paula agrees to it, it will happen; and if she does not agree to it, it will not. Here the choice is up to Paula, but notice that her choice only concerns whether or not to do something her doctor has already determined is beneficial for her. If she chooses to have it, her doctor will perform it because he thinks this is what is best for her (not because it is something she has autonomously chosen). We will consider the reasons that a patient should have this kind of more circumscribed choice in the next section.
8. As in the case of *Bang v Charles T Miller Hospital*, 251 Minn. 427, 88 N.W. 2d 186 (1958). That case concerned consent, not choice, and we will return to the issues it raised in chapter five.
9. This argument concerns patient choice, and has nothing to say about consent. As such, nothing said here challenges the idea that it would be wrong to give competent patients' treatment they have not consented to (that is, have not made permissible) because doing so would fail to respect their autonomy.
10. As we will see the issue is not really one of consent, it is one of choice, but the same issues arise.

5 Consent and the Treatment of Chronic Illness

5.1 Introduction

The previous three chapters have all been about choosing. But choosing is not an end in itself. Unless the choice is to do nothing, someone or more frequently several people, need to act. Who that is, and what they need to do, depends on the choice made. Where a healthcare professional needs to act, doing so will sometimes be wrong unless her patient has consented.[1] The mere fact that she is enacting her patient's choice is not sufficient to avoid this wrong. As we have seen, choosing and consenting are not the same. While ethicists have tended to focus on consent for treatment or research, when it comes to patients with chronic illnesses consent may also be needed for other things—including carrying out tests (such as taking a blood sample or carrying out a physical examination), assisting the patient to carry out everyday tasks (like washing or going to the toilet), entering the patient's home or living space (as part of a home visit), and passing on information about the patient to others (including family members and people working for other support services). In some of these cases formal written consent procedures will be in place, in others they will not. What we say about consent will need to accommodate this variety.

When we are concerned, as people often are, with what those formal procedures should say (or with assessing the adequacy of existing regulations governing consent) it is reasonable to start by asking what purpose they serve. As we saw in chapter one, when it comes to informed consent regulations there are several ways of answering that question—to ensure autonomy is respected, to promote patient well-being, or to protect healthcare professionals. However, when, as here, we are concerned with what healthcare professionals should do in the world in which they work, a world governed by existing regulations, three different questions take precedence—what I will call the 'when', 'who', and 'how' questions.

First, when do healthcare professionals need consent? Consent makes permissible what was previously impermissible. As such, healthcare professionals only need consent where: 1. they have reason to do something,

2. doing it would currently be wrong, and 3. someone else (but not the healthcare professional) can bring it about that it would not be wrong. We might put it this way: consent raises a normative barrier in the way of doing something the healthcare professional has some reason to do. Once that barrier is lifted she will normally have a reason to act. However, this is always a reason that exists before the consent was given (it is the reason she needed consent in the first place). It is not created by the act of consenting. That is, consent does not give anyone a reason to act; it removes a reason not to act.

Second, when healthcare professionals need consent, who do they need it from? The obvious answer is that consent is needed from the patient. He, and he alone, can make it permissible for them to act. But that is only sometimes the right answer—either the patient or his spouse, for example, could consent to a nurse entering his house. To the extent that the patient alone can consent, his authority is absolute (Feinberg, 1986, pp. 47–97). To act would always be wrong unless he has consented. However, given the way I am using 'consent' it does not follow either that it would be wrong all things considered, or that his consent makes acting all things considered permissible. To consent, as I explained in chapter one, is to bring it about that something that would have been wrong for some reason is no longer wrong for that reason. That an act is wrong for *some* reason does not mean it is wrong all things considered, and that an act is not wrong for some reason does not mean that it is not wrong *simpliciter*.

Third, how do healthcare professionals know that they have got consent, and so know that it is permissible for them to proceed? When consenting people communicate their consent in different ways. In the context of consenting to medical treatment, for example, a patient might do so by signing a consent form, by saying he agrees to what his doctor proposes, or by rolling up his sleeve so she can give him an injection. Colloquially we might call such acts consenting. But, of course, not all acts that look like consent (that involve doing the things that people do, or saying the things people say, when they consent) are in fact consent. For an act to be consent it must meet certain criteria, what we can call the constitutive rules for consent (Searle, 1969, pp. 33–42). These criteria may not be the only rules that govern consent. There may also be what Searle refers to as 'regulative rules'. While an act that meets the constitutive but not the regulative rules for consent changes the normative landscape in the required way, there is a sense in which it is defective—just as while an insincere promise is a promise there is something wrong with it as a promise (for example, because to make such a promise is morally wrong; see Kant, 2005, pp. 98–99).

In healthcare ethics three constitutive rules for consent have been prominent: 1. the individual consenting must be competent, 2. the act by which he consents must be voluntary, and 3. he must at the time he consents have substantial understanding of what is proposed. According to this set of constitutive rules, to determine whether her patient has consented a healthcare professional needs to determine whether he is competent, is acting voluntarily, and has the required level of understanding.

However, while discussions of consent have focused on voluntariness, competence, and understanding, these cannot be the only constitutive rules for consent. Consent must also be intentional (Raz, 1986, p. 81; Beauchamp, 2005, p. 314; Owens, 2012, p. 165). That is, for an act to constitute consent it must be done with the intention of making something permissible. To see why, consider an actor playing a patient. He does the same things that a real patient would do when giving consent. He is also competent, is acting voluntarily and has the relevant understanding (the actress playing his doctor has explained it to him just as a real doctor would). But he has not consented. And the reason he has not consented is that he was not acting with the right intention. That consent has to be intentional in this sense will play an important role in what follows.

Even with this addition there is still something missing. Consider the following situation. Joe (a competent adult) signs a consent form on behalf of his sister Mary (also a competent adult). He does so voluntarily, and he has the required level of understanding. His intention is to make it permissible for Mary's doctor to give her treatment. Joe seems to meet all the constitutive rules for consent, but he has not consented—his signing the form does not make it permissible to give Mary the treatment. Why not? The obvious answer is that Mary, and Mary alone, can give the necessary consent (taking us back to the 'who' question). As such, we need another constitutive rule for consent—the person acting must have the standing, or authority, to consent (to bring it about that what was wrong for some reason is no longer wrong for that reason).[2] Who has this standing, or authority, will depend on why it would be wrong to act without consent. To see why, consider the consent healthcare professionals need to avoid the wrong of failing to comply with regulations they ought to comply with (what in chapter one I called regulatory consent). Informed consent regulations are of this type. But they are not the only such regulations. Property laws, for example, mean that healthcare professionals should not enter a patient's house without consent. Both informed consent regulations and property laws stipulate whose consent is needed to avoid failure to comply with them—the patient (if he is competent) in the case of informed consent regulations, the owner or occupier of the property in the case of property laws. Because these are different it follows that who has the standing or authority to consent varies depending on whether consent is needed to avoid the wrong of failing to comply with informed consent regulations or to avoid the wrong of trespassing.

Regulatory consent is not the only type of consent that healthcare professionals need if they are to avoid wrongdoing. Some things would be wrong if done without consent even in the absence of regulations.

102 *Consent and Treatment of Chronic Illness*

There is likely to be considerable overlap between what is needed for this non-regulatory consent and what is needed for regulatory consent—particularly where regulations attempt to capture pre-existing moral requirements. But we should not expect the two to be identical. Indeed, that they are not identical is behind many critiques of existing informed consent regulations (as we saw in chapter one). This means that to get a full picture of healthcare professionals' obligations when treating those with chronic illness we need to investigate both regulatory and non-regulatory consent. How we answer the three questions with which we started (when, who, and how) when it comes to one cannot safely be assumed to give us the answer to those questions when it comes to the other. In principle, though not always in practice, what is needed for regulatory consent is relatively straightforward. We will, therefore, deal with it first.

5.2 Regulatory Consent

There are regulations (including, but not limited to, informed consent regulations) that healthcare professionals ought to comply with. What those regulations require varies from country to country. There is no way to cover them all here, and it would be problematic to focus on the regulations that exist in one country (treating them as though they are a model for everywhere else). Instead in this section I want to clarify in general terms the ways in which regulations governing healthcare professionals impose obligations on them. That is partly because these obligations matter in practice. But it is also because it is easy to run the requirements for regulatory and non-regulatory consent together unless the former are explicitly separated out and addressed on their own terms.

As explained in chapter one, 'regulations' (unlike 'guidelines') do not simply reflect the obligations people have, they create obligations. They can do so in different ways. For example, where someone has voluntarily agreed to do something, they ought to do it. This is required if they are to keep their word (a requirement of fidelity in W.D. Ross's sense [Ross, 1930; Audi, 2004], though as Margaret Gilbert has pointed out philosophers have paid less attention to agreements than to promises under this heading [Gilbert, 2014, p. 28]). As such, if a healthcare professional has voluntarily agreed to abide by a professional code of conduct, and her licence to practice is given to her on the basis that she will do so, she thereby has an obligation to abide by it. If that code of conduct says she must obtain a patient's consent before acting, then she would be acting wrongly if she does not obtain his consent (and would be doing so even if this would not be wrong in the absence of that code of conduct). Healthcare professionals, like everyone else, also have obligations to obey the law (Gert, Culver, and Clouser, 2006, p. 36)—though whether there is a moral obligation to do so in all circumstances may be questioned. Finally, regulations in healthcare typically include penalties for non-adherence. These can be severe—loss of employment and/or licence to practice, fines, or imprisonment (depending on the details of the regulations that have been broken). As such, those working in healthcare have prudential reasons to comply with whatever the regulations say. But they may also have non-prudential reasons to avoid these penalties. Breaking the regulations to help one patient may mean they are unable to benefit many others in the future because they are no longer licensed to do so.

It is a feature of what I am calling regulations that they proscribe certain acts. Which acts they proscribe will be specified by the regulations themselves. But, depending on how they are written, those regulations might also allow specified individuals to change this—to bring it about that those acts would not be wrong in particular instances. That is, they may create the possibility for regulatory consent. Which individuals can consent in this way and what they can consent to will depend on what exactly the regulations say. For example, the regulations may stipulate that only competent adults can consent. In which case there is nothing those who are not adults, or who are not competent, can do to make acting permissible. Those regulations may also stipulate that while competent adults can make some things proscribed by the regulations permissible, there are other things proscribed by those regulations that they cannot make permissible (for example, certain types of very dangerous research). In that case there are some things that it would always be wrong for healthcare professionals to do. Whatever their patient says or does, acting in those ways is something the healthcare professional should not do because it would be a failure to comply with regulations she ought to comply with.

When it comes to regulatory consent, that is, the answers to the 'when' and 'who' questions depend on how the relevant regulations are written. How they are written will also typically provide an answer to the 'how' question. Regulations that incorporate consent clauses normally spell out (at least in general terms) what criteria need to be met for a patient's act to make it permissible under the regulations for a healthcare professional to do things like perform surgery or give an injection. As such, if healthcare professionals are to avoid acting wrongly they need to know what is required by the regulations governing their practice. That will vary from place to place depending on local laws and institutional requirements. There is, therefore, nothing general that can be said about it here—and it would take us too far from our aims to analyse all the various regulations that govern healthcare in different places. I do however want to stress that what is required for regulatory consent is dependent on both the context and the location. This can sometimes be missed if we focus on the idea that consent is needed in order to respect autonomy—simply because it might be thought that the requirement to respect autonomy is the same everywhere.

Healthcare professionals ought to comply with regulations for the reasons explained above, but there is also something else they should do. They have an obligation to benefit their patients, and some things that would benefit patients (such as giving medical treatment) are frequently proscribed by regulations healthcare professionals ought to comply with unless the patient has consented to them. As such, healthcare professionals need to seek their patients' consent. Doing so can require more than merely asking for it. A patient may (depending on what the regulations say) not be *able* to give regulatory consent unless he either has or understands certain information. Alternatively, he may not be *willing* to consent unless he has that information. In either case, given her obligations his doctor (or other healthcare professional) ought to give the information to him. Unless she does so, she will not be able to do what she ought to do (benefit him) without acting wrongly (by failing to comply with regulations she should comply with). It is worth saying a bit more about what this requires.

The idea that a patient cannot consent unless he has, or understands, certain information is a familiar one. The explanation, when it comes to regulatory consent, is that the regulations do not allow it. Informed consent regulations often say something along these lines: an individual, T, must not do X unless 1. S has been told about the nature, benefits, and potential risks of X; 2. S has been given time to consider that information and consult with others should he choose to do so; and 3. T has obtained S's voluntary agreement to T doing X. If this is what the regulations say, then unless S has been told about the 'nature, benefits and potential risks of X' he cannot consent to T doing X. Whatever S says or does, T would be failing to comply with the regulations were she to do so. As such, an uninformed patient is in the same position as a child or incompetent adult. There is nothing he can do to bring it about that it is permissible to give him treatment. That is, in this context at least,

> If a patient or research subject remains uninformed or under-informed about what others (researchers, clinicians) propose or request, then however eagerly or fully he appears to agree to their proposals, those indications of agreement do not count as giving consent, and do not licence others to act as they propose.
> (Manson and O'Neill, 2007, p. 89)

The healthcare professionals treating a patient can change this simply by giving him the specified information in an understandable form. He is now able to consent. Because they need his consent healthcare professionals thus ought to give him that information. This is necessary if they are to be able to do what they ought to do (benefit their patients) without breaching regulations they ought to comply with. What information they ought to provide depends on what the regulations say, and on how they should be interpreted (Raz, 2009)—something that will vary from place to place.

There are two conclusions we can draw at this point. First, a point sometimes neglected in the healthcare ethics literature is that laws and other regulations create reasons for healthcare professionals to provide information to their patients that would not exist in their absence. That there are these reasons can, and should, influence our judgments about what information is needed for a patient to be able to consent to medical treatment—that is, they can, and should, influence our judgments about the constitutive rules for consent in this context. However, it is important to recognise that these judgments are about the constitutive rules for regulatory consent. Because they are shaped by what the regulations say they may not capture what is needed for non-regulatory consent. Second, informed consent regulations frequently say that informed consent, in the sense of an autonomous authorisation (an authorisation made voluntarily by a competent and substantially informed person; Beauchamp, 2005, pp. 314–317), is needed before giving treatment (though the details will vary from place to place). This tells us what the constitutive rules for regulatory consent are—only an autonomous authorisation can bring it about that giving medical treatment is not contrary to regulations healthcare professionals ought to comply with. It does not tell us that the reason it would be wrong to give treatment without consent is that doing so would fail to respect the patient's autonomy (see Walker, 2018). The idea of autonomy potentially plays a double role here, one that can be missed if we are not careful. Of course, the regulations may have been shaped at least in part by the idea that healthcare professionals should respect their patients' autonomy. But, the obligation both to give patients information and to obtain their consent would exist even if this were not the case.

While, as we have just seen, healthcare professionals ought to give patients whatever information is needed for regulatory consent, doing so may not be enough. In some cases a patient will not be willing to consent unless he has additional information (he may phrase this by saying that he needs more information but this does not mean he cannot consent without that information). In this situation the healthcare professionals treating him have reason to give him that information whatever it turns out to be (Walker, 2012b). Doing so is required if they are to get the consent they need. What this means in practice will vary from patient to patient—some patients may be happy to grant consent on the basis of very little information, while others require a fairly detailed explanation before being willing to do so. In many cases this information will have been given to the patient at the time treatment was chosen. But sometimes he will have forgotten it in the interim and so want it explained to him again, and at others things may have come to mind during that interim that he wants clarified before proceeding. Because the reason for providing this information is that the patient is not willing to consent unless he has it, not that he cannot consent unless he has it, we are not here talking about the subjective standard for information disclosure (Beauchamp and Childress, 2009, pp. 123–124). That standard is part of an account of what is needed to avoid failing to respect the patient's autonomy. The proposal presented here concerns something different—what information healthcare professionals ought to provide to patients who are not prepared to decide whether or not to consent to treatment without it. And the source of this obligation is not primarily the obligation to respect autonomy; it is the obligation to do what benefits the patient.

It might be objected that such an open ended requirement could place large, and unreasonable, demands on healthcare professionals—to provide whatever information (however abstruse) a patient wants.[3] However, in practice the requirements are unlikely to be excessive. Patients typically want treatment (Jonson, Siegler, and Winslade, 2002; Richman, 2004). It is because they want treatment that they take time out of their schedules to attend their doctor's surgery, the local clinic, or the nearest hospital. As such, in many, perhaps most, cases the patient is not trying to put barriers in their doctor's way. This can be lost in discussions of both medical ethics and healthcare ethics simply because these straightforward cases are rarely discussed there. Furthermore, the obligation here is not as open ended as it may appear. The purpose of seeking consent is to resolve a conflict between obligations. There are good reasons to try to do that. But at some point, and where that point is will vary from case to case, the effort to do so will cease to be worth it. This is easiest to see in the case of research. Suppose a potential research participant will not consent unless he has more and more information. In this situation the researcher might reasonably decide to move on and not include him—she needs N participants, but for her purposes it does not matter if he is one of those N. Once she does this, she no longer has any reason to give him the information he wants. Things are not so simple when it comes to treatment a healthcare professional judges is best for her patient—she has an obligation to do what is prospectively best for him. But that does not mean this point will never be reached. She has other obligations—including obligations to her other patients—that she will not be able to fulfil if she spends lots of time finding out information just for him. In that situation she should treat the patient as if he had refused consent. If the obligation to obey the law, or comply with relevant professional or institutional codes of conduct, outweighs the obligation to do what is best for him, she should not provide the treatment.

As we have seen laws, codes of conduct, and institutional rules sometimes create obligations to obtain consent. They do so even if they are flawed—and there are important questions about what the regulations should say that take us beyond the remit of this book. The obligation to comply with these regulations means healthcare professionals should seek this (regulatory) consent. That requires more than just asking for it. It involves telling the patient what the treatment involves. This could be because only those to whom it has been explained can consent to it. Or it could be because the patient is not willing to consent unless this is done. What is required for the former will be set out in the regulations; what is required for the latter will not and will in fact vary from patient to patient. Having said that, there may be some information that many patients would want before consenting, but that is not needed in order to be able to consent. If that is the case, it would be useful to have that information available in a readily understandable form to give to patients. The role of that information, however, needs to be borne in mind. It will not follow from the fact that a patient has not taken it in that he has not consented—by stipulation this is not information that a person needs to understand in order to consent.

5.3 When Is Non-Regulatory Consent Needed and Who Is It Needed From?

In the previous section our focus was on regulatory consent—the idea that sometimes acting without consent would be wrong because it would be a failure to comply with regulations healthcare professionals ought to comply with. But that is not the only reason consent might be needed, and is not what most writers in this area have focused on. There are reasons an act might be wrong if done without consent that are independent of any such regulations. It is to what is required for this non-regulatory consent that we now turn.

Within healthcare ethics the most widely discussed, and accepted, account of non-regulatory consent says that acting without consent would be a failure to respect autonomy (see, for example, Beauchamp and Childress, 2009, ch.4; Harris, 1985, ch.10). This gives us an answer to the 'when' question—healthcare professionals need consent when what they are proposing would fail to respect a patient's autonomy if done without his consent, but would not be a failure to respect his autonomy if done with his consent. That however does not get us very far. We need to know which acts would involve a failure to respect autonomy if done without consent. One way to proceed here would be to provide, and defend, an account of what 'autonomy' is (as we have seen there are many accounts of this; see Dworkin, 1988, pp. 3–6; Arpaly, 2003, pp. 117–148; Taylor, 2005b; Stoljar, 2007; Wilson, 2007, pp. 353–356). We could then work out what is called for by the fact that someone is autonomous, and hence when acting would be inconsistent with doing so.

That is not the way I intend to proceed for three reasons. First, doing so can take us away from what really matters. There is a danger of getting hung up on details that make no difference given the issues we are concerned with; or our enquiry can start to become untied from the real world (becoming the pursuit of an unrealistic ideal). It can, and sometimes does, subtly shift so that instead of thinking about what is needed to avoid the wrong of failing to respect someone else's autonomy, we start to focus on what is needed for them to be truly autonomous. We start saying that the patient who makes a choice without understanding much is not acting as autonomously as he could, and that a patient who does not want to make decisions for himself is failing to be autonomous. That may be right, but what does any of this matter when our concern is with when consent is needed? It may be argued that it matters because acts that constitute consent need to be autonomous or given by a person who is autonomous (in some sense). But that is to change the topic. It concerns the constitutive rules for consent, not why it would be wrong to act without consent.

This takes us to my second reason for not starting with an account of autonomy—doing so risks considerable confusion. What is needed for an act to constitute consent can, and sometimes is, captured by saying that it must be autonomous. As such, it may turn out that healthcare professionals need an autonomous authorisation to avoid the wrong of failing to respect autonomy (indeed that looks like a pretty standard account). But the words 'autonomous' and 'autonomy' here refer to different things—the former to an act that has certain features (it is intentional, voluntary, informed), the latter to a person who has different features (a certain capacity, or standing) (Walker, 2018). Using the same word to refer to both in what follows would be a recipe for confusion.

Finally, starting with the idea that non-regulatory consent is needed to avoid the wrong of failing to respect autonomy assumes that this is the only reason it would be wrong to act without consent. There are times when that might be reasonable. However, when our concern is with the treatment of chronic illness it is not. We could avoid this by defining 'respect for autonomy' so that anything that would be wrong if done without consent, is wrong on the grounds of failing to respect autonomy (excluding those cases where it would be wrong for regulatory reasons). Anything can be located within such a category, just as perhaps any wrong can be fitted into the four principles framework (Sokal, 2009). But it is unclear what the advantage of doing so would be. Any such move would mean that we cannot determine when consent is needed by starting from the idea that it is needed to respect autonomy. What will count as 'respecting autonomy' will be shaped by our analysis of when consent is needed, and so cannot be used to determine when it is needed.[4]

For these reasons I intend to take a different approach. We want to know when it would be wrong (independently of any regulations) for healthcare professionals to act without consent. One way to do this is to start with a list of the types of thing that would be wrong if done without consent—for example, acts that in the absence of consent would breach confidentiality, invade privacy, cause wrongful harm, or violate bodily integrity. Any act that fits into one of these categories is one for which non-regulatory consent is needed. Intellectually that may be unsatisfactory. We want to know why it would be wrong to do these things without consent. This is where accounts that explain the need for consent in terms of respect for autonomy come in. They attempt to tell us why, for example, it would be wrong to do something to a person's body without his consent. But for our purposes here we do not need to delve into this—our concern is not primarily with why consent is needed, but with when it is needed. Furthermore, delving into why consent is needed will take us into debates that are not relevant given our purposes. This all requires a bit of explanation.

Sometimes the reason something would be wrong if done without consent is relatively uncomplicated. Consider a breach of confidence. Where a healthcare professional has been told something in confidence it would be wrong for her to tell other people what she has learnt because doing so would break an agreement she voluntarily entered. Information was given to her on the understanding, which she accepted, that it would not be passed on without consent—and where she accepts information from someone on that basis, it would be wrong to pass it on unless they have consented.

In other cases the reason consent is needed to avoid acting wrongly may be a matter of some dispute (even where there is no dispute over whether it is needed). It is, for example, widely accepted that doing things to (or inserting things into) a competent person's body is wrong if done without his consent.[5] One explanation for this is that a person's body is something over which they are sovereign (Mill, 1859/1974; Feinberg, 1986; Ripstein, 2006). Those working on sovereignty, when it comes to states, make a distinction between internal and external sovereignty (Feinberg, 1986, p. 48; Philpott, 2010; Grimm, 2015). Internal sovereignty concerns the authority the sovereign has within his realm—in the personal case this would include the authority a person has over what he does to, or puts into, his own body. External sovereignty, in contrast, concerns the authority the sovereign has *vis-a-vis* other sovereigns. While in some relationships people may have authority over what others do, the relationship between healthcare professional and patient is not one of them. Healthcare professionals are not the vassals, or hand servants, of their patients (Jackson, 2012, p. 239). What patients' external sovereignty gives them, and what it must give them if their internal sovereignty is to be absolute, is authority over what it is permissible for others to do to their body. On this account, then, the reason it would be wrong for a healthcare professional to do something to a patient's body without his consent is that this would violate his sovereignty (if we think of autonomy as sovereignty, it would thus be a failure to respect his autonomy). The reason he and he alone can consent is that this is a realm over which he, and he alone, is sovereign.

A different account of why it would be wrong to do something to a person's body without his consent starts from the idea that a person's body is his property (Thomson, 1990, p. 225). As such, doing things to his body is wrong because it is a trespass on his property (though it should be noted that not all accounts of violations of bodily integrity as a trespass start from a strong claim of ownership in the body, see Archard, 2008). The patient can alter this by consenting. When he does so he brings it about that acting on his body is no longer a trespass, and hence no longer wrong for that reason. Of course, that it is his property and he gives permission for someone to do something to it does not mean that they have any obligation to do so. But just as on the sovereignty account, it seems that if he has consented then it is permissible—this is something over which he has absolute authority. The reason that the patient and the patient alone can consent on this account is that he is the sole owner of the property.

Finally, according to yet another account, doing something to a person's body without his consent is wrong because it sets back his permissive interests (Owens, 2011, 2012, chapter 7). On this account, it would be bad for an individual if other people were allowed to do whatever they wanted to his body. But equally it would be bad for him if no-one was ever allowed to do anything to his body—that would prevent him from getting, or engaging in, things that he values. As such, each individual has an interest in being able to make it permissible for other people to do things to his or her body. There is an important reciprocal element here. If a person wants to claim that this is an interest other people should respect, they must also acknowledge and respect other people's interest in being the one to determine what it is permissible to do to their body. On this account, the reason that the patient and the patient alone can consent is that it is his permissive interests that would be set back by acting without consent.

A lot more can, and has, been said about all three of these accounts. Each has faced considerable criticism. But for now I want to focus on what they have in common. They all agree that it is wrong to touch, insert things into, or cut things out of a competent adult's body without his consent. This should not be surprising. That doing these things is wrong is not something discovered on the basis of these theories. Nor is it something anyone is trying to prove using them. Instead the theories are an attempt to make sense of, or to explain, something people are already committed to (this is not something anyone need shy away from, see Waldron, 2017, p. 66). Indeed one way the theories are challenged is by arguing that they fail to adequately account for why certain things would be wrong (for an example see the arguments that property accounts do not adequately account for the wrong of rape in Archard, 2008 and Phillips, 2013). We can all agree, that is, that certain things are wrong even if we disagree about why they are wrong. Given our purposes here it is thus not necessary for us to adjudicate between these accounts. Our concern is with what healthcare professionals ought to do, not with why they ought to do those things. While the latter is an important theoretical question, it is one we can safely leave to one side for now. It may be that there are cases where we are unsure whether or not consent is needed, and where the different theories give conflicting answers. To deal with such cases more detailed work would be needed. But we do not need to undertake that work here. We can instead proceed on the basis that if healthcare professionals are going to do things to a competent patient's body they need his consent if they are to avoid acting wrongly.

Just as there are different ways of explaining why it is wrong to do something to a person's body without his consent, there are different ways of explaining why it would be wrong to harm him without his consent. The idea that consented to harms are not wrong is captured by the law in the principle of *volenti non fit injuria* (for a discussion tracing this back as far as Aristotle see Feinberg, 1984, pp. 114–116). However, not everything that might harm someone, wrongs them if done without their consent (Dworkin, 2011, pp. 285–299; O'Neill, 2002, p. 162; Thomson, 1990, pp. 229–245—for an alternative view see Zimmerman, 2008, pp. 80–83). We might seek to explain when consent is needed to avoid wrongful harm by building on the sovereignty account outlined above. Alternatively we might seek to explain it, as Ronald Dworkin does, in terms of the ability to live one's own life (Dworkin, 2011, pp. 285–299).[6] Suppose someone sets back your interests by marrying the person you wanted to marry or fairly winning the tournament you were trying to win. On some accounts they have harmed you. But they have not normally wronged you. As Dworkin argues none of us could live our own life if it was impermissible for us to act in these ways. This should be familiar from our discussion in chapter four. But equally none of us could make our life our own, we could not plan for the future and work towards it, if other people were able to interfere directly in our life whenever they chose. If they were to interfere in this way they would be both harming us (by setting back our interests) and wronging us (by setting back our autonomy). So far we have not got to consent—the category of wrongless harms that Dworkin is referring to here (competitive harms) are not ones that are relevant for our purposes. However, we can easily do so by incorporating ideas gleaned from Owens' account of permissive interests outlined above. Just as I could not live my life if other people were allowed to interfere with my plans whenever it suited them, I could not do so if they were never allowed to do things that might harm me. That would rule out being able to play certain sports, and more relevantly for our purposes it would rule out getting certain types of medical treatment. Because of this I have an interest in being able to make it permissible for others to do things that might harm me (one they should respect, just as I should respect their similar interest). That is, on this account, there are some harms someone might cause me that would always wrong me, some that would never wrong me, and some that would wrong me unless I have consented to them.

As was the case when it came to the body, for our purposes here we do not need to adjudicate between these accounts of when it is wrong to harm someone without his consent. That might look too quick. It is not always clear when consent is needed to avoid wrongful harm. To see why, consider harms that are minor or very unlikely. Consent is not always needed to make it permissible to act in ways that might produce these harms. To explain why, we might argue that in these cases acting is justified by the benefits produced (Zimmerman, 2008, p. 83, Gert, Culver, and Clouser, 2006, pp. 36–37). That is how people attempt to justify giving medical treatment to children that could harm them (even where the potential harm is fairly large). However, doing so looks problematic in other cases. It implies that as long as healthcare professionals do what is prospectively best for their patients they never need consent to avoid wrongfully harming those patients. That would be inconsistent with both the 'sovereignty' or 'ability to live our own life' accounts outlined above. As such, a different approach is needed. That approach starts from the fact that both accounts involve a reciprocal recognition of others. What it would be wrong for you to do to me without my consent must be the same as what it would be wrong for me to do to you without your consent. As such, none of us are likely to want to insist that to respect us, our interests, or our sovereignty other people need our consent before doing things that would impose only minor (or very unlikely) harms on us. Doing so would impose significant restrictions on what we can permissibly do. Where the line is drawn here, on either account, is not clear. As such, turning to the extant theories will not necessarily help us to overcome the problem we started with—our uncertainty about when consent is needed to avoid wrongfully harming others.

Given the above, we can see that untangling the reasons an act might be wrong if done without consent is largely unnecessary given our purposes. As such, in what follows I will proceed on the basis of the following set of mid-level principles. Consent is needed where what healthcare professionals take themselves to have reason to do would involve one or more of the following: 1. doing something to the patient's body, 2. harming or potentially harming the patient in a way that would wrong him if done without consent, 3. invading a person's privacy, or 4. breaching a duty of confidentiality. No-one (not even those who are sceptical about the role autonomy plays in bioethics) seriously denies that consent is needed for such acts where the patient is a competent adult, nor that it is needed from the patient himself. By proceeding in this way we can avoid getting sucked into debates that while theoretically important take us away from the issues that matter for our purposes here. It is also easier, in most cases, to determine that an act involves something like touching the body or passing on confidential information, than that it fails to respect autonomy or sets back a permissive interest.

If this is what consent is needed for (the answer to the 'when' question), what is needed for something to be consent? It is to this that we now turn. Before doing so, however, it is worth explaining why 'treatment' was not included on the above list. Surely it is something for which consent is needed? Often it is. But where it is, the reason is not that it is treatment—at least when our concern is with non-regulatory consent, things may be different for regulatory consent. That is, its status as treatment is not doing the work.[7] The reason non-regulatory consent is needed for treatment, where it is, is that it involves doing one or more of the things indicated above. If a healthcare professional intends to give me an injection, she would need my non-regulatory consent. That is because she is intending to insert something into my body (both the needle and the substance injected), and in doing so potentially harms me. It is these features that mean it would be wrong to act without my consent, not that the injection constitutes treatment. It is easiest to see that treatment itself is not the relevant issue by considering treatments that are not invasive—things such as prescribing an arts participation or a course of medication to take at home. These are treatments. But in writing the prescription the doctor involved is not doing anything that would be wrong if done without consent (unless there are regulations that require consent for such acts) (Walker, 2017). All that she does is give the patient an opportunity to access resources that may benefit him. He does not have to take that opportunity. Giving someone such an opportunity may sometimes be wrong—if I were to give an alcoholic a gift of alcohol, I cannot defend myself by saying that all I did was give him an opportunity, one he did not need to take. But where it is wrong this is not because consent was not given. It is wrong because it exposes the other person to a risk of harm. We will return to this point below.

5.4 The Constitutive Rules for Non-Regulatory Consent and What They Mean for Healthcare Professionals' Obligations

Having addressed when non-regulatory consent is required, we now turn to what is required for someone to give it.[8] With regulatory consent, as we have just seen, this depends on what the regulations say—informed consent regulations, for example, stipulate that the person consenting must be competent, have sufficient understanding, and be acting voluntarily. They say this, at least in part, to protect patients from being wronged by those treating them. As such, we should expect there to be similarities between the constitutive rules for non-regulatory consent and those for regulatory consent. There are, however, two reasons for looking specifically at the constitutive rules for non-regulatory consent. First, in the context of chronic illness some of the things for which healthcare professionals need consent do not fall under informed consent regulations, and we need to know what is required in those cases. Second, the requirements for regulatory consent and those for non-regulatory consent may not be identical (and even if they are identical in some countries, they may not be identical in all). As such, an act that satisfies all the constitutive rules for regulatory consent may not satisfy all the constitutive rules for non-regulatory consent—for example, some informed consent regulations may allow acts that would be wrong on the grounds of failing to respect autonomy (Beauchamp, 2011; Levy, 2014).

In investigating the constitutive rules for non-regulatory consent we will look at voluntariness, understanding, and competence in that order. The first can be dealt with quickly, however the other two require more detailed investigation as here differences between regulatory and non-regulatory consent often open up.

Voluntariness

When writers in healthcare refer to consent being voluntary they standardly mean that it was not obtained by either coercion or manipulation (see, for example, Beauchamp and Childress, 2009, pp. 132–135).[9] This means that consent can be voluntary even if there is no reasonable alternative available. Were that not the case it is hard to see how patients could consent to life prolonging treatment. But patients can, it seems, make it permissible for their doctor to give them such treatment—treatment that would be wrong in the absence of consent. Our account of the constitutive rules for consent must acknowledge this. However, while a patient's agreement to treatment that is necessary to prevent his illness killing him can constitute consent, his agreement to treatment that is necessary to prevent his doctor killing him cannot. In part this is because both coercion and manipulation are wrong in themselves (O'Neill, 2002; Cave, 2007). As such, they are not things that healthcare professionals should do. But that is not the whole story. Acts that are coerced or manipulated cannot make the required change in the normative landscape. To see this, imagine a patient who has been coerced into signing a consent form by someone other than the healthcare professional treating him. In this case it would still be wrong to give him the treatment. This follows from two things we established earlier—the patient and the patient alone can consent, and consent must be intentional. If someone else could make it permissible for a healthcare professional, Mary, to do something to one of her patients, Bill, by coercing him into signing a consent form (say), then Bill does not control whether or not it is permissible for Mary to act in that way. The other person, any other person, could do so. But that is inconsistent with our response to the 'who' question. More importantly, if Bill is coerced into saying he agrees to have a certain treatment, it is implausible to think that his intention when he does so is to make it permissible for Mary to give him that treatment. His intention is to avoid the threatened harm for not doing as he is told (for a similar point in a different context see McGregor, 1994). Things are different when someone agrees to life prolonging treatment. Their doctor will not give them that treatment unless it is permissible for her to do so (something the patient will usually understand). As such, while the patient's reason for agreeing to the treatment may be to avoid harm, their intention is likely to be to make giving the treatment permissible. Doing so is necessary to obtain what they want—the treatment—and it is this that means they act in the way that they do. What all this means is that only acts that are voluntary (in the sense that the actor was neither coerced nor manipulated into performing them) can constitute non-regulatory consent.

Understanding

As we have seen, in many cases regulatory consent can only be given by those who understand what is proposed in some detail. Informed consent regulations, for example, typically require that the person consenting has been told about, or understands, "the nature, risks, costs, benefits, [and] side-effects" of what is being proposed (Manson, 2007, p. 299). The extent of understanding required has both grown and become more finely specified as new regulations have been introduced (Walker, 2012b, p. 50). However, to say that a patient must understand certain things to be able to consent, is to say that a patient who does not understand those things is not able to consent. Whatever he says or does will not make it permissible for a healthcare professional, or anyone else, to act (for example, to do something to his body). As such, it is not up to him whether acting in that way is permissible. That creates a tension with our answer to the 'who' question earlier in this chapter. We said there that healthcare professionals need consent specifically from their patients because the patient and the patient alone can make it permissible to act. But now it seems that if the patient lacks understanding he cannot do this. This raises two questions. First, what explains why a person's ability to consent is constrained by his lack of understanding—for example, why would the mere fact that he does not understand the benefits of a proposed action mean he cannot make it permissible? Second, what explains how it is that simply by coming to have more understanding—by learning something—he comes to have a power he previously lacked (the power to make it permissible for others to act)? Similarly, what explains why forgetting something, so he no longer understands it, means he loses a power he currently has? With regulatory consent the answers to these questions are simple—only a person with the specified understanding fits the description of who can consent written into the regulations. But when our concern is with non-regulatory consent that answer is not available.

Because giving non-regulatory consent is something that people do, and must do both voluntarily and with the right intention, there are clearly some things they need to understand before they can consent (Walker, 2012b). To act with the intention of making something permissible a patient must believe that whether it is permissible is up to him. He also needs to believe that he has a choice about whether it happens. That is, he needs to believe both that it is at least partly up to him what happens, and that his granting permission affects this (Manson and O'Neill, 2007, p. 93). If he does not, there is little point in him spending time deciding whether to consent. Instead what he needs to decide is whether he will go along with, or resist, what is being proposed. As such, his agreement will at best only indicate acquiescence. But mere acquiescence is not sufficient for consent. That I go along with, rather than struggling against, something I think will happen whatever I do cannot safely be interpreted as my voluntarily acting with the intention of making it permissible—something that has been at the heart of criticisms of some rape statutes (see, for example, McGregor, 1994).

To consent, people also need to know something about what it is they are consenting to. They are making something permissible and to do that they must pick out what it is they are making permissible (Manson, 2007, p. 299). As Onora O'Neill has argued not just any way of doing so will suffice (O'Neill, 2002, p. 42, 2003; Manson and O'Neill, 2007, pp. 12–15). Even if someone can pick out an act under one description, they may not understand that it has features not included in that description (including some that are logically entailed by it). For example, they may know that what is proposed is an operation on their prostate, but not realise that what is proposed will make them sterile. As such, while they may appear to have given the needed consent, they have not (they have not consented to being made sterile).[10] O'Neill's argument for this rests on her characterisation of consent as a propositional attitude, and in particular on the fact that propositional attitudes are opaque. That is not how I have been characterising consent. I have been taking it that consent is something that people do—they give it, withhold it, withdraw it—not just an attitude they have to a proposition. As such, I cannot rely on O'Neill's argument here. There is, however, an alternative way of arguing to the same conclusion—one that rests, not on the idea that propositional attitudes are opaque, but on the idea that consent has to be intentional.

Suppose that while a patient can pick out a treatment, call it X, under some description he is unaware that it involves inserting something into his body (the description does not mention this). Assume also that the only reason it would be wrong to do X without consent is that it involves inserting something into the patient's body. Were this patient to voluntarily agree to a healthcare professional doing X, it is implausible to think that his intention is to make inserting something into his body permissible. He cannot be acting with that intention because he does not understand that this is what X involves. Similarly if he misunderstands what X involves doing to his body, he cannot be thought to have acted with the intention of making doing what X actually involves permissible. To see this, consider a patient who thinks his surgeon is going to replace the joint in his right hip, where in fact she is planning to replace the joint in his left hip. In this situation it is implausible to think that when he agreed to the operation he was acting with the intention of making it permissible for her to cut open his body on the left hand side, remove part of it and insert an artificial joint at that point. He can in this situation reasonably complain that he did not consent to *that*, even though he has consented to something.

Because of this, in any given situation there are certain things a patient needs to understand before he can give the necessary consent. If acting without consent would be wrong for some reason, R, then a patient can only consent if he understands that what is proposed has those features that mean it would be wrong for reason R. For example, if R is that acting involves inserting something into his body he needs to understand that what is proposed involves inserting something into his body. If an act would be wrong for more than one reason were it done without consent, he will need to understand that it has the features that mean it would be wrong for each of those reasons. So, if giving treatment without consent would be wrong both because it involves doing something to his body and because it might wrongfully harm him, it is not sufficient that he understands that something will be done to his body. That would at best enable him to remove the first reason. It would not affect the second. To be able do that, he would also need to understand that the treatment potentially harms him. We can now answer the two questions raised earlier. The reason gaining understanding enables a patient to consent is that he can only act with the intention of making what is proposed permissible if he has that understanding. Similarly, the reason it is not up to him whether giving treatment is permissible where he lacks understanding is that in that situation he cannot act with the intention of making it permissible.

We now have an account of what a person needs to understand if he is to be able to give non-regulatory consent. What this is will vary with the reasons it would be wrong to act in the proposed way without that consent. It will not, however, include everything contained in most informed consent regulations. For example, while non-regulatory consent is sometimes needed for acts that benefit patients, the reason it is needed is not that it provides this benefit. It is implausible to think that benefitting a patient without consent is wrong on the grounds that it benefits him. As such, he does not need to understand the benefits if he is to give the needed non-regulatory consent. There is also, according to this account, no requirement that a patient understands what is proposed in any detail. To be able to consent he needs to understand that what is proposed has those features that mean it would be wrong if done without his consent. These can be specified in greater or lesser detail—treatment involves doing something to his body, or replacing the joint in his left hip, or a female surgeon replacing the joint in his left hip, and so on. As long as what is proposed fits under the relevant description, any of these is sufficient when it comes to non-regulatory consent (though the requirements for regulatory consent are likely to be more prescriptive). Of course, a patient may not be willing to consent unless things are explained to him in some detail. In that situation the healthcare professionals treating him should provide a suitably detailed account. But as we saw in section 5.2 this is a different issue. The reason they should provide that information is not that the patient *cannot* consent unless he has these details, it is that he *will not* consent unless he has them.

On the account developed here there are some things a patient needs to understand if he is to be able to give non-regulatory consent. But this is less than might have been thought, and less than is typically required by informed consent regulations. Some readers are likely to raise an objection at this point. There is something, they will argue, that has been missed. The patient requires more extensive understanding before consenting if giving treatment is not to constitute a failure to respect autonomy—by moving away from the language of autonomy I have, it might be argued, missed what is really important. I will address this objection below. Before doing so, however, I want to draw out some of the implications of what has just been argued for.

Suppose an act would be wrong for reason R if done without consent. A patient can only change this if he understands that the act has those features that mean it would be wrong for reason R. Where his doctor should perform this act (because it is what is best for the patient) she should ensure that he has the relevant understanding. This may involve explaining to her patient that what is proposed has those features. Unless she does this there is no way for her to get the consent she needs. In doing this, and assessing whether she has the needed consent, the pragmatics of communication need to be borne in mind—something stressed by Neil Manson and Onora O'Neill (Manson and O'Neill, 2007). As such, context matters. If Bill consents to Mary doing whatever she wants to his body, what it is permissible for her to do will vary depending on whether he is in her consulting room or her bed. Because of this there is considerable potential for misunderstanding between healthcare professional and patient to occur. Because the healthcare professional needs to ascertain whether she has consent, the onus is on her to clarify what the patient understands where this may be in doubt.

That does not mean she has to check everything. If she reasonably believes that her (competent) patient has the required understanding, there is nothing wrong with her taking his voluntary agreement to constitute the consent she needs. This is the case even though he may not in fact have taken account of the relevant information when giving his agreement (that he took account of it does not follow from the fact that he understands it). To return to an earlier example, suppose I give you permission to remove all the books from my front room, but it has slipped my mind that I left a book I want to keep in that room. Have I consented to you taking that book? I said earlier that I have. I acted with the intention of making it permissible for you to take the books in that room, and this is one of the books in that room. I will also say, when I discover what has happened, that I did not intend to make it permissible for you to take it—implying that I did in fact make it permissible. However, someone might dispute that. Suppose they are right and no consent has been given. It will still be the case that, in taking the book, you did nothing blameworthy. Given the situation, you could reasonably take it that you had permission to do so. The same will be true when it comes to consent to medical treatment.[11] One thing that this case reveals is that where healthcare professionals have reason to doubt that a patient has taken account of all the relevant information, they should require him to take his time. Even if that is not needed to ensure they have his consent, it will help to avoid the situation where he regrets giving it.

We now need to consider the objection outlined above. The standard reason for thinking that it would be wrong to give medical treatment without consent is that doing so fails to respect autonomy. The account developed here appears to challenge that position but does not directly engage with it. Appearances however might be deceptive. I argued above that where an act would be wrong for some reason if done without consent, only someone who understands that it has those features in virtue of which it would be wrong for that reason can consent. It follows that where giving treatment without consent would be wrong because it fails to respect autonomy, only a patient who understands that it has the features that would make it wrong on the grounds that it fails to respect autonomy can consent. What features are those? As we saw in section 5.3 above they include that the treatment involves doing something to the patient's body, or would harm him by setting back his ability to live his own life, or would violate his privacy. As such, the account here might be thought of as a clarification of the standard account, rather than a challenge to it.

That, however, is unlikely to be satisfying. It does not acknowledge the extent to which the position defended here challenges the idea that informed consent (in the sense of an autonomous authorisation) is needed before giving medical treatment. In both medical ethics and healthcare ethics an authorisation typically only counts as autonomous if the person giving it has substantial understanding of what is proposed (including its possible consequences) (see Beauchamp, 2005, pp. 314–317). As Jukka Varelius puts it, "Accepting that decisions made in ignorance of relevant facts can be autonomous would . . . be incompatible with the understanding of the nature of autonomy commonly accepted in medical ethics" (Varelius, 2006, p. 456). If that is what it is to be autonomous, the argument of this section is that non-regulatory consent does not require an autonomous authorisation as that is usually conceptualised (depending as it does on a particular interpretation of 'relevant facts'). That is perhaps less radical than it appears. First, it does not, in itself, challenge those informed consent regulations that stipulate patients must give an autonomous authorisation before receiving treatment. As we saw in chapter one these regulations frequently have several aims. Because patients are both autonomous and vulnerable, requiring an autonomous authorisation could be defended as a way to protect patients while also respecting their autonomy (though assessing that proposal would take us too far from the aims of this book). Second, while it may sound odd to say that an act which is not autonomous could nevertheless constitute consent, we should not be misled by language here. This only follows if we interpret 'autonomous' in a certain way—such that only well informed acts can count as autonomous. On other interpretations of what it is for an act to be autonomous, the argument here would not challenge the idea that only an autonomous act can constitute consent.

Having said that, there are important differences between the account defended here and the standard account. In particular, the former requires less understanding for consent than the latter. A competent patient who voluntarily agrees to medical treatment without understanding much about what is proposed may on my account have given consent. But in doing so he will not have acted as autonomously (at least on some accounts of autonomy) as he could. Were he to be better informed his act would be more autonomous. That may be desirable. But it does not follow that his less autonomous act has not made giving treatment permissible. Our concern here is with whether when a healthcare professional gives him an injection, bathes him, or uses an anal probe to inspect his prostate she wrongs him. It is unclear why performing these acts would wrong him if, when voluntarily agreeing to them, he was not acting as autonomously as he could, but would not wrong him if he becomes more (though still not fully) autonomous. To argue that it would, and hence argue that non-regulatory consent requires greater understanding than I have allowed, requires adopting one of two approaches (which differ in where they draw the threshold for being autonomous). As we will see neither succeeds.

The first option is to argue that only those with substantial understanding are autonomous. If that were the case, only a person with substantial understanding could consent—could bring it about that in acting someone else does not wrong him by failing to respect his autonomy. This is because a person who lacks substantial understanding would not be autonomous. There is thus nothing that could constitute a failure to respect his autonomy. Hence there is nothing he could do to bring it about that he is not wronged for that reason—it is already the case that nothing would wrong him for that reason. He could, of course, agree to what is proposed (and do so voluntarily). But his doing so would make no normative difference. In contrast, a patient who has substantial understanding is autonomous (assuming that he is also competent). To treat him without his consent would thus be to fail to respect his autonomy, whereas to do so with his consent would not.

While this would explain how simply by gaining understanding patients gain the power to give non-regulatory consent, it faces two serious problems. First, on this account a healthcare professional would not be acting wrongly, on the grounds of failing to respect her patient's autonomy, were she to give an uninformed patient treatment without his consent. As such, her obligation to do what is best for him (given her expertise and available resources) does not come into conflict with her other obligations—except those created by regulations. There is thus no reason for her to seek non-regulatory consent as a way to dissolve such a conflict (though she may still have reason to seek regulatory consent). Second, if only patients with substantial understanding are autonomous, giving them relevant information can make them autonomous. When it does, it creates a situation where the patient's consent is needed to avoid the wrong of failing to respect his autonomy. However, it seems to be a rule of practical reasoning that, all else being equal, if someone ought to do A (here do what is best for their patient given their expertise and available resources) and doing B (here giving him information) might prevent them from being able to do A (by making it the case that it would be wrong to act without consent—consent that may not be given), then they ought not to do B. As such, if substantial understanding is needed to be autonomous, healthcare professionals ought not to tell their patients about what treatment involves.

Such a conclusion looks deeply problematic. It can be avoided by dropping the idea that to be autonomous one must have substantial understanding. Indeed it is rare to find any such requirement in the medical or healthcare ethics literature (for a possible exception see Coggon and Miola, 2011). Those working in this area standardly take it that 'autonomy' has to be characterised in such a way that the vast majority of adults count as autonomous (Dworkin, 1988, p. 111; Beauchamp and Childress, 2009, pp. 101 and 113; Manson and O'Neill, 2007, p. 21). The reason for this is the one we have just seen. If the bar for being autonomous is set too high, it would not be wrong on the grounds of failing to respect autonomy to give at least some competent adults treatment without their consent. Because of this, as we saw earlier, Tom Beauchamp and James Childress argue that when it comes to healthcare, "the characteristics of a competent person are also the properties possessed by [an] autonomous person" (Beauchamp and Childress, 2009, p. 113).

However, drawing the threshold for being autonomous at this point makes it much harder to see why considerable understanding is needed for non-regulatory consent. Those competent adults who lack understanding are still, on this account, autonomous. And their autonomy must be respected. Arguing that they cannot consent—that is, cannot make it the case that a healthcare professional's actions are not wrong on the grounds of failing to respect their autonomy—seems incompatible with this. Suppose a patient in this situation voluntarily agrees to treatment. Why would giving him that treatment be a failure to treat him in the way called for by the fact that he is autonomous? Similarly, why would his gaining understanding make a difference here? It may be true that if he gains understanding he becomes more autonomous (in some sense). But that is irrelevant for two reasons. First, when we are talking about respecting autonomy in healthcare the relevant sense of 'respect' is what Darwall calls recognition respect (1977)—respect due to the patient because he has some feature (here that he is autonomous). We are not talking about what Darwall calls appraisal respect. But only the latter could vary with how well the patient uses his autonomy. Second, the argument here involves a shift in the meaning of 'autonomy'. When it comes to consent what is important is a person's standing to consent (autonomy as sovereignty). And this does not alter as a person gains understanding. A person's sovereignty, if he has it, does not come in degrees—either he is sovereign or he is not.

Before leaving the understanding requirements for non-regulatory consent I want to stress three things. First, if what has been said here does not seem to capture everything needed to respect patient autonomy, that is because it does not. No account of consent can do that. There are, as we saw in chapter four, more ways to fail to respect someone's autonomy than to act without their consent. Second, on the account developed here if a competent but uninformed patient agrees voluntarily to his doctor doing X, it would not be a failure to respect his autonomy to do X. But that does not mean she should do X. His consent makes it permissible, it does not make it obligatory. Furthermore, where informed consent regulations impose obligations on her, it does not even make it all things considered permissible. In the absence of consent there were two ways in which it would have been wrong to act. The patient's consent has only removed one of these, it leaves the other unaffected. As such, acting would still be at least *pro tanto* wrong. Third, and following on from this, that a patient does not need to understand certain information to give non-regulatory consent, does not mean there is no reason to give him that information. In some cases, as we saw above, this is required if the patient is to be able to give regulatory consent. In addition, patients may not be willing to give even non-regulatory consent unless what is proposed is explained to them in some detail. In that situation those treating them have good reason (and in some cases a *pro tanto* obligation) to provide that explanation. Finally, it is worth bearing in mind that healthcare professionals typically provide information to patients as part of seeking their consent for something the healthcare professional ought to do (what is best for the patient given her expertise and the available resources). They would be doing this badly if they do not tell their patients about the benefits or potential benefits of the proposed treatment. That in itself gives them a reason to provide that information. This in turn may create risks for patients—unscrupulous healthcare professionals (or researchers) may try to obtain agreement by stressing the benefits and downplaying the risks. For that reason it may be reasonable to introduce regulations that impose an obligation to provide a more balanced picture before obtaining consent (I make no claims here about what those regulations should say).

Competence

Informed consent regulations standardly specify that only the competent can consent—where to be competent a person must be able to understand relevant information, retain it long enough to use it, make decisions on the basis of it, and communicate his decision to others (see, for example, Beauchamp and Childress, 2009, pp. 112–117). Because a person's ability to do this can vary, competence in this sense is task specific. Typically only those who are competent can affect whether healthcare professionals would be breaking regulations they ought to comply with. Competence is also required for non-regulatory consent. There are two possible explanations for this. One explanation starts from the fact that consenting requires a certain intention. To act with that intention there are some things a person must understand. A person who cannot understand that what is proposed involves doing something to his body, for example, cannot act with the intention of making it permissible to do something to his body. Equally, a person who understands this information but cannot retain or use it, cannot act with the required intention. Finally, a person who cannot communicate cannot let anyone know that the act is permissible, and so cannot act in a way that makes it permissible. As such, a person who is not competent (in very much the sense outlined above) would not be able to give non-regulatory consent. The second explanation starts from the wrong that would be done in the absence of consent. It argues that whereas it would be wrong to do things to a competent patient without his consent, things are different if the patient is incompetent. This will be the case, for example, with the wrong of failing to respect autonomy if, as suggested above, only the competent are autonomous in the relevant sense. If those who are incompetent are not autonomous, then nothing anyone does could constitute a failure to respect their autonomy. There is thus no way they can bring it about that an act would not be wrong for that reason. It is already not wrong for that reason.

There is an important difference between these two explanations that affects what healthcare professionals should do. According to the first explanation acting in certain ways is *always pro tanto* wrong where the patient is incompetent. This includes all acts that would normally be wrong if done without consent. Because the incompetent patient, unlike the competent patient, cannot consent there no way to remove the normative barrier in the way of acting (as there is when the patient is competent). In contrast according to the second explanation it is *never* wrong to do these things to an incompetent patient. The reason consent is needed from a competent person to avoid acting wrongly does not exist where the patient is incompetent. There is thus no normative barrier in the way of acting in these cases (whereas if the patient were competent there would be).

As such, determining healthcare professionals' obligations to their incompetent patients would appear to require ascertaining which of these explanations is correct. Doing so may be particularly pressing in the context of treating patients with chronic illness (simply because the ages at which chronic illness is most prevalent are also the ages at which dementia is most prevalent, though of course most patients at these ages are fully competent). That in turn might seem to require clarifying the reasons it would be wrong to act without consent (contrary to what I argued in section 5.3 above). To see why, consider acts that involve inserting something into a patient's body. If we explain why acts of this type are wrong (where the patient is competent) in terms of a permissive interest—the interest a person has in controlling whether it is permissible to insert things into their body—we should adopt the second explanation above.[12] Those who are incompetent have no such interest. Remember that the reason for thinking people have this interest is that it enables them to avoid two dangers: that it would always be permissible for other people to do things to their body, and that it would never be permissible for other people to do things to their body. It will only avoid the second danger, however, if the individual concerned is able to consent, something the incompetent cannot do. While the incompetent have an interest in it sometimes being permissible to insert things into their body (as part of medical treatment), they do not have an interest in it being up to them whether this is permissible. That those who are not competent do not have the same permissive interests as those who are competent does not mean that they have no relevant interests. They have, for example, an interest in there being restrictions on what may permissibly be done to their body—including an interest in it never being permissible to do some things to their body—but not this interest. As such, if the reason healthcare professionals need the consent of competent adults is that acting without it would set back the latter's permissive interests, where the patient is incompetent there will be no such need (simply because in that case the patient does not have the relevant permissive interest).

On the other hand, if it is wrong to insert things into a person's body either because it violates his sovereignty or trespasses on his property, things are less clear. While sovereignty accounts do not normally explain how a person comes to be sovereign over a certain realm, there is little reason to think that it is depends on his competence (though for a different

Consent and Treatment of Chronic Illness 125

view see Feinberg, 1986, pp. 28–31 and p. 48).[13] Certainly when it comes to the political realm, from which this account is derived, incompetence is no barrier to sovereignty. There have been sovereigns who ascended the throne while still a young child (Henry VI became king of England in 1422 at nine months, Mary became queen of Scotland in 1542 at just six days) (Ross, 2016; Wormald, 1988). There have also been sovereigns who were unable to govern their realm due to illness (Friedrich Wilhelm IV of Prussia became incapable of ruling in 1858 but remained on the throne until 1861 [Evans, 2016, p. 250], George III of Britain's mental illness meant he was unable to govern for the last ten years of his reign [from 1810 to 1820] [Black, 2008]). Similarly being incompetent is not in general a barrier to being a property owner.

However, while important theoretical differences exist between these accounts, given our concerns they make little difference in practice. In the examples above, while the sovereign may not have been able to understand enough, or reason well enough, to actually rule his or her realm, decisions still needed to be made. If they were not, the realm itself would have been under threat. As such, those decisions (including decisions about what it is permissible for others to do) were typically taken on the sovereign's behalf by someone else—a regent. In practice this was often a family member (in the case of Friedrich Wilhelm IV of Prussia, for example, his son Prince Wilhelm; in the case of Henry VI of England, his uncles the Dukes of Bedford and Gloucester). Something similar occurs when it comes to managing the property, for example the land, of those who are incompetent. We should not push the analogy between individuals and political entities too far. The underlying point, however, remains. Those who are competent can, if they choose, make it permissible for others to act on their body. Because of that they can control (at least to some extent) what is done to them. Those who are incompetent cannot. They are thus vulnerable in ways that the competent are not, and we need a way to avoid that. As such, there must be a way, on either sovereignty or property accounts, that inserting something into an incompetent person's body is sometimes all things considered permissible, despite the fact that normally only the sovereign or owner could make it permissible. If there is not, these accounts would simply be implausible. Of course not just any trespass or violation of sovereignty would be permissible. But those that are needed either to prevent harm or to significantly benefit the incompetent person would be.[14] In practice, therefore, despite the important theoretical differences between them, what the sovereignty, property, and permissive interest accounts require of healthcare professionals (if they are to be plausible) is the same. If the patient is competent (and this is decision specific) the patient's consent is needed to avoid wrongdoing. If he is incompetent it is not. But acting on the incompetent patient's body without his consent will only be morally permissible where doing so is needed either to benefit him or to prevent him being harmed.

Before completing this look at consent there is one more point I want to consider—what happens when the requirements for regulatory and non-regulatory consent come apart. This is most likely to happen where the patient is a child whose cognitive capacity is above the level needed for competence, sometimes known as mature minors (Archard, 2007; Dickenson, 1994; Manson, 2015; Parekh, 2007; Walker, 2016). While such children may constitute only a relatively small proportion of those living with chronic illness, they cannot be ignored. There are children of all ages living with asthma, diabetes, or cancer (among other chronic illnesses) and an account of healthcare professionals' obligations must cover them. When we think about the whole range of situations where consent is needed, it should be obvious that children can sometimes give non-regulatory consent. A child (even a very young child) can release someone from an obligation arising from a duty of confidence. In doing so he is consenting—making it permissible to do something that would otherwise have been *pro tanto* wrong. However, it is not unusual for regulations that require consent to include an age-based cut-off. This means regulations can diverge from what is required in their absence in one of two ways. First, where regulations specify that to consent a person must be over some specified age, someone under that age cannot give regulatory consent even if their cognitive and communicative abilities are above the threshold for competence. They could, however, give non-regulatory consent. Second, there may be things for which regulatory consent is not needed when the patient is a child, but which would nevertheless be wrong if done without non-regulatory consent. Informed consent regulations, for example, may permit giving treatment to children without their consent, irrespective of whether the child is competent. On the account developed here, however, providing that treatment will sometimes be wrong if done without the child's (non-regulatory) consent. In this way informed consent regulations may allow healthcare professionals to do things that are morally wrong.[15]

Once we acknowledge that healthcare professionals need both regulatory and non-regulatory consent there is no way to avoid this (unless regulations exactly capture all and only the pre-existing non-regulatory requirements). It follows from this that there may be situations in which it would be wrong to give treatment to a competent and informed person who voluntarily agrees to that treatment. That will be the case where the patient is a child and regulations prohibit giving this treatment to children. More frequently, perhaps, it will mean that healthcare professionals sometimes need consent to avoid acting wrongly even where informed consent regulations do not require it. For example, where a nurse has to carry out a test for testicular cancer on a fifteen-year-old boy, or has to help him take a bath, she should seek his permission beforehand. To proceed without it would be wrong, in much the same way that it would be wrong if he were a few years older. In such cases what is needed for consent is not determined by what the regulations say. It is solely determined by the constitutive rules for non-regulatory consent.

This requirement for non-regulatory consent may seem to create challenges for healthcare professionals. The problem is not that children, though competent, might consent to things that would be bad for them. Consenting at most makes it permissible to do what has been consented to—it does not provide a reason to act, and certainly would not make doing so obligatory. Rather it is that a child might not consent to treatment that would be very beneficial. If that happens, the healthcare professionals involved would be acting wrongly were they to provide that treatment. If the reason it would be wrong to act without consent is that doing so violates the patient's bodily integrity, he and he alone can bring it about that it is not wrong for that reason. And he has not done so. It does not follow from that, however, that giving the treatment is necessarily wrong all things considered. It is wrong for one reason (it would violate the patient's bodily integrity). But that is not the only thing that is morally relevant here. If the treatment would prevent the child suffering serious harm or would significantly benefit him, that also needs to be taken into account. Where these harms or benefits are sufficiently large, giving the treatment might be all things considered morally permissible. That should not be surprising. If the reason violating bodily integrity is wrong is that it is a failure to respect autonomy, what we have here is a clash between respecting autonomy and benefitting the patient. Where these are independent moral requirements there is no reason to think that the former will always outweigh the latter (see Beauchamp and Childress, 2009; Gillon, 2003; Dawson and Garrard, 2006).

If that is right in the case of a competent child, then it must also be right in the case of a competent adult. When it comes to the need for non-regulatory consent these are on a par (though where the patient is an adult there are likely to be additional reasons, stemming from the regulations in force, against acting if the patient has not consented). At this point an objection will be raised—overriding a competent adult's informed and voluntary refusal is wrong because it would be paternalistic. There is no space to go into whether paternalism is always wrong here (and given our concerns little need to do so). I do, however, want to make the following points. First, whether it would be morally permissible to override a competent patient's refusal is in many cases of purely academic interest (whatever the patient's age). Successful treatment of chronic illness standardly requires the patient's co-operation, and where consent has been refused this co-operation is unlikely to be forthcoming. In that case the refusal means treatment cannot be given. So whether or not it would be permissible need not detain us. Second, nothing said here contradicts the claim that patients have absolute authority to determine whether acting is wrong on the grounds that it violates their sovereignty, trespasses on their property, would fail to respect their autonomy, or would set back their permissive interests. It concerns whether acts which would be wrong on those grounds are sometimes permissible. There is no reason to think that this is something that patients, and patients alone, have authority to determine—something that those opposed to paternalism accept (for example, when acting is needed to prevent serious harm to third parties). Third, to the extent that paternalism is thought to be wrong on the grounds that individuals know best what is in their own interests, as it sometimes is (see discussion in Young, 2008), this was addressed in chapters two and three. As we saw there, this empirical claim is problematic. Fourth, nothing said here challenges the idea that the law should prohibit giving medical treatment to competent adults unless they have given their consent. That is, it does not challenge the idea that the law should be anti-paternalist (which is the primary concern of at least some of those arguing against paternalism, see Feinberg, 1986). Such laws might be supported on a variety of grounds. For example, it might be argued that the risks of allowing paternalistic acts in a particular context, or the benefits of prohibiting them, are sufficiently high that they should be prohibited across the board. Or it might be argued that there are broad social benefits from prohibiting paternalism. Such arguments need not rely on the idea that paternalism is always morally wrong. I take no position on whether such laws are justified, but nothing said here challenges the idea that they are.

5.5 Conclusion

In this chapter we have been concerned with what healthcare professionals need to do to navigate the normative landscape in which they operate. As we have seen that landscape is a complex one—shaped both by regulations (laws, professional codes, institutional rules) and normative requirements that are independent of those regulations. There are important questions about what the regulations, in all their different forms, should say. Debates about informed consent, as we saw in chapter one, are frequently focused on those questions. That has not been our task here. Our concern has been with what healthcare professionals should do in the world in which they work, not with what the regulations that govern that world should say (though the two are no doubt linked). This is a world in which sometimes doing what would benefit a patient is wrong, but where the patient can change this by consenting to it. In such situations healthcare professionals should seek their patients' consent. That requires more than just asking for it. It requires ensuring that the patient understands relevant information (where what he needs to understand varies with what is proposed). The obligation to do this, however, is limited.

Due to the complexity of the normative landscape we have not been able to draw any simple conclusions. What is needed to comply with regulations healthcare professionals ought to comply with (the requirements for regulatory consent) often differs from what is needed to avoid acting wrongly for other reasons (the requirements for non-regulatory consent). Some of these differences are ones of scope—regulatory consent may be needed in cases where non-regulatory consent is not, and vice versa. Recognising this is particularly important where, as if often the case, our focus is on informed consent regulations. Not everything for which healthcare professionals need consent falls under those regulations (nor should it). Other differences concern what is required for something to count as consent. As we have seen, informed consent regulations frequently require a greater level of understanding than that needed for non-regulatory consent. That may look surprising, and is certainly out of line with other arguments in the literature. But it should not. To see why, think about a simple case of non-regulatory consent. I told you something in confidence, but now agree to you making that information public. Intuitively I can do this even though I am unaware of the possible consequences of your doing so. Should those turn out to be harmful I may regret allowing you to make the information public. I may also say that I would not have consented had I known that this would (or could) happen. But none of that means I did not consent. Making the information public was not a breach of confidence. It might, of course, still be morally wrong. For example, if you knew that making the information public was likely to harm me, then that itself may have made disclosure wrong. I will have much more to say about cases like this, ones where we know that harm to others could result from our actions, in chapter seven.

Having considered cases where treatment is delivered by healthcare professionals, it is now time to turn to those where it is primarily delivered by either the patient or a member of his family. In doing so we move away from topics, like choice and consent, that have been at the heart of healthcare ethics for some time. Those topics needed to be dealt with. But in investigating them our focus has sometimes had to move away from chronic illness. This was to ensure that the account being developed was defensible across the board—what is needed for consent in the treatment of chronic illness, for example, must be in line with what is needed for consent in other areas of healthcare. In the next chapter we home in on features that are much more specific to chronic illness—starting with healthcare professionals' obligations where the patient is largely treating himself.

Notes

1 For the reasons outlined in chapter one I will be using the term 'consent' here, rather than 'informed consent' or 'valid consent' (the more usual terms in healthcare ethics). The term 'consent' as I am using it refers to an act that makes something that would have been wrong for some reason no longer wrong for that reason.
2 It might be thought that this standing to consent can be subsumed under the 'competence' condition. A person is only competent to consent, it might be

argued, if he has the standing to consent. That may well be right. However, this is not the way the term 'competence' is standardly used in healthcare ethics, as we will see in more detail below. In that context it refers solely to a person's cognitive capacity.

3   I would like to thank Angus Dawson for pressing me on this point.
4   A similar problem arises if we draw the line between what is counted as autonomous and what is not at a certain point for practical reasons (Beauchamp, 2005, p. 316). If we do that, we cannot argue that the reason we should treat people on one side of the line differently than those on the other is that the former are autonomous and the latter are not.
5   I will focus on doing things to the body and doing things that might harm the patient in this chapter. The topic of consent to disclosing information about the patient will be dealt with in more detail in chapter seven.
6   Dworkin phrases this in terms of autonomy. In doing so he is not using that term to refer to sovereignty. He is using it in the way it was used in chapter four—that is, to refer to a person's ability to live their own life. Characterising both of these accounts in terms of respecting autonomy would not be wrong, but would be misleading.
7   This does not in itself mean that treatment is not a significant category when designing regulations. There may be features of medical treatment—such as the imbalance in knowledge and power between doctors and patients—that mean regulations specifically requiring consent for treatment are justified.
8   Just as with regulatory consent, non-regulatory consent is something healthcare professionals must seek. That may require more than just asking for it. It may, for example, require giving information to the patient where he is either unable or unwilling to consent unless he has it.
9   This may create problems in a few areas—such as those where a person has a compulsion or addiction that may affect his ability to refuse an offered intervention (Charland, 2002; Foddy and Savulescu, 2006; Walker, 2008).
10 This example is based on a legal case: *Bang v Charles T Miller Hospital*, 251 Minn. 427, 88 N.W. 2d 186 (1958). For a different explanation of why consent was not given in this case see Beauchamp and Childress, 2009, pp. 127–128.
11 There is a potential difference between these cases. In the book example it may seem that you should return it to me. There is no parallel to this in the case of consent to treatment.
12 In Owens' account of permissive interests (2011, 2012) he does not consider this kind of case, so what is said here is an extrapolation from his account.
13 Given that sovereignty is one way of characterising autonomy, that may look inconsistent with the view, outlined earlier, that what it is to be competent and what it is to be autonomous are the same. However, it is not. The account of 'autonomy' being used by those who link competence and autonomy is not a sovereignty account—it takes 'autonomy' to be a capacity people have. From the fact that 'autonomy' in that sense is linked to competence, it does not follow that 'autonomy' in any other sense is also linked to competence.
14 I will not attempt to provide a full account of this here as my intention is not to defend a particular account of bodily integrity. I am concerned only with what healthcare professionals should do, not with the details of why they should do it.
15 This should not be taken to be a criticism of the regulations—there is no reason to think that they should map exactly onto what is morally required in their absence.

6 How to Respond to Non-Adherence

6.1 Introduction

In chapter five we focused on situations where healthcare professionals need to act—specifically where they need to do something for which consent is required. But when it comes to chronic illness they are not the only ones who need to act. Frequently the patient herself must do so—the Parkinson's patient must take her medication according to the required schedule, the diabetic must manage her diet and give herself the right dose of insulin, the patient with asthma must use her inhaler on a daily basis. The success of the treatment depends on this. These are not things for which consent is needed. Where a patient gives herself medication (by swallowing, injecting, or inhaling it) she does not need anyone's consent to do so. In such situations the role of healthcare professionals is not (as it would be in the case of surgery) to provide treatment directly, it is to support and enable the patient to treat herself. That in turn affects their moral obligations.

For patients to successfully manage their illness they require two things: knowledge and resources. They may have neither unless healthcare professionals provide them. As such, if the latter are to fulfil their obligations to benefit and not harm their patients there are certain things they must do. To successfully follow a course of medication, for example, a patient needs to know what medication to take, when, and in what amounts. She must also have access to that medication. While what medication is to be taken will normally have been agreed at the choice stage, merely knowing that is not enough. If the patient does not know how much to take and when to take it, she may end up taking either too much (potentially exposing herself to harm) or too little (potentially missing out on the benefits altogether). Those providing the medication thus have an obligation to explain all this to her (for further discussion see Walker, 2017).[1] If the medication is prescription only, the patient's doctor will need to write out a prescription to enable his patient to access the medication. Unless he does this (and it is filled by a pharmacist) his patient cannot do what she needs to do. In turn that means that he will not have benefitted her at all. Finally, in some cases knowing *what* to do is not enough, the patient also needs to know *how* to do it—that might include knowing how to use equipment such as an asthma inhaler or insulin pump, or how to perform particular tasks such as testing blood glucose levels.

Healthcare professionals should provide this knowledge and these resources because they have an obligation to benefit their patients. Given what is needed they cannot fulfil that obligation directly, but must proceed indirectly—by enabling the patient to benefit herself. That can create a problem. The patient may not, and as we saw in chapter one sometimes does not, do what is required. If she does not, the healthcare professional treating her has not benefitted her. What are his obligations in this situation? What should he do when faced with a non-adherent patient? This chapter will address these questions. Doing so requires getting clearer on the benefit being aimed at when treating patients with chronic illness. It also requires getting clearer about why patients do not always adhere to their treatment. Once that is done two challenges to the idea that healthcare professionals have any obligations in such cases emerge: that further intervention would be unacceptably paternalistic, and that any further harms are the patient's own responsibility. I will argue that we should reject both these challenges.

The focus of this chapter is patient non-adherence. Patients are not, however, the only people who can fail to adhere. Sometimes treatment is delivered by other people, such as family members. That could be because the patient is unable to do what is required (she lacks competence in the sense outlined in chapter five, or is physically unable to do so). Alternatively it could be because what needs to be done requires coordinated activity and support. Consider, for example, the situation where a patient's diet needs to be managed as part of treating her chronic illness. If the patient does not cook her own meals, the person cooking them needs to adhere to the patient's dietary requirements. These other people may not do what is required. This need not be intentional (though that is a possibility). Instead, just as with the patient herself, those members of her family involved in her care may fail to do what is required unintentionally—they forget to do things, they get into bad habits, or they mistakenly think they are doing it right when they are not. The role of other people, such as family members, in the treatment of patients with chronic illness is an important topic in its own right. Chapter seven is devoted to it. As such, I will leave consideration of non-adherence by people other than the patient to that chapter.

6.2 Clarifying the Benefits of Treatment for Chronic Illness

As we saw in chapters one and two there is a common understanding that healthcare professionals will use their skills and knowledge to benefit their patients. Where our focus is on acute illness this benefit can be characterised in terms of cure—healthcare professionals benefit their patients by curing them. But where, as here, our focus is on chronic illness this will not do. Chronic illness often cannot be cured—however successful their treatment a diabetic remains a diabetic and a patient with asthma still has asthma. In chapter one I argued that in these cases treatment typically aims at one or more of the following: 1. alleviating or relieving the underlying disease's symptoms, 2. preventing those symptoms from occurring, 3. reducing the severity of future symptoms, 4. preventing or reducing any risks the underlying disease poses to the patient's future health.[2] Intuitively meeting these aims benefits the patient. However for our purposes here we need to dig a bit deeper. That is the aim of this section.

It will be useful to start with an example. So, consider pain. Pain is a feature of many, but not all, chronic diseases. It is, for example, one of the main symptoms of arthritis. In addition, chronic pain is itself a chronic illness. At first sight the benefit of treatments that alleviate pain is simply that they alleviate pain, something intrinsically bad (Nagel, 1986, pp. 156–162). Pain is unpleasant in itself, and all accounts of well-being hold that (all else being equal) alleviating or preventing unpleasant sensations makes a person's life go better. But that is only part of the picture. Pain also negatively affects people's lives by making it harder for them to do the things that matter to them. It is a visceral factor, something that grabs their attention (for a general account of visceral factors see Loewenstein, 1996). As such, it makes it harder to attend to other things, such as what their spouse is saying, the work they are doing, or the road on which they are driving. The more severe and long lasting the pain, the greater the interference with a person's ability to live their life on their own terms. There is therefore another way in which someone's life goes better, all else being equal, when they are not in pain. Alleviating their pain can benefit them precisely because, and to the extent that, it removes this interference. Because of this, treatment to alleviate a patient's pain can benefit her in two distinct ways: removing both an unpleasant sensation and something that interferes with her ability to live her life (see Molyneux, 2009, p. 246). It will not always do so. Sometimes a patient's pain does not really interfere with her life at all—it is at most a minor irritant. In that case alleviating her pain only produces the first benefit.

Pain is not the only symptom of chronic illness that has this dual nature. The breathlessness and difficulty breathing associated with asthma, for example, both makes it harder to do other things and is subjectively unpleasant. In some cases alleviating unpleasant sensations is the main benefit of treatment. In others alleviating, or preventing, things that make it harder for the patient to live her life is more important. Consider in this regard treatment for Parkinson's disease, the main symptoms of which are (as we have seen) tremor, slow movement, and muscle stiffness. Each of these symptoms can, depending on its severity, interfere with a patient's ability to live her life. They make it harder for her to go to work, harder to complete her work when she gets there, harder to go to the shops, harder to look after herself at home, harder to play with her children or grandchildren, harder to get dressed in the morning and harder to get undressed in the evening. Treatments for Parkinson's disease include medications that counteract these symptoms, though their effectiveness decreases over time. By doing so they allow the patient to perform these everyday tasks, and at least for a time to live her life as she did before becoming ill. Other treatments may also be available as the disease progresses to help minimise its impact on the patient's ability to live her life—including physiotherapy to help relieve muscle stiffness and thus enable her to remain active, occupational therapy to help her manage everyday activities despite the symptoms she is experiencing, and speech and language therapy to mitigate the effects of her difficulties speaking or swallowing. To the extent that these treatments benefit the patient they do so by counteracting the negative effects of her illness on her ability to do the things that matter to her, and to perform the everyday tasks that are an important part of her life.

At first sight things might look different when the aim of treatment is prevention (as it often is in chronic illness). As we saw in chapter one high blood glucose levels over a prolonged period can cause diabetic ketoacidosis (which is life-threatening) or diabetic retinopathy (loss of vision). They also increase the risk of heart disease, stroke, and kidney disease (among other things). Treatment for diabetes is designed to avoid this happening. Here it looks as if the treatment's benefit is a reduced risk of serious illness or premature mortality. But, just as with pain relief, we can ask why this is a benefit. When we do, we see that the answer relates to the patient's future ability to live her life. Take for example the way treatment prevents a patient's diabetes increasing her risk of having a stroke, something that could have a significant negative effect on her ability to do a whole range of things (for a detailed first-hand account of the effects of a stroke see McCrum, 1998). In doing this, the treatment helps to ensure her diabetes does not compromise her ability to live her life in these ways. That is the benefit it produces. Similarly, where treatment reduces the risk of premature mortality associated with illness the benefit it gives is a potentially longer life. And, at least one way in which living longer benefits people is that it enables them to continue to do the things that matter to them. They cannot do that if they are dead (Nagel, 1979; Nussbaum, 2006, pp. 76–77).[3]

We are now in a position to specify more clearly the main benefits aimed at in the treatment of those with chronic illness. These fall into one, or both, of two distinct categories: 1. alleviating or preventing subjectively unpleasant experiences, and 2. counteracting the ways in which the patient's illness negatively affects, or would if untreated negatively affect, her ability to live her life on her own terms (either now or in the future). The latter will play the largest role in what follows.[4]

However, the idea that this is the benefit aimed at may seem problematic to some readers. For a person to be able to live their own life—to shape it in the light of their goals, values, and commitments—is for them to be autonomous (on at least some accounts of autonomy, see Dworkin, 1988; Gillon, 1986, 2003). As such, the account developed here could be characterised as saying that the aim of treatment is to counteract the ways in which chronic illness undermines a person's autonomy. Where it is successful, treatment enables the patient to be more autonomous (either now or in the future) than she would otherwise have been. That it does this, I have argued, is the benefit provided by the treatment. Such an account might seem to unhelpfully conflate two values normally kept apart, particularly in medical ethics: beneficence and autonomy (see, for example, Beauchamp and Childress' criticism of Pellegrino and Thomasma in Beauchamp and Childress, 2009, p. 207). If it does, so be it—what else could the benefit of Parkinson's medication be? However we should note that this conflation depends on how we characterise what it is to respect autonomy. First, it will only occur if we characterise autonomy as a capacity. Were we to adopt a different account, such as the sovereignty account outlined in chapter five, chronic illness would not interfere with a patient's autonomy. Having diabetes or arthritis does not reduce anyone's authority over what is done to their body. As such, treatment could not be characterised in these cases as enabling the patient to be more autonomous in that sense. Second, it will only occur if we interpret what it is to respect autonomy broadly, so that it includes a requirement to enable patients to be more autonomous. As we have seen, this is an interpretation favoured by some writers. Doing so may follow from other commitments these writers have—for example, that the sole reason for having institutional informed consent procedures is to ensure autonomy is respected and that those procedures should require healthcare professionals to enable their patients to be more autonomous. However, it is not obvious that we should accept this (and in chapter eight I will argue that we should not). Why not say that the aim of informed consent procedures is both to ensure autonomy is respected and to ensure that it is enabled? In that case there remains a clear gap between the requirement to respect autonomy and the requirement to benefit patients. It also avoids expanding the sense of 'respect' in ways that are potentially confusing.

In this section the focus has been on getting a clearer picture of the benefits aimed at in treating chronic illness. Doing so was necessary for the argument in the rest of the chapter. Before continuing, however, it is worth pausing briefly to relate what has been said here to the epistemic argument in chapters two and three. The starting point of that argument was that healthcare professionals have no special expertise in determining what is best for their patients. We can now see more clearly why this is. Treatment for chronic illness benefits the patient where it prevents, minimizes, or alleviates symptoms that make it harder for her to live her life on her own terms. Healthcare professionals will typically know what will have these effects on a patient's symptoms—that is where their expertise lies. How much benefit a treatment provides is partly dependent on that. But it is also partly dependent on two other things: 1. what the patient's commitments, values, and goals are, and 2. the effects of the treatment on her ability to live her life in accordance with those commitments, values, and goals. The patient is not a blank slate when illness strikes. She will, in many cases, already have made her life her own—there are things and people that are important to her, that are closely tied to her identity, and that she values. It is not easy to change these, nor should it be. Having lasting, relatively fixed, commitments is for most people part of what makes their life go well (Williams, 1981). Things that negatively affect a patient's ability to pursue those commitments will have a particularly significant effect on her wellbeing. Because people have different commitments, how an illness affects one person's ability to live her life is likely to be different from its effects on other people's ability to live their lives. Suppose, for example, that Mary is a photographer. She has spent the last twenty years honing and developing her skills—photography is her life. Something that would damage her sight would thus have a significant detrimental effect for her. Her doctor might recognise that, but he may not be in a good position to assess its extent.[5] That matters because chronic illness is not the only thing that can interfere with a person's life. Treatment can too. To return to an earlier example, Freud's cancer of the jaw would have caused him significant pain. As a result it would have made it harder for him to do things that were valuable to him (because it would have made it harder for him to concentrate on them). He would for this reason, among others, have benefitted from pain relief. But the available pain relief in 1930s Britain would also have made it difficult for him to do the things he valued—in particular, his work. As with the illness itself, the extent to which treatment affects a person's ability to live her life (either positively or negatively) will vary depending on her values, commitments, and goals. For this reason it will often be difficult for healthcare professionals to accurately assess whether a treatment would all things considered benefit a patient—they may be able to assess what its effects are, but assessing the extent or size of those effects is a different matter.[6]

6.3 Two Reasons for Non-adherence

Sometimes treatment for chronic illness is provided directly by healthcare professionals—a surgical team carries out a bronchial thermoplasty that will stop the patient's airways narrowing, or a hip replacement that means the patient's osteoarthritis no longer impedes her ability to walk. But often it is not. Instead treatment is indirect. The healthcare professional concerned gives his patient knowledge and resources so that she can counteract the negative effects of her illness on her ability to live her life (either now or in the future). Non-adherence occurs where she does not do so. As such, the benefit aimed at (the reason for giving her this knowledge and these resources in the first place) has not been achieved. At first sight there may not appear to be much of an ethical problem here. In other cases where treatment is not benefitting the patient, for example where medication is not proving as effective as expected, it seems clear that the healthcare professional involved should intervene. He cannot just shrug his shoulders and say that he has given treatment and so has done what he should do. Something similar might seem to be the case when the reason treatment is not working is that the patient is non-adherent. We need to work out how to increase adherence, perhaps, but that does not fall within the ethicist's area of expertise—it might more appropriately be addressed by psychologists (investigating why patients do not adhere, and how to change their behaviour) or by sociologists (investigating the social structures that influence the extent to which patients adhere).

Things are not, however, as ethically straightforward as this might suggest. To show why, I need to say a bit more about non-adherence. In medicine, as we saw in chapter one, a distinction is made between cases where non-adherence is intentional and cases where it is not. For our purposes here a different distinction (one that cuts across the intentional/non-intentional divide) will be more important: sometimes a patient does not adhere because she is not able to do so, in other cases she does not adhere despite being able to do so. The latter might be intentional—as when Freud in our earlier example chooses not to take painkillers—but it might not. It is important not to over-intellectualise things here (something that is, perhaps, an occupational hazard for ethicists). People, including those with chronic illness, have busy lives. As such, they forget to do things they intended to do. They get caught up in problems at work, in their grandchild's difficulties at school, and in celebrating with family and friends when things go well. In doing so they may lose sight, at least for a time, of other things. They get into bad habits and as a result perform tasks poorly even though they have everything they need to perform them well. For all these reasons a patient may non-intentionally fail to adhere despite being able to do so.

The distinction I am pointing to here aligns with one stressed by Amartya Sen in his work on capabilities (Sen, 1982, 1999). Pulling out the similarities with, and incorporating some of the terminology of, the capabilities approach will be helpful in revealing the ethical challenges raised by patient non-adherence. But in doing so it is important to bear in mind that my concern here is not with justice at the level of either the health service or society more broadly—as has been the focus of most of those working on capabilities and health (for two book length accounts see Ruger, 2010 and Venkatapuram, 2011). It is on the obligations of healthcare professionals as individuals. This, of course, includes an obligation to treat patients fairly. And, while it is certainly possible that a doctor who does not give his patients treatment that will help them function effectively has acted unfairly, he need not have. Perhaps more importantly I am not concerned here with what the currency for egalitarian justice should be (which was Sen's initial concern, see Sen, 1982). What is required by an individual's obligation to benefit others, and what is required by a State's obligation to act justly, are not necessarily the same thing.

Those working within the capabilities approach make a distinction between capabilities and functionings. We can think of functionings as achievements—what a person does or what they are—whereas capabilities are the effective freedom, or opportunity, to do or be those things. Similarity at the level of functioning can mask differences at the level of capabilities. Someone fasting and someone starving may eat the same amount of food, for example, but the former has an effective freedom the latter lacks (Sen, 1999, p. 76). People need to have a minimum level of health if they are to have the effective freedom to live the life they choose (whatever that is). As such, Martha Nussbaum argues that health is a core capability (Nussbaum, 2006, pp. 76–77), and Sridhar Venkatapuram argues that it is a meta-capability (Venkatapuram, 2011). Given this, treatment for chronic illness can be conceptualised as counteracting the ways in which a patient's illness does (or might) reduce her capabilities.

But health is not just a capability, it can also be thought of as a functioning. People differ in their capability, their effective freedom, to be healthy (something stressed by Ruger, see Ruger, 2010, pp. 81–88). Being in pain, for example, affects a person's capability (their effective freedom) to do a whole range of things (by making it harder to do them). But, just as people differ in the amount of pain they are experiencing, they also differ in their capability to be pain free. Someone with easy access to cheap and effective painkillers can effectively alleviate her pain should it occur. Someone with no such access—because painkillers are not available or are too expensive—does not. The latter lacks a capability to be pain free the former has. The person with access to painkillers may not use them, in which case these two people may experience the same amount of pain. As with the amount people eat, similarity of functioning can co-exist with differences in capability.

Because health can be thought of as either a capability or a functioning, there are two ways in which healthcare professionals can try to increase a person's effective freedom (their capability) when they are ill. They can do so directly, or they can do so indirectly (by giving them the resources to increase their own effective freedom). Consider in this regard different ways of treating osteoarthritis in the hip—something that limits a person's effective freedom to move around by making it more difficult and painful to do so. If a patient's doctor were to replace her hip, he would be directly increasing her effective freedom to move around. In contrast, if he were to give her medication (including painkillers) to take at home, he would be giving her the effective freedom to control the extent to which she is effectively free to move around. In one case his actions directly affect the patient's effective freedom to move around, in the other they give her control over that freedom. This distinction is related to that which Ruger draws between 'effective freedom' and 'control freedom', though the context is very different (see Ruger, 2010, p. 55).

In the cases we are concerned with here, treatment (where it is successful) gives patients the effective freedom to control whether their condition negatively affects their capability to live their life on their own terms (whatever that is). Merely providing them with relevant knowledge and resources may not do this. As those working on capabilities have stressed, for resources to increase a person's capability, her effective freedom, she must be able to convert them into increased functioning (Sen, 1982, 1999; Venkatapuram, 2011, pp. 121–122). A patient who can do this, can adhere to the treatment plan; a patient who cannot, cannot. The latter is one potential source of patient non-adherence. Consider in this context a patient who does not know how to use her asthma inhaler correctly (errors in using inhalers are common among those with asthma; see, for example, Brocklebank et al., 2001, pp. 85–98; Melani et al., 2011). The inhaler, let us suppose, could effectively control the patient's asthma so that it does not interfere with her ability to life her life. For patients who know how to use it, being given this inhaler increases their effective freedom. But for this patient it does not. As a result her symptoms will be poorly managed, and it is easy to classify the reason for this as patient non-adherence. She is not adhering. But that is because she cannot adhere. In this example the patient has the resources she needs, but lacks the skill to use them effectively. In other cases she may have the needed skills, but lack the resources. A diabetic who must manage her diet may know what to do, but lack the effective freedom to do it—for example, because she cannot afford to, or because the shops she can get to only stock high salt, high fat, high sugar convenience foods and ready meals. Explaining to her what she needs to do in this situation will not increase her effective freedom to manage her condition, though it may well increase the effective freedom of other patients (ones who have more resources or live in a different area).

Neither the asthmatic patient who does not know how to use her inhaler, nor the diabetic who cannot realistically access the right types of food, will adhere to their treatment plan. They lack the ability, the effective freedom, to do so. Ethically, cases like these are very similar to those where prescribed medication proves ineffective. There too the healthcare professional involved has given his patient a resource, but in doing so has not increased her effective freedom to control her illness (and hence the extent to which it interferes with her life). As such, he has not benefited her. As we saw in chapter one, it may not have been possible to determine this in advance. The treatment had to be tried to discover that for this patient, unlike others, it is not effective. But now the healthcare professional knows this, he must try something else. Failing to do so means failing to fulfil his obligation to do what, of the things he can do, is prospectively best for his patient. Similarly, where the patient is unable to adhere, more may need to be done if healthcare professionals are to fulfil their obligations. In the case of the asthmatic patient this means doing what is necessary to ensure that she knows how to use her inhaler—whether that be a practical demonstration, hands on training, or the use of multimedia (in some places training in technique is now included in asthma management guidelines; see, for example, British Thoracic Society [BTS] and Scottish Intercollegiate Guidelines Network [SIGN], 2016, p. 87). Doing this is as much part of enabling the patient to control whether her asthma limits her effective freedom to live her life as is providing the inhaler itself. Of course, there are limits to what healthcare professionals can do. They cannot change what food is stocked by shops near their diabetic patients, for example, and are unlikely to be able to directly provide that food or the means to access it. But that does not necessarily mean there is nothing they can do even in cases like this. There may be ways to help their patients work around the problem, or other services that could help patients get to appropriate shops if they knew about them. Where even this is not possible, the healthcare professional is in the same position as a doctor who discovers that the medication he has prescribed is ineffective but no other medication is available. In that case his ability to benefit his patient is extremely limited. As are his obligations—we saw in chapter two that healthcare professionals' obligations to do what is prospectively best for their patients are limited to what they can do given their expertise and the resources available to them (something that will vary considerably from place to place).

Cases where patients do not adhere because they cannot adhere are ethically relatively straightforward (though given that what a patient is able to do varies from patient to patient identifying them in practice may be difficult). But not all cases of non-adherence are like this. Sometimes a patient does not adhere even though she has everything she needs to control whether her illness interferes with her effective freedom to live her life on her own terms. In that case it might be doubted whether those treating her have any further obligations. As Ruger puts it in a slightly different context, "once capabilities are assured people must be free to make the choices they like" (Ruger, 2010, p. 45). There are two reasons for this. First, any further intervention may seem unacceptably paternalistic. The patient has the capability to control how her illness affects her life, but does not use it. Were her doctor to try to bring it about that she adheres he would be intervening in her life, and the reason he would be doing so is that he thinks it would benefit her. Given that she is a competent adult, that may well look morally wrong. Second, if the patient does not adhere (despite being able to do so), any resulting ill health might seem to be her responsibility (not that of the healthcare professionals treating her). As such, it might be argued, those treating her have no further obligation to help her—they have put her in a position where she can control her illness, and that is all they have an obligation to do. We will look at these two arguments in turn over the next two sections.

6.4 Is Intervention in the Face of Non-Adherence Permissible?

The situation we are concerned with is this. Healthcare professionals have given a patient everything she needs to manage her illness. For example, she has been given an inhaler and trained in how and when to use it. Were this patient to do what her healthcare professionals have enabled her to do, her illness would not interfere with her ability to live her life to the extent that it does. But she does not do these things. That does not mean those healthcare professionals have not benefitted her. She is now able to prevent her illness interfering with her ability to live her life—she can at least to some extent mitigate its effects on her ability to go to work, play with her grandchildren, visit her friends, or look after herself at home. Just knowing that she can do this, should she choose, may make her illness easier to deal with. That itself looks like a benefit (for a related point see Sen, 1999, p. 76). As such, if healthcare professionals' obligations were simply to benefit their patients, enabling those patients to control their illness would be sufficient to fulfil their obligations. But, as I argued in chapter two, that is not the right way to characterise the obligation of beneficence. In practice, it requires doing what, of the things that can be done given the healthcare professional's expertise and available resources, is prospectively best for the patient. Normally following a treatment plan provides greater benefits than simply being able to follow it. If that is right, healthcare professionals need to do more than enable their patients to adhere. They should, where they can, act to ensure that their patients do adhere. Sometimes they cannot do this. But even in that situation there is often more they can do. They could, for example, switch the patient onto a different treatment plan, one she is more likely to adhere to. This is not, however, likely to be the best option. While it may be better for the patient than doing nothing, if the original treatment was preferred at the choice stage it is unlikely to be as beneficial as bringing it about that the patient adheres.[7]

Bringing it about that she adheres, however, means attempting to bring it about that the patient acts in certain ways—that she does what the healthcare professionals treating her have enabled her to do. That creates a problem. To see why, consider the situation where a healthcare professional increases his patient's effective freedom (her capability) to do things like go to work, or play with her grandchildren, directly—for example, by replacing her hip joint. The patient's life will, let us suppose, go better if she does these things. But she does not. It would be an unacceptable intrusion into this patient's life were her surgeon to attempt to bring it about that she does what his surgery has enabled her to do (go to work or play with her grandchildren). He has enabled her to do these things, but whether or not she does them is rightly up to her (and her alone). In the cases we are concerned with in this section healthcare professionals have also increased their patient's effective freedom—albeit the effective freedom in these cases is the freedom to bring it about that her illness does not interfere with her ability to live her life. If intervening to make sure that she uses her effective freedom to act in ways that benefit her would be wrong in one case, why would it be any less wrong in the other? Unless there is a way of satisfactorily answering this question we will need to conclude that only two things are morally permissible when faced with a non-adherent patient: 1. taking steps to enable her to adhere, or 2. switching her onto a different treatment.

In this situation it will not do to say that at least where non-adherence is non-intentional intervening would be at worst soft paternalism, and thus not morally wrong.[8] It may be that soft paternalism does not involve a failure to respect autonomy and so is not wrong on that ground (Beauchamp and Childress, 2009, pp. 209–213). Indeed it may not even be paternalism (Feinberg, 1986, p. 12). But even leaving aside cases of intentional non-adherence (where intervention would be hard paternalism), drawing a distinction between hard and soft paternalism will not enable us to draw the line in the right place. Consider a patient who has her hip replaced. Her effective freedom to go to work or play with her grandchildren is enhanced, and that may be why she chose the operation in the first place. Now suppose that, despite still intending to do those things, she does not do them. Like everyone else she has a lot going on in her life. Sometimes things do not work out the way she intended, sometimes she forgets to do what she fully intends to do, and sometimes despite her intentions life gets in the way of acting on them. In this situation intervening to bring it about that she does the things she intends (such as playing with her grandchildren) would be on a par with intervening to bring it about that the non-intentionally non-adherent patient follows her treatment plan. If the latter is soft paternalism so is the former. But, the former would still be morally wrong. To see why, imagine that someone else (perhaps a parent) intervenes without your asking in the way you bring up your children or do your job. Even if they are trying to bring it about that you do this well (as you yourself might see it), the intervention is troubling and may well be resisted. The reason for this is that it can send a message—'you are not up to it', 'you are doing a bad job', 'you are a failure'. It shows a lack of appreciation for the fact that you are living your life and are doing it on your own terms—even if given your circumstances this involves stumbling from one decision to another (to use Jeremy Waldron's apt description, Waldron, 2017, p. 113) rather than following a worked out plan. Treating patients in this way, as we saw in chapter four, is not consistent with treating them with respect.[9] As such, it is something that healthcare professionals should not do.

One response to this concern would be to draw on work on mental health problems (including addiction and bipolar disorder) which make adherence particularly difficult (see, for example, Elster, 2003; Robertson, 2003; Andreou, 2008; Brock, 2003; Dresser, 1982; Davis, 2008; Spellecy, 2003; Walker, 2012a).[10] This work focuses on patients who have voluntarily agreed to do certain things (such as refraining from drinking alcohol), but who realise they are unlikely to stick to that agreement. In some cases it looks backward to the agreement, focusing specifically on pre-commitment devices or Ulysses contracts—where the patient authorises healthcare professionals to give her treatment in the future even if she refuses it at that time (Elster, 2003; Robertson, 2003; Brock, 2003; Dresser, 1982; Walker, 2012a). That is not likely to be relevant here, though such devices may be a way of dealing with foreseeable non-adherence in some cases. However, in other cases it is forward looking, focusing on the way that treatment can enhance the patient's future autonomy (Davis, 2002, 2008; Spellecy, 2003). Given that this is also one of the aims of treatment for chronic illness, this work does look relevant. The basic idea is as follows. While in the short term intervention to bring about adherence interferes with the patient's autonomy, in the longer term it enhances her autonomy. As long as the latter is larger than the former then all things considered the intervention does not undermine the patient's autonomy. Those treating her are restricting her autonomy in order to enhance it (Levy, 2014). It is unclear that that would count as acting paternalistically.

Whatever the merits of this argument in the specific cases it was developed to address, when it comes to non-adherence more generally we should resist it. Chronic illness can interfere with a person's autonomy, either now or in the future, by making it harder (perhaps impossible) for her to shape her life in accordance with her goals, aims, and commitments—that is, it can interfere with her personal autonomy, the extent to which she can make her life her own. Treatment aims, at least in part, to counteract this. Where it succeeds the patient will be more autonomous, in this sense, than she would have been in its absence. Given all this, intervening to bring it about that she adheres will in some cases make her more autonomous (taking a long term view). It may thus appear to be justified. Far from being a failure to respect autonomy, it is an enhancement of autonomy. However, focusing only on personal autonomy is to miss something important. An example will show why.

Consider a patient with cancer, who requires a course of chemotherapy. If she has it she will continue to live; if she does not her cancer will kill her. Further suppose that on completing the course of chemotherapy she will be able to do many of the things she values. In this situation the overall effect on the patient's personal autonomy of having chemotherapy would be positive. This is likely to be the case even if she is forced to have it. But that in no way justifies forcing her to have chemotherapy. To do so, as we saw in chapter five, would be a failure to respect her autonomy in the sense of sovereignty (her standing to control the permissibility of doing things to her body). That is, while imposing treatment might enable her to be (all things considered) more autonomous in one sense of 'autonomy', it would be a failure to respect her autonomy in a different sense of 'autonomy'. There are two distinct values here and we should not let the fact that we use the same word to refer to both mislead us into thinking there is only one. To argue that interventions that enhance a patient's future personal autonomy (such as those that would bring it about that she adheres) are all things considered justified we would need to show that they are justified despite the failure of respect involved. Such an argument would need to take a familiar form—it would need to show that the benefit in terms of enhanced personal autonomy is more pressing or important than the wrong done by failing to respect the patient or her autonomy (in the sense of sovereignty).

I do not think that this is a promising way to go. Instead I want to argue that the concern that acting to ensure patient adherence is objectionably paternalistic stems from taking too narrow a perspective. When we focus on what healthcare professionals need to do to provide treatment, or on what patients need to do to deliver it, we look at particular parts of the treatment plan—the healthcare professional does this part, the patient does that part. That forces us to look closely at what each person's role is, something that matters ethically. But it can also obscure the fact that these different actions are part of a whole that neither the patient nor the healthcare professional does on their own. Instead, it is something they do together. By this I mean more than that the patient does it and the healthcare professional does it. I mean that they collaborate to do it, and that the success of the treatment is dependent on each doing their part. That is, this is a shared project or activity.

In healthcare the idea of a shared activity is most familiar from discussions of shared decision making (see, for example, Coulter and Collins, 2011; Cribbs and Donetto, 2013; Edwards and Elwyn, 2009; Elwyn, Tilburt, and Montori, 2013; Godolphin, 2009; Friesen-Storms et al., 2015). This, it is sometimes argued, should be how decisions are made—rather than it being the case either that the healthcare professional should decide, or that the patient should decide. Chapters two to four can be read as arguing for this conclusion when it comes to some, but not all, treatment decisions. They do so on the basis of the healthcare professional's obligations—he has no obligation to do what his patient wants just because she wants it, he has an obligation to treat her in a way that is not demeaning or belittling, and he has an obligation to take the option that is prospectively best for her. To fulfil these obligations he must in many cases involve his patient in choosing what to do, but should not cede decision-making authority entirely to her. If decision making *should* sometimes be shared, treatment provision (in the cases we are concerned with here) *must* be shared. Healthcare professionals can make treatment decisions on their own (even if they should not), they cannot provide these treatments on their own. As such, we do not need to argue that treatment should be a shared activity, we need to recognise that it is a shared activity. Doing so has implications for what healthcare professionals ought to do. It also, as we will see, has implications for what patients ought to do (and for what their responsibilities are). To draw these out, and to see how they relate to patient non-adherence, it will be useful to look briefly at some points in the philosophical literature on shared action (see, for example, Bratman, 1993, 2014; Gilbert, 2014; Searle, 1990; Velleman, 2000).

We can start by looking at how shared actions are initiated. A shared action is something that one or more people do together. It can appropriately be characterised by saying 'we are doing this' (where that is not reducible to 'I am doing this and you are doing it too'). While shared action in this sense is philosophically puzzling,[11] no-one seriously denies that it exists. Common examples in the literature include going for a walk together (Gilbert, 2014), painting the house together (see Bratman, 1993), and executing a pass in (American) football (see Searle, 1990). While these examples are all simple, and that is important given the authors' aims, other cases will be more complex. That people are doing something together does not mean that they are doing the same thing, or acting at the same time. Sometimes the things people do together extend over a long period (in these cases it may be clearer to talk of a shared activity rather than a shared action). For example, where a couple is bringing up their child together this is a shared activity. It is not that he is bringing up his child, and she is bringing up her child. Putting it that way would fail to capture the fact that bringing up their child is something they do together.

According to Margaret Gilbert a shared action exists wherever one person, S, indicates a willingness to do something with someone else, T, and T indicates a willingness to do it with S (by, for example, agreeing to do it with S) (Gilbert, 2014, pp. 47–48). In contrast, David Velleman takes it that shared action requires reciprocal conditional intentions—S intends to do something, say paint the room, if and only if T intends to do so; and T intends to paint the room if and only if S intends to do so (Velleman, 2000). For our purposes here we need not enter this debate. All those involved agree that a voluntary agreement,[12] whether explicit or tacit, to do something together means that this is something people are doing together. If this is how shared activity begins, then healthcare professional and patient are acting together whenever they agree to a treatment plan that requires both to act. They may also be acting together in the absence of any such formal agreement. As I pointed out in chapter one, before prescribing medication a doctor should determine (to the extent that this is possible) whether the patient is likely to take it. By seeking his patient's agreement to take the medication the doctor indicates that he has a conditional intention—he intends to provide the medication if (and only if) the patient intends to take it. In agreeing the patient indicates that she also has a conditional intention—she intends to take the medication if her doctor provides it. Alternatively, by proposing a treatment a doctor indicates a willingness to work with his patient to treat her illness, and in agreeing to take the medicine the patient indicates her willingness to work with him to treat her illness.[13]

It might be objected that this moves too quickly because the patient may have neither the intention nor the willingness I have ascribed to them. While that is certainly possible, it would be unusual. Why would a patient in this situation agree to treatment if at that time she does not intend, or is not willing, to take it? No doubt there are scenarios where there is a good answer to this question. But any such scenario involves the patient acting insincerely—she voluntarily agrees to do something while having no intention, or willingness, to do it even as she agrees to do so. Normally it will also involve her being irrational. For the most part patients visit a healthcare professional (indeed seek out that healthcare professional) because they want something to help with their illness. That is now on offer. Agreeing to what is offered means other options will not be explored. Thus agreeing to treatment while not intending to take it, or not being willing to take it, effectively rules out any chance of getting effective treatment. And that would be inconsistent with the patient achieving her own aims.

Having said all that, the patient may not realise that she is engaged in a shared activity with a particular healthcare professional. The latter should, therefore, take the steps necessary to ensure that she does—particularly as entering a shared activity imposes obligations on those involved. In healthcare there are advantages in making sure that all those involved in delivering treatment are aware of what their part involves. We would, for example, expect this in the case of other members of the treatment delivery team. There is no reason to think that things should be any different when it comes to the patient. With treatment for chronic illness she is as much part of the treatment team as anyone else. In this context we need to get away from the idea that the patient is simply a patient to whom treatment is given. She is the patient, but she is also, must also be, an agent. Furthermore, there is some evidence to suggest that making such agreements more explicit helps to increase patient adherence (Nunes et al., 2009).

Having argued that treatment for chronic illness is a shared activity, we now need to consider the implications of this for those involved. It must be acknowledged that there is considerable disagreement about this in the literature on shared action. However, that disagreement is much less where the shared action is initiated by an agreement (either explicit or tacit), simply because the agreement itself plays an important role. Acting with others typically involves a commitment to them. According to Gilbert, for example, this must be the case if we are to distinguish two people going for a walk together from two people who happen to be walking along a path at the same time (Gilbert, 2014, pp. 24–26). The former, but not the latter, have at least some obligation to each other. They cannot, for example, unilaterally leave the walk with no explanation. Indeed on Gilbert's account they cannot permissibly cease acting together without the permission of those with whom they are acting. The only exception is where the initiating agreement either explicitly or tacitly gives one person authority to cancel the shared activity on their own initiative (Gilbert, 2014, p. 40). Healthcare is one such exception (patients can generally withdraw from treatment any time they choose, whereas healthcare professionals generally cannot). Furthermore, on Gilbert's account this commitment means those with whom a person is acting can reasonably demand of her that she fulfil that commitment, and can hold her accountable (and even rebuke her) if she does not (Gilbert, 2014, pp. 88–89, p. 120). Suppose you and I have voluntarily agreed to do something together. Given my agreement, you have a reasonable expectation that I will do my part. If I do not, you have grounds for complaint against me. I have at the very least let you down. The idea that an agreement to do something together binds us in this way, is not a feature of Gilbert's account alone. It is also a feature of accounts that conceptualise agreement as an exchange of promises (see, for example, Bach (1995)). If in agreeing to do something with you I am implicitly promising to do it (or more precisely to do my part in it if you do your part), then you can reasonably hold me to that. I cannot legitimately pull out of our agreement without your permission—to do so would be to break my promise. I am also bound to act in the way agreed, simply because that is something I have promised to do so.[14]

According to these accounts, doing something together places obligations on everyone involved—particularly when, as in the case of treatment for chronic illness, it is initiated by a voluntary agreement. However, such accounts have been challenged. First, it can be argued that in some cases nothing as demanding as an obligation is created simply from the mere fact that people are acting together (Bratman, 1993). If we think of shared action as being initiated by mutual conditional intentions, for example, the link will be both weaker and easier to get out of than that. Second, the idea that when acting together people have an obligation to do what has been agreed creates problems where the shared action would be morally wrong (see Bratman, 1999). Were we robbing a bank together, for example, it looks wrong to say that each of us has an obligation to do our part, or that we can be held accountable (and rightly rebuked) if we fail to do so. It is worth addressing these points briefly.

In response to the first of these objections I want to stress something stated earlier. Whatever the case with less formal arrangements, shared actions initiated by a voluntary agreement do seem to impose obligations on those involved (and it is these that will be important in what follows). Suppose we have agreed to cook a meal together tomorrow. Having agreed, I should make the effort to turn up, or at the very least let you know if I cannot do so. You could justifiably criticise me if I do not. I have let you down, and that is something I should not do. In contrast, if we have made no such agreement, but have left it open whether I will join you or not, none of this applies. In that situation it would be unreasonable to criticise me for failing to show up (even if I did not let you know I would not be coming). We might disagree about whether it is appropriate to characterise the obligations I have here, where I have them, as moral obligations (on Bach's account they are, on Gilbert's they are not). But it is hard to see how the agreement could make no difference to what I ought to do.

The second objection cannot be dealt with in this way. Gilbert responds to it by stressing that on her account the obligations created by shared intentions are not moral obligations (they are things people owe each other in virtue of the fact that they are doing something together) (Gilbert, 2014, pp. 121–122). As such, where they are doing something morally wrong together these obligations can be outweighed by relevant moral obligations—for example, Bill's obligation to rob the bank stemming from his agreement to do so is outweighed by his moral obligation not to steal. But that may not seem adequate. The objection outlined above was that someone cannot have any obligation to rob a bank just because they voluntarily agreed to rob it, not that they cannot have such an obligation all things considered. An alternative way to respond to this objection draws on work in a related area—promising. Bill could certainly say 'I promise to help you rob the bank' in a way that seems to fit the standard requirements for promises to be binding. If this is a binding promise, then it would follow (contrary to the objection we are considering) that he could have an obligation to do something morally wrong. But suppose it is not. We would not then conclude that promises cannot impose obligations on those who make them. Instead we would attempt to explain why this is an exception to that general rule, something that is both complex and a matter of considerable debate (see, for example, Altham, 1985; Gilbert, 2014, pp. 296–323; Owens, 2012, pp. 245–249; Searle, 2001, pp. 193–200; Shiffrin, 2011; Smith, 1997; Watson, 2009). To have a full account of promising we would need to resolve that debate. But where our concern is with the practical implications of promising to do something that is not morally wrong, we do not. The same is true when we turn our attention to obligations that stem from an agreement to do something together (indeed if agreements are reciprocal promises they are the same thing). If doing something wrong together does not generate obligations to do what those involved agreed to do, that needs to be explained. But, the existence of such cases should not lead us to conclude that where people are doing something together that is not morally wrong (for example, treating a patient's illness) their agreement does not create any obligations either.

With this theoretical account in place we can now return to the problem of patient non-adherence. Where treatment is something healthcare professional(s) and patient do together, both have obligations stemming from the fact that this is something they are doing together. In such cases the patient is not just a patient—someone to whom treatment is given. She is as much a part of the treatment team as anyone else (something that discriminatory social norms may make it harder to see in the case of older patients or those with cognitive and/or physical limitations that affect what they can do). Treating her with the respect she is due requires acknowledging that fact. She has chosen to work with one or more healthcare professionals on managing her illness. Just like them she has her reasons for doing so. They are working with her because this is the way to fulfil their obligation to do what is prospectively best for her; she is working with them because this is a way for her to manage her illness most effectively. For none of them is this thing they are doing together the only thing that matters in their life. Because of this patients will sometimes decide they do not want to continue with the treatment they are on (and have agreed to). They are entitled to do so. When that happens healthcare professionals and patient are no longer acting together, the patient has unilaterally cancelled their shared activity. She should, if what I argued above is correct, tell the healthcare professionals involved that she has done so—they, as people with whom she was working, have a reasonable complaint against her if she does not. In this situation it would be inappropriate for a healthcare professional to try to bring it about that his patient adheres to the previously agreed treatment. To do so would be to attempt to impose on her something she has decided not to do. That, as we have seen in previous chapters, would be wrong. This does not mean there is nothing more the healthcare professional should do. He still has an obligation to do what, of the things that he can do given his expertise and the resources available to him, is prospectively best for his patient. That is not affected by his patient's decision not to continue with the agreed treatment. But her decision does change what he can permissibly do. The original treatment is now no longer an available option. As such, he should consider which of his remaining options would be prospectively best for his patient and draw up a new treatment plan with her on that basis.

Things are different, however, when the patient's non-adherence is not intentional. In that case she has not changed her mind about the treatment, and has not cancelled the agreed treatment plan. As such, healthcare professional and patient are still engaged in a shared activity. They are not doing it well, given the patient's non-adherence, but that in itself does not mean they are no longer doing it together. Taking steps to bring it about that the patient adheres would, in this situation, be an attempt to put this shared activity back on track. Doing that does not look morally problematic. The healthcare professional would be trying to bring it about that his patient does what she herself is committed to doing in virtue of the fact that they are acting together. That is not paternalistic on most accounts of paternalism. He is not imposing anything on her, something required for paternalism (see, Archard, 1990; Bullock, 2015; Coons and Weber, 2013).[15] He is holding her to what she has herself voluntarily agreed to do. That does not mean that just anything that could increase patient adherence is permissible. The method used must, as we have seen, treat the patient with the respect she is owed as an equal, and vital, participant in the shared activity—something that rules out interventions that are demeaning or belittling.

Thinking about things in this way enables us to answer the question posed at the start of this section—if it would be morally wrong for a healthcare professional who has directly increased his patient's effective freedom to do some things (like go to work or play with her grandchildren) to intervene to bring it about that she does them, why would it be permissible for him to intervene where he has increased his patient's effective freedom to do other things (those required to manage her illness)? We can now see that the relevant difference is that in the latter, but not the former, the healthcare professional's actions are part of a shared activity, something that healthcare professional and patient do together. For that shared activity to succeed the patient must use the effective freedom gained by having access to medical resources and expertise to counteract the ways in which her illness compromises her ability to live her life. That is, she must adhere to the agreed treatment plan. Because this is a shared activity, the healthcare professionals with whom she is working can reasonably hold her to this (up to the point where she withdraws from, and thus cancels, the shared activity). They can also reasonably intervene to help her do what she needs to do. In doing so, they do not impose on her to achieve their own goals, they act to help her fulfil her commitments towards their joint goals. None of that is true where a healthcare professional has acted directly to increase his patient's effective freedom to live her life (as is the case where he replaces her hip joint). The shared activity, to the extent that it exists in this case, only extends to the activities needed to successfully perform the operation. The patient may have agreed to that operation because she thought having it would improve her life by making it easier to do a whole range of things. But she did not agree to do those things when she agreed to have the surgery, and doing them is no part of anything she is doing with her surgeon. For this reason it would be inappropriate for him to try to bring it about that his patient uses the increased freedom provided by her operation.

I have argued that treatment for chronic illness is something that healthcare professional and patient do together—it is a shared activity. While recognising that fact has been helpful, it may be thought to raise problems of its own. Where people are acting together each can be held accountable for doing their part. That means patients can be held accountable for following, or failing to follow, their treatment plan. Because following the plan is their responsibility, patients who do not adhere despite being able to do so (and as we have seen not all can) would seem to be responsible for any ill health that results from their non-adherence. That, in turn, might suggest that such patients have at best a lower claim on treatment. That is, it might be argued that non-adherent patients who experience health problems as a result of their non-adherence are not owed the same priority for treatment as others (such as adherent patients or those who are unable to adhere). If this is right, then non-adherence would affect healthcare professionals' future obligations to their patients. It is to this argument that we now need to turn.

6.5 Patient Responsibility and the Obligations of Healthcare Professionals

The argument that patient responsibility has implications for what they are owed is familiar in healthcare—including discussions of non-adherence (see, for example, Buetow and Elwyn, 2006; Draper and Sorell, 2002; Galvin, 2002; Morreim, 1995). Having put a patient into a position where she can (to the extent possible with current technology and medication) manage her illness, it might be thought that it is up to her what she does with that opportunity. She may take it, or she may not. Where she does not, her health may suffer (perhaps seriously). In some, but not all, cases it will be apparent that those health problems stem from her failure to adhere. It would be hard to deny, for example, that the breathing difficulties of a non-adherent patient with severe asthma are at least in part a consequence of her failure to control her asthma.[16] Because patients who experience these health problems have been given the resources and knowledge to prevent them, is any more owed to them? Or should we hold that because their ill health is their own responsibility, it is not? In other contexts, a common response to these questions is to challenge the idea that patients are ever really responsible for their ill health. Given what I argued above, that response is not available to us here. In this section I want to hold onto the idea that it is often appropriate to hold patients responsible for their failures to adhere (see, also, Draper and Sorell, 2002), and I will provide additional arguments to support that claim. But I will also argue, drawing on work by Yascha Mounk (2017), that this has no implications for what healthcare professionals ought to do in cases where a patient does not adhere despite being able to do so.

Decisions about resource allocation in healthcare are taken at several levels. Some concern what policy should be, or what should be funded. While important in practice, these are not our concern here. Others are matters of what an individual healthcare professional should do in the face of competing demands on his resources, including his time. Time spent helping one patient, is time that cannot be used to help others. Resources used to help one person, are not available to help other people. In deciding what to do a healthcare professional must work with what he has, and that may require prioritising some patients over others. His obligation to benefit his patients must be seen in this context. This was implicitly recognised in the account developed earlier (by restricting it to what is prospectively best *given* the healthcare professional's expertise and *available resources*). Where a healthcare professional cannot, through lack of resources (including time), benefit everyone equally, he must decide who to treat first. There are many different ways in which he could do this. One option, that is at least initially appealing for many people, is to take account of the patient's responsibility for her illness. For example, to argue that healthcare professionals' obligations do not extend to rescuing patients from the consequences of their own actions. This idea has been investigated, and challenged, in relation to the allocation both of healthcare resources in general (see, for example, Cappelan and Norheim, 2005; Dietrich, 2002; Feiring, 2008; Harris, 1995; Martin, 2001; Resnik, 2007; Walker, 2010; Wikler, 2002; Wilkinson, 1999), and of liver transplants in particular (see, for example, Brudney, 2007; Glannon, 1998; Ho, 2008; Smart, 1994).

The case we are concerned with here is distinct in that, somewhat unusually in this context, the non-adherent patient has already received treatment for her illness.[17] Her doctor (and other healthcare professionals) have done what they can to benefit her. They have given her the resources she needs, and have devoted time to her care. As such, the issue is not whether she should be given treatment, but whether she should be given *more* treatment—treatment that is only needed because of her non-adherence. Doing so takes resources that could be used to benefit others, including those who have not yet been treated. That, the argument we are considering here says, would be unfair. She has had her chance, though she did not take it. Those other patients have not. To give her a second chance at their expense would thus be to deny them an equal chance of treatment. That would be wrong. The only way to avoid this wrong is for the non-adherent patient to be given lower priority (which, given the pressure on resources, may mean she gets nothing). We might put the point this way, the obligation to help others is affected by how they came to be in a position where they need help. If their being in that position is a consequence of something they were able to avoid but did not (particularly where they had previously been given everything needed to avoid it), they have a lower claim on our assistance than they otherwise would. That is, the strength of our obligations to benefit others tracks their responsibility for the position they are in—something that is as true for healthcare professionals as anyone else.

Arguments of this form within political philosophy have faced considerable criticism. This is particularly the case for the most prominent political theory of this type, luck egalitarianism (for accounts of luck egalitarianism see Arneson, 1999, 2001; Cohen, 2011; Dworkin, 1981a, 1981b, 2002; Segall, 2010). Readers familiar with that theory will recognise that the account just outlined is not strictly a form of luck egalitarianism as that has usually been developed. This allows it to avoid some criticisms that might otherwise prove challenging. For example, one prominent and influential objection to luck egalitarianism is that it is too harsh (Anderson, 1999; Voigt, 2007). At least in some versions, it says that if someone is in a life-threatening situation as a result of something they chose, there is no obligation to rescue them even where that could easily be done. That is likely to look morally troubling, particularly in the context of healthcare. Whatever the validity of this as an objection to luck egalitarianism (and for a luck egalitarian response to it see Segall, 2010, ch.4), it is not an objection to the position outlined here. That position does not deny that where resources are available every patient should be helped, irrespective of how they came to need help (something required by healthcare professionals' obligation to do what is prospectively best for their patients). What it says is that while non-adherent patients have a claim on the resources that would benefit them, they have less of a claim on those resources than other patients (see, Smart, 1994; Walker, 2010—for a response, see, Wilkinson, 1999). Where resources are scarce someone will miss out, the question is who. Saying that this should be those who have previously received benefits they did not use, does not on the face of it look unduly harsh. Furthermore, such an approach does not (as is sometimes claimed in the applied ethics literature) inappropriately punish patients, perhaps capitally, for their past actions (see Harris, 1995; Brudney, 2007). It is not a punishment for resources that would benefit you to be given to someone else who has a greater claim on them.

That it can avoid these criticisms does not, however, mean we should accept it. Other challenges remain, and have yet to be considered. Perhaps the most common, at least in applied contexts, is that those who need help are not really responsible for being in that position. That is the case whether our concern is with welfare in general (see discussion in Mounk, 2017, pp. 13–16, 99–109), or healthcare in particular. Opponents of using patient responsibility as a criterion when allocating liver transplants, for example, have argued that the patient may not be responsible for her drinking (because she is addicted, or started drinking while a child, or never chose to be a heavy drinker, or had no access to centres that could treat her addiction) (see, for example, Glannon, 1998; Ho, 2008). More broadly in public health ethics there is considerable resistance to the idea that patients are responsible for their ill health, even where it apparently results from their behaviour, with much attention being focused on the social determinants of health (Commission on the Social Determinants of Health, 2008; Marmot and Wilkinson, 2005; Venkatpuram, 2011). As Mounk points out, arguments of this type (unlike Anderson's) do not challenge the idea that resource allocation should track responsibility, they focus on who is responsible (Mounk, 2017, p. 14). He goes on to argue that that may be problematic in the context of welfare provision. We should instead, or so he argues, directly challenge the link between responsibility and what people are owed.

It is this response that I want to explore in some detail here. This is because when it comes to patient non-adherence denying that the patient is ever responsible is particularly problematic. Earlier I distinguished between cases of non-adherence where the patient could not in practice adhere from those where the patient could adhere. The former can be dealt with easily—the patient in these cases cannot reasonably be thought to be responsible for any ill effects stemming from her non-adherence. The problem is with the latter. There are three reasons for this. First, denying that the patient is responsible in these cases is inconsistent with the way we treat other people. Consider two cases. In the first a patient forgets to take her medication, and as a result her health suffers. In the second a doctor forgets to do something, and as a result his patient's health suffers. Whatever reason is used to deny that the patient is responsible—she has a busy life that demands her attention, she is not responsible for being a forgetful person—could equally well apply to the doctor. But people are unlikely to accept that the doctor is not responsible here (at least on these grounds). There are, of course, exceptions. Were they to learn that this doctor has had to work excessive hours without adequate support they might shift their judgment of who is responsible onto the hospital or practice management. In doing so they are not giving up on the idea that someone is responsible for what happened, they are adjusting their account of who is responsible (for a related point see Mounk, 2017, pp. 191–192). The basic point here is that we regularly hold some people, healthcare professionals, responsible for their failures to follow agreed treatment plans (particularly where this is due to forgetfulness, falling into bad habits, or misunderstanding what to do despite being shown—that is, for the things that cause non-intentional non-adherence). We also hold them responsible for any harm to the patient's health that results. As such, it seems inconsistent to deny that other people, patients, who are equally involved in providing treatment are responsible for similar failures. It might be objected that there is an important difference between healthcare professional and patient here. The former, but not the latter, has a duty of care and that is why we hold him responsible. That difference is likely to be relevant if our concern is with the law (particularly where it comes to negligence). But it is not relevant here. That the doctor has a duty of care means he has certain responsibilities that his patient does not. Where he fails to fulfil them he can in most cases be held responsible. However, as I argued above, the patient also has responsibilities stemming from her active role in treatment. Where she does not fulfil them, the failure of the treatment is attributable to her. As such, she is responsible for it. What we are concerned with here are the conditions under which it would be appropriate to attribute responsibility in this way. The existence of a duty of care is not the only thing that does that.

Second, denying that the patient is ever responsible in cases of non-adherence would be inconsistent with the rationale for giving her medication in the first place. Remember the situation we are concerned with here. A healthcare professional aims to benefit his patient by giving her resources (such as medication) to take at home, along with the knowledge needed to use it appropriately. He does this precisely to enable his patient to effectively manage her illness. This is only reasonable where she could in fact manage her illness once he has acted (by giving her any necessary medication, information, or training). As such, we cannot turn around later, when the patient does not take her medication, and say that taking it was outwith her control. If it was not something that she could control (even when she has the appropriate medication and skills), there was no point in giving her the means to control it. That is not to deny that sometimes healthcare professionals only discover that a patient is unable to do what is required after providing treatment. As we have already seen, such cases are ones where despite being given resources or information the patient lacks the effective freedom to manage her condition. But not all cases are like that—if they were, it would never make sense to provide patients with treatments of this type.

These first two reasons for thinking non-adherent patients should be held responsible for their failures to adhere rely on claims about consistency. It is a weakness of such arguments that there are always two ways to resolve an inconsistency (one could, for example, accept that the forgetful doctor is not responsible for the consequences of his forgetfulness). The third reason does not face this problem. It rests on the idea that by denying the patient's responsibility we fail to recognise her as an agent—someone who can look after herself, can manage her life, and can do things like take a tablet every day. As such, it fails to treat her with the respect she is owed. That failure to respect her as an agent, in turn, constitutes a failure to treat her as an equal (Dworkin, 1981b; Waldron, 2017, p. 13). For this reason it is not something that healthcare professionals should do. There are a variety of ways we might argue for this. One option is to draw on Peter Strawson's work on reactive attitudes

(Strawson, 1962—for discussion see Mounk, 2017, pp. 161–164 and essays in McKenna and Russell, 2008). According to Strawson holding people responsible is an integral part of seeing them as agents, as subjects rather than mere objects. As such, to deny that it is ever appropriate to hold someone responsible, as some of the more enthusiastic advocates of the social determinants of health come close to doing, is to deny that she is an agent. It is to treat what happens to her as being determined by forces over which she has no control—forces of which she is the mere plaything. Another option, is to argue that treating some people as incapable of being responsible is to deny them equal status within society (Mounk, 2017, pp. 164–168). A third option, and one that is more relevant given our purposes, takes us back to something we looked at earlier—the value of being the one to choose (Scanlon, 1986, 1998, pp. 253–256; Mounk, 2017, pp. 147–156). When thinking about our own life we at least sometimes value being treated as responsible both for what we do, and for its consequences. This is particularly the case where other people are held responsible in similar circumstances. If we are treated differently from them it conveys a message about how we are seen, one that is likely to be demeaning or belittling. To see this, suppose that a patient is being treated by a team of healthcare professionals. Were one of them to fail to do his part in providing the treatment (without good reason), his colleagues would hold him responsible for that and for any problems that result from it. There would be something odd if they did not. If that is right, then refusing to attribute responsibility to the patient where she is the one who does not adhere is to treat her differently from the other members of the team. They treat each other as people who can do things, remember what needs to be done, and stick to a plan. They treat her as if it is not reasonable to expect her to do any of that. There is clear message here—their colleagues are competent and responsible adults who can be relied on to do what they have agreed to do, their patient is not. To deny her agency in this way is demeaning, and a failure of respect. She is ill, but that does not mean she cannot do things for herself. As such, if healthcare professionals are to treat their patients with the respect they are due, patients must be held responsible for their failures to adhere where they could in fact do so. That may be particularly important where the patient is an older adult and/or has some cognitive or physical impairment (as is not uncommon in cases of chronic illness). Widespread discriminatory norms mean such patients are at particular risk of being treated with failures of respect of this type. Ageism, for example, can show itself in a failure to treat older patients as agents, instead relegating them to a purely passive role. In doing this the patient's agency, and responsibility, is being denied. She is being treated as someone who cannot be expected to remember to do things for herself, or cannot do them if she does remember, even though she can in fact do these things. And that constitutes a failure of respect.

Given all this, we cannot avoid the argument outlined at the start of this section by denying non-adherent patients are ever responsible for their non-adherence. If we want to challenge that argument, we must look elsewhere. That means challenging the idea that what healthcare professionals should do is affected by whether their patients are responsible for the situation they, the patients, are in. As Mounk points out, in the political realm ideas of this type stem from adopting a pre-institutional, or pre-political, approach—that is, one that starts with an account of what justice requires independently of any political or institutional arrangements (Mounk, 2017, pp. 174–183). For example, the account referred to earlier holds, roughly, that it would be unjust if someone were to lose out as a result of things outwith her control (this is the egalitarian thought), but it would not be unjust if she were to lose out as a result of her own choices (this is what ensures justice tracks responsibility). If that is right, we should as far as possible ensure that people do not lose out because of factors for which they are not responsible, but have no obligation to ensure that they do not lose out because of factors for which they are. There is, however, another way to think about what justice requires (see Mounk, 2017, p. 175). We could, following theorists like John Rawls, adopt a post-political or post-institutional approach. On Rawls' account just institutions are those that would be agreed under a fair decision procedure (behind the veil of ignorance), not ones that ensure some pre-existing pattern of just distribution is achieved (Rawls, 1971). Furthermore, the institutions that emerge from this procedure have specific aims. What justice requires, then, is that there be institutions with those aims, and that they operate in ways that achieve those ends. Thinking about justice in this way affects what we should say about the link between what people are owed and their responsibility. Rather than looking back to some pre-institutional notion of desert, we should instead focus on whether practices of giving lower priority to those responsible for their condition furthers or sets back the aims of the relevant institution (Mounk, 2017, pp. 184–206). Where it sets them back, it would be counter-productive to engage in those practices. For example, if a just political system requires that the State ensure no citizen falls below a certain level of well-being, then justice requires that as far as possible the State operates its welfare system in a way that achieves that aim. Having a policy of not helping those whose well-being falls below that level because of choices they have made will in many cases not do so. As such, those policies would be unjust.

Which of these is the right way to think about justice, even in healthcare, is a matter of considerable debate (Norman Daniels, for example, takes a post-institutional approach, whereas Sridhar Venkatapuram advocates a pre-institutional one; Daniels, 2008; Venkatapuram, 2011). The idea, common to both, that we should start with an ideal account of justice (rather than with where we are) has also been challenged (see

Sen, 2009; Gaus, 2016). While for our purposes here we do not need to enter these debates, they force us to consider our starting point—is it a world of individuals as yet lacking any institutional or political structures, or is it a world in which those individuals exist within a particular institutional and political context that shapes what they owe others. It should be clear that we are firmly in the latter. Our focus throughout has been on what healthcare professionals ought to do in the world as it is, a world containing healthcare providers (for whom they work), professional codes, and legal rules. Healthcare professionals as individuals are only able to do many of the things they do to benefit patients because this institutional structure (or something like it) is already in place. That structure, and the regulations it creates, in turn affects what healthcare professionals' obligations are (as we saw in chapters two and five). In addition, as I argued above, when treating chronic illness healthcare professionals are typically working with their patients. That itself takes us away from a pre-political or pre-institutional world.

Recognising this means we need to take account of the context in which healthcare professionals operate when thinking about their obligations towards non-adherent patients. Typically this is one in which they are employed by a service provider (either publicly or privately funded) that has particular aims, and that employs them to perform a particular role. That role, as we saw in chapter two, is to use their expertise and the resources made available to them to benefit their patients. It would be incompatible with fulfilling this role, and with meeting the aims of the institutions for which he works, for a healthcare professional to deny his patients treatment on the grounds that they are responsible for their own condition. If he were to do so, he is almost guaranteed not to have benefitted them. As such, he will not have fulfilled his obligations to either his patient or his employers. On the other hand, were he to intervene perhaps he could help his patient do what is required, and so pull things back on track. It will be objected that this misses the point. The situation we are concerned with is one in which healthcare professionals lack the time (and other resources) to benefit all their patients effectively. As such, choices need to be made. But we can now see that the relevant criterion for making these choices is not which patients are responsible for their own condition (something that may be difficult to determine in any case). It is how well different options enable the healthcare professional to fulfil his obligations to all his patients, including the obligation to benefit each of them, taking account of what he can do and the aims of the institution for which he works. Sometimes the patient's responsibility for her condition will be relevant when determining that. At other times it will not. That will depend on the details of the case, and on both the current and future impact of not intervening in different cases.

Something else is also important here. Focusing just on the patient's responsibility for non-adherence risks treating her as an isolated individual, and assumes no prior relationship between healthcare professional and patient. But, as I argued earlier, treatment for chronic illness once it has started involves healthcare professional and patient working together. Because of this (as we saw in section 6.4 above) healthcare professionals can appropriately hold patients accountable for their part of the shared activity. They can, and should, attribute responsibility for any failures stemming from patient non-adherence to the patient (assuming she is in fact able to adhere). The patient can extract herself from this shared activity by withdrawing from the treatment. Given the nature of healthcare it is at least implicit in any agreed treatment plan that she has the authority to do so. But the patient is not the only one bound by the agreement. The healthcare professional is too. He has either a directed duty to his patient to work with her to counteract the extent to which her illness limits her ability to live her life, or has implicitly promised to do so.[18] Unlike the patient the healthcare professional cannot get out of this commitment by choosing to do so. Just as with his obligation to benefit his patients, it is simply incompatible with these commitments for him to stop treating a patient simply because she has failed to do her part (or is doing it poorly). A person's agreements, including healthcare professionals' agreements with their patients, place obligations on them that they cannot get out of that easily. In this context stopping treatment for these reasons would also be counterproductive. It ensures that the shared project of which the healthcare professional is a part will not succeed.

To summarise, I have argued that when it comes to the treatment of chronic illness we should accept that non-adherent patients are sometimes responsible for their non-adherence. In such cases any health problems that stem from that non-adherence are appropriately attributed to them. To deny this would be to deny patients the respect they are owed. But I have also argued that not much follows from this when thinking about what healthcare professionals should do. To think that it does, would be to ignore the context in which treatment for chronic illness is provided. In particular, it would be to ignore both the extent to which a healthcare professional's obligations are shaped by the professional and institutional roles he fills, and the prior commitments he has made to his non-adherent patients. That does not mean that healthcare professionals must always help their non-adherent patients, even where they can. But it does mean that typically whether the patient is responsible for that non-adherence should not determine this.

6.6 Conclusion

In this chapter we have been focusing on the ways healthcare professionals support and help their patients care for themselves—something that is particularly important in the treatment of chronic illness. We have seen that in fulfilling this role ethical questions arise. To a large extent these revolve around the value of autonomy (conceptualised, as in chapter four, as the ability to shape one's life in accordance with one's own values, goals, and commitments). But they do so in a way that is not captured by a narrow focus on informed consent and patient choice (important as they are). We have also seen that there are close links, at least when it comes to the treatment of chronic illness, between enabling patients to be more autonomous and benefitting them.

I have argued that patent non-adherence can occur for a range of reasons. Sometimes it is because the patient cannot adhere (despite everything the healthcare professionals treating her have done). Identifying such cases can be difficult, depending as it does on the details of each patient's situation. Where this is the reason for non-adherence there is more healthcare professionals must do if they are to benefit their patients. In other cases the patient can adhere, but does not. This is not necessarily because she has changed her mind about having the treatment, though that can happen. Patients sometimes forget to do things, make mistakes, or get into bad habits. Other things happen that squeeze out the required action or distract them from what they need to do to manage their illness. Where patients could adhere but do not, it might be thought that healthcare professionals should not intervene for one of two reasons: 1. to do so would be to try to bring it about that the patient does what the healthcare professional thinks she should do, and that would be objectionable; or 2. non-adherence in these cases is the patient's responsibility and so nothing more is owed to her. I have argued that we should resist both these arguments because they ignore the context in which treatment occurs. Healthcare professional and patient are acting together to treat the latter's illness. As such, there are things each should do arising from that shared action (and the broader institutional structure in which healthcare is provided). This applies to the patient as much as to the healthcare professionals involved. She has to be seen as part of the treatment team, not just as the person being treated. To refuse to hold her responsible or accountable for her part would, in this context, constitute a failure of respect. But that she can and should be held responsible does not mean she should have lower priority for treatment.

If the patient is part of the treatment team, so too in many cases are members of her family or those close to her. We have not yet said anything about these people. It is to them that we now turn.

Notes

1 They should also make sure their patient knows of any risks involved in taking the medication—for example, whether it is likely to make her drowsy so that driving after taking it would be dangerous. Untangling the reasons for this will take some time. As such, I will leave discussion of it to chapter eight below.

2 It should be acknowledged that this list is not complete. Poorly controlled asthma during pregnancy, for example, can lead to low birth weight and premature birth, and high blood glucose levels in early pregnancy can increase the risk of miscarriage and birth defects. As such, during pregnancy the benefits of effective treatment may extend beyond the benefit to the woman being treated to incorporate benefits to her unborn child. These benefits, where they are part of what is being aimed at, are not well captured by the account given here. While important in practice, they do not affect the argument of this chapter.
3 There may be other ways in which being kept alive benefits a person. It may, for example, also be intrinsically beneficial. Nothing said here rules out that possibility. It is however not a possibility that plays any part in the argument of this chapter.
4 We can now see why the choice of a naturalistic, rather than a normative, account of chronic illness does not make any substantial difference given our concerns. On a normative account, such as Nordenfelt's, how healthy a person is depends on the extent to which they can realise their vital goals. Chronic illness would thus compromise their health precisely because it makes it harder to achieve those goals. As such, treatment should aim to prevent this happening, or if that is not possible to counteract the ways in which the illness makes it harder. That is, the requirement is largely the same as that we have arrived at starting from a naturalistic account.
5 This does not imply anything about the life of those who are blind. It is simply to say that given who Mary is, given the commitments she has, losing her sight would be particularly devastating for her. She may be able to develop new commitments should she lose her sight, but doing so is not easy and would inevitably involve a somewhat lengthy period of transition.
6 That does not mean they can never do this. As we saw in chapter three the effects of illness or treatment are sometimes either so large or so small that differences between people are effectively swamped. Furthermore, recognising that this is the source of the epistemic difficulty healthcare professionals face, reveals that this difficulty will be considerably less where the patient is a young child—a young child will not yet have developed the commitments that create it.
7 This assumes that the reason for non-adherence is not that new information about the effects of the treatment on the patient's well-being, such as the severity of experienced side effects, has come to light.
8 The distinction between hard and soft paternalism centres on the extent to which the choices or behaviour imposed on by the paternalist are truly voluntary: if they are, it is hard paternalism; if they are not, it is soft paternalism (Feinberg, 1971, 1986, pp. 12–16).
9 While this could be phrased in terms of a failure to respect autonomy, that language may be misleading. It is not their autonomy, but them as a person, that is not being treated with respect.
10 Given the account of chronic illness outlined in chapter one, both addiction and bipolar disorder are chronic diseases.
11 For example, on most accounts action requires an intention, so shared action would seem to require a shared intention. But the idea of a shared intention risks ontological extravagance—positing a shared mind over and above the minds of the individuals who are engaged in the shared action.
12 Throughout the rest of this chapter when I refer to an agreement I mean a voluntary agreement unless stated otherwise.
13 Having the appropriate intention, or willingness, at the time she agrees does not of course mean she will in fact do it.

14 By placing these accounts together I am passing over some important differences between them (though these do not affect what follows). One such difference concerns the nature of the obligation. On Gilbert's account this is a structural feature of the shared activity—it is a directed duty, one people owe to those they are acting with simply because they are acting with them. On Bach's account it is a moral obligation—a promise—which is not a directed duty in the same sense.

15 It should be noted that this is not required on all accounts of paternalism, for example it is not a requirement for libertarian paternalism (see Thaler and Sunstein, 2008).

16 Other cases will be less straightforward. Consider a diabetic who has a stroke after a long period during which she has not kept her blood glucose under control. In this case it is tempting to think that, because she might have had a stroke anyway, we cannot be sure that her stroke was caused by her uncontrolled diabetes (even though uncontrolled diabetes increases the risk of stroke). That, though, might well be a mistake. The relevant consideration here is not whether she might have had *a* stroke even if she had controlled her diabetes well, it is whether she might have had *this* stroke if she had controlled it well. That is, the issue is whether we can reasonably hold that her high blood glucose level played *no* causal role in the stroke she actually experienced. It is important in such cases to make a distinction between the type of event (having a stroke) and a particular token of that type (having this particular stroke). When it comes to responsibility it is tokens, not types, that matter. If I shoot Bill I cannot argue that I am not responsible for his death because if I had not shot him someone else would have (even if that is true).

17 This is a feature of some liver transplant cases and has been discussed in that context. A patient who has had a transplant may sometimes require a second transplant as a result of her continued drinking. These are cases of non-adherence which raise the issue here in particularly stark form.

18 He does not have a directed duty to provide a specific treatment where that is not working. Doing so is not a way to further the shared activity in which healthcare professional and patient are engaged.

7 Broadening Our Vision
The Role of Families and Others

7.1 Introduction

Successful treatment for chronic illness does not cure the patient, it makes it easier for him to live his life despite being ill: either by counteracting his illness' negative effects on his ability to do so, or by alleviating or preventing unpleasant symptoms. In many cases success depends on the patient doing his share of the work. But, as we have seen, sometimes he is not really able to do that. Where that is due to a lack of either knowledge or skill in using the resources he has been given, there is a fairly obvious way for healthcare professionals to respond—they can take steps to enable him to do what he needs to do. However, there are other reasons a patient may struggle to do what is needed. Living with a chronic illness can make everyday activities difficult unless a broader infrastructure is in place. Consider, for example, Robert McCrum's description of living with a stroke (for a more detailed description of his experience in the immediate aftermath of his stroke see McCrum, 1998):

> The upshot is that even the smallest journey each day has to be planned in advance. If I drive to the shops for milk or bread, shall I also go to the bank? Can I park close enough to Barclays to be able to cross the road to Sainsbury's afterwards? If I arrange to meet a friend in the West End can I drive to the rendezvous, or shall I find a 'Disabled' parking bay and take a bus or taxi for the last mile? . . . On and on it goes: every day becomes an accumulation of a thousand internal transactions in which nothing can be taken for granted.
> (McCrum, 2017, pp. 25–26)

What would make it easier for McCrum to visit the shops, or meet his friend, are things like better public transport, or more parking spaces. While this is not itself an example of difficulties adhering to treatment, suppose (what is not in fact the case) that in addition to having had a stroke McCrum was diabetic (it is worth recalling that diabetics are at increased risk of having a stroke). Further suppose that these shops are the nearest ones that stock the kinds of food he needs to manage his blood glucose levels effectively. In that case his stroke in conjunction with the transport system would make it hard for him to adhere. Furthermore, with only a few alterations McCrum's account might easily be a description of the effects of poverty. As such, a poor diabetic may also have problems adhering for the same reason.

More generally, a whole host of things can affect how much a patient's illness negatively affects his ability to live his life, including: the architecture of his living space and of other spaces he may visit (including the realistic potential for these spaces to be adapted to meet his needs), the availability of social care or assisted living arrangements (and the money to take advantage of those), the safety and layout of public areas (including availability of seats or public toilets), and the financial resources available to the patient (to adapt his home or buy in support services) (World Health Organization, 2015). The exact mix will, of course, vary from person to person, and from place to place. The social, cultural, financial, and built environment not only affects a patient's ability to manage his illness, it is also changing and will continue to change. This all matters when it comes to developing policies to tackle chronic illness. However, where our concern, as here, is not with policy but the obligations of healthcare professionals we can largely put much of this to one side. Healthcare professionals need to be aware of how these things affect what patients can do. But there is little that individual healthcare professionals, in their role as healthcare professionals, can do about transport systems, poverty, architecture, or planning.

The same is not true when it comes to another factor that can affect the success of treatment for chronic illness. This is the role of other people, whether non-professionals (spouses, partners, children, parents, friends, shopkeepers, volunteers) or professionals working for other services (social workers, care assistants). The importance of that role is perhaps most obvious in cases where the patient is unable to manage his illness himself (as will be the case with some older patients and with patients who are young children). But, as we have already seen, the involvement of other people is not restricted to such cases. This creates three ethical challenges for the healthcare professionals involved. First, where the success of a particular treatment depends on other people, their ability and willingness to do what is needed has to be assessed. To do that they must be told something about the patient's illness—his diagnosis, what treatment might involve, and what they might need to do. At first sight telling them this looks wrong, at least if done without consent, because much of this information is either confidential or private. Whether this is always the case is doubtful—for example, a young child cannot consent to information being passed to his parents but that does not mean it would always be wrong to do so. More importantly, it is not unusual for private or confidential information to be shared among healthcare professionals treating a patient where this is necessary for the treatment's success—even if no explicit consent has been given. If this practice is not wrong, and I will argue that it is not, why would it be wrong to share patient information with all those who are heavily involved in a patient's treatment (including those who are not healthcare professionals)?

Second, where these other people are willing to help, and have agreed to do so, they are effectively a part of the treatment team (and in many cases an essential part of that team). As with other members of the team, including the patient, these people may not do what they said they would. Again, as with others, this failure may be either intentional or non-intentional. In such cases something needs to be done, though what that is may be unclear. However, that is not all. These people may also act in ways that thwart or set back the effectiveness of treatment. In some cases they do so intentionally (as in cases of abuse). Where a healthcare professional suspects this is happening she has an obligation to do something, she cannot simply ignore evidence of harm. What she should do will vary depending on the details of the case. Reporting her suspicions, for example, means telling others about the patient's illness, and so may breach confidentiality or privacy—something that may or may not be justified. But as we will see below, getting in the way of successful treatment can also be non-intentional. That may be hard to pick up, but where it is, what, if anything, should healthcare professionals do about it?

Third, the ability and willingness of other people to help changes over time. This can affect how well treatment works. For example, suppose that a patient with Parkinson's disease has been helped with the activities of daily living by his wife, but she has now become ill and so cannot do everything he needs. Or, he has been supported by his daughter but she now needs to work additional hours to provide for her children, to advance her career, or to cover her mortgage. She thus does not have time to do everything she was doing, or that in an ideal world she would want to do. This is an example of a bigger issue—that the world in which the patient's chronic illness is being treated is not static, but shifts in a variety of ways over time. If healthcare professionals are to provide the best treatment for their patients they need to both be aware of, and respond to, this changing world.

In this chapter we will address the first and second of these three issues—leaving the challenges of responding to a changing world to chapter eight. The focus will thus be on the role of other people. Because we have just been looking at non-adherence I will start, in section 7.2, with problems that arise when someone other than the patient does not do what they said they would. The important topic of what is required to avoid violating confidentiality or privacy will be dealt with in section 7.3. While this topic has been mentioned in passing in chapters two and five, much more needs to be said if we are to have a full account of healthcare professionals' obligations in this area when it comes to patients with chronic illness.

7.2 Other People as Helpers or Obstacles

Typically to successfully counteract the effects of chronic illness on a person's effective freedom to live his life several people need to act, including in most cases the patient and one or more healthcare professionals. Those actions do not take place in a vacuum. Sometimes for them to be effective other people also need to act, or to refrain from acting, in certain ways. The involvement of these other people should not be thought of as an optional extra. Nor should it be thought of as an independent factor, one that can be treated in isolation from the actions of the patient and the healthcare professionals treating him. Some of these people can reasonably be thought of as part of the treatment team. They are people together with whom the doctor and her patient are working to manage the latter's illness and restrict the extent to which it negatively effects his life. Where the patient is very young, for example, it is natural to think of his parents as working with the healthcare professionals treating him to benefit their child. In other cases the involvement of others is not as direct as this—the local shopkeepers may have a significant effect on a diabetic patient's ability to manage his diabetes but it would be odd to characterise them as working with the patient and those treating him on a shared project. Either way, the potential impact of these other people on a patient's health, means their role must be considered. Where they are uncooperative or where they act in ways that thwart a patient's treatment plan, they render treatment less effective than it could be. That is not something that healthcare professionals can ignore if they are to fulfil their obligation to do what (of the things they can do given their expertise and the available resources) is prospectively best for their patient. What healthcare professionals' obligations are in this situation is the focus of this section.

Before getting to that, however, there are two preliminary points I want to make in order to put them to one side. First, I will not be concerned with what these other people—the patient's family, friends, neighbours, etc.—ought to do. Their actions have the potential to benefit or harm the patient. As such, it is easy to slip into making moral judgments about them, or their actions. However, doing so would distract us from our main concern, which is with the moral obligations of healthcare professionals. Even if a family member has a moral obligation to help those in his family, healthcare professionals have no authority to force him to do what he is morally obligated to do. If the patient's son is not willing to help his father, for example, the healthcare professionals involved may deplore this and judge the son harshly, but there is not really anything they can do about it. There is a parallel here to the debate about consent and respecting patient autonomy. When our concern is with what healthcare professionals should do to respect their patient's autonomy, our focus is on them not on whether the patient is acting as autonomously as he could. It is not about how he should act, but about how they should act if they are to treat him in the way called for by the fact that he is autonomous. It can, however, be easy to lose sight of this unless we link everything back specifically to the question of what healthcare professionals should do.

Second, in this section I will be concerned with what healthcare professionals should do when they become aware that the actions, or omissions, of others are negatively affecting the success of their patient's treatment. In practice they may lack this awareness. Furthermore, while other people will sometimes tell them what is going on, these sources are not always reliable—they make mistakes and have their own agendas. Because of this, healthcare professionals face a tricky epistemic problem when trying to work out what is happening and why (one that can get missed if we stick to clear-cut cases). When trying to solve that epistemic problem they can, at least in some cases, directly ask either the patient or those involved in his care for information. But, perhaps for very good reasons, these people may not be entirely forthcoming, or may lack the necessary knowledge themselves. When it comes to asking people other than the patient two other concerns are likely to arise: one concerning privacy (to be dealt with in the next section) and the other concerning transparency and respecting the patient's wishes (to be dealt with later in this section). The challenge of working out what is going on and why is particularly acute when trying to determine why treatment is no longer as effective as it once was. Because this is part of a broader challenge connected to treating patients in a changing world, we will return to it in chapter eight.

With these preliminaries out of the way we are now in a position to focus on what healthcare professionals' obligations are where a patient's treatment is being negatively affected by other people. Suppose that a patient's family have at least tacitly agreed that they will help manage his illness. For example, suppose that the wife of a patient with Parkinson's disease is actively involved in helping him manage the activities of daily living as his condition worsens, or a young diabetic's parents have committed to giving him his insulin every day and managing his diet as required. Suppose further that in both these cases the non-professionals involved, the patient's wife and parents respectively, are not doing what they have agreed to do. As a result the patient's illness is not being as effectively managed as it could be. What should the healthcare professionals treating these patients do when they become aware of this?

To answer this question we need to start by drawing a distinction (paralleling one drawn in the last chapter) between cases where the person concerned cannot in practice do what is required, and those where they could. The former is the easiest to deal with. Just as a patient may not be able to convert his resources into improved health, those who are helping him may not be able to do so either. In most of the cases we have looked at the patient's inability to adhere is not a consequence of his illness (though, of course, sometimes it is). It is due to a lack of know-how, or a lack of resources, or an unsupportive environment. These can be just as much a problem for other people as they are for the patient himself. Where the success of the patient's treatment depends on other people, and those people, while willing, are not effectively able to do what is required, the position is ethically the same as that where the patient cannot in practice adhere. In some cases there will be little that healthcare professionals can do to alleviate this problem. If the patient's daughter has to work longer shifts and so no longer has time to do what is needed, or has lost her driving licence and so can no longer take her father to the shops, healthcare professionals cannot do anything about that—they cannot alter the daughter's shifts or restore her driving licence. But in other cases there will be things that the healthcare professionals involved can do. In such cases they would seem to have an obligation to do them. Not doing so would constitute a failure to do what, given available resources, is prospectively best for the patient. For example, there is little point providing a patient with the equipment his family needs to manage his illness effectively, if they do not have the skill required to operate that equipment. If the young diabetic patient's parents in our earlier example do not know how to give the needed injections, they may well make mistakes. As such, they need to be shown what to do, not merely provided with the means to do it. Just as enabling those working with the patient to manage his illness can involve providing them with necessary skills, it can also involve providing them with information. That can be information about the patient's illness, and about how to respond to problems that might occur given that illness. But it can also include information about where and how to access support services—whether these are provided by the health service, by voluntary organisations, or by patient support groups. What is available and how to get it is not always clear, particularly in the early stages of dealing with a serious chronic illness affecting a family member. To the extent that there is an obligation to provide this information it cannot be captured by the idea that healthcare professionals should provide information to patients as a way to respect their autonomy—the information we are concerned with here is going to someone other than the patient.

When thinking about what someone can effectively do it is easy, and tempting, to focus on the individual acts involved—for example, can they give an injection, or can they help the patient get dressed. However, it is also important to take account of the cumulative effects of doing these acts day after day over a period of several months or years. While each step may be within the ability of the care-giver, the ongoing requirements may nevertheless take it out of them (for a detailed description see Gawande, 2014, pp. 82–87)—particularly if, as is often the case, they are also caring for other people (such as, their children, their spouse, or their parents) (Brannan, Moss, and Mooney, 2004). Given their resources (material and emotional) they may come to a point where doing any more becomes a real struggle. Alternatively they may end up not doing everything that is needed because the cumulative effects are too much for them. To the extent that the care giver's involvement is an essential part of a patient's treatment, without which it would not be as effective, in this situation healthcare professionals have an obligation to do what they can to enable the care-giver to continue. The reason for this is the same as the reason for providing equipment or resources that will benefit the patient. It is part of what the healthcare professional needs to do in order to fulfil her obligations to her patient. What that calls for in practice will both vary from case to case, and depend on what resources if any, are available (which they might not be). It might, for example, involve providing temporary cover to give the care-giver a break (perhaps on a regular basis). To the extent that resources are available for this the healthcare professional should help (to the extent she can) those working with her and her patient to access them. It is not for her to make cost/benefit calculations in this, any more than in any other, case. Of course, those resources may not be available. Difficult decisions about what should be funded and why need to be taken when we move to a policy level. Addressing that topic would take us too far from our aim—the obligations of healthcare professionals as individuals in the world in which they work. However, it is worth pointing out that if the assessment here is correct, support to care-givers is in some cases as much a part of effective treatment as providing medication or equipment.

These cases of long term support create problems when drawing a line between what a person can and cannot do. It has been useful to deal with them as examples of the latter because they are cases where care-givers need additional support to help the patient. But such cases could also be thought of as ones where the care-giver does not do what is required despite (in some sense) being able to do so. There is a continuum of cases here from ones that are clearly in one category to ones that are clearly in the other, with a significant grey area between them. That makes it harder in practice for healthcare professionals to work out what they should do. Nevertheless drawing this distinction is conceptually important because it affects what healthcare professionals' obligations are. Where the people involved are not doing what is needed despite being able to do so, there cannot be an obligation to enable them to act (they can already do that). It is now time to look at what healthcare professionals should do in such cases.

As we saw when looking at patient non-adherence, failure to do what was agreed can be either intentional or non-intentional. From the outside distinguishing between these can be hard. There is an additional complication where someone other than the patient intentionally stops doing what they were doing—sometimes this happens because the patient has asked them to stop. That could happen for a variety of reasons. Suppose, for example, that the patient is a child who is now growing into an adult. At some point he is likely to want to start doing things for himself, rather than his parents doing them for him. There will, and should, come a point where his parents take that step back. In this case they have intentionally stopped doing what they were doing in order to respect the patient's wishes. This is entirely appropriate (assuming he can in fact do what is needed). Cases like this pose no particular challenge for the healthcare professionals involved, though they do affect the way treatment is being delivered. Of course, not all cases where a third party intentionally stops doing, or does not do, what would benefit the patient are of this type. Members of a patient's family or support network might choose to stop doing what they have been doing, or what they agreed to do, for a whole range of reasons. In such cases there would seem little that the healthcare professionals involved can do about it—except (as was the case where the patient intentionally does not adhere to the treatment plan) try to work out a way round the problem that would keep everyone on board.

It would be a mistake, however, to think that every failure by third parties to help the patient, or to do what was agreed, is intentional. There can be a tendency when we look at things from the outside to over-intellectualise them, and to treat what people do (or do not do) as being the result of their conscious choices. Even if we think this is what people should do, reflection on our own lives will reveal that it is not that common (Goldman, 2009, pp. 1–5; Kay, 2010, pp. 89–97). Expecting it of others may be appropriate when our focus is on healthcare professionals. This is their job and they have an obligation to think about it carefully. But the people we are concerned with here (family members, friends, neighbours) are in a different position. They have their own lives to lead. While helping the patient is part, and in some cases a very important part, of that, it is not the whole of their life. They have other commitments (to the rest of their family, to their employer, to their friends, and to themselves) and face other pressures (financial, emotional, and social). These can crowd out what they had said they were going to do. Their lives may be well organised or somewhat chaotic. They may have too much to do, and not enough time or money to do it. Their children may be having trouble at school, their boss wants them to work at the weekend and they can't get a babysitter, their sister is getting married next month, and they need to get someone in to repair the faulty boiler. They may just need a break and a chance to relax at times. Given all that, it would not be surprising if they sometimes forget to do what is needed to help their relative or friend who has a chronic illness, or if they sometimes rush things and so do them poorly. In such cases the failure to help is non-intentional. The person involved is still committed to helping, it is just that other things sometimes get in the way of doing so.

It is not only that other people may forget to do what would benefit the patient, they may also inadvertently do things that make it harder for him to manage his condition. For example, they know what triggers his asthma but nevertheless act in ways that trigger it, or they know that the patient is trying (and perhaps struggling) to stick to a new diet to manage his illness but take home the wrong kinds of food because they need a pick-me-up themselves. In these cases it is not that the people involved do not know that their actions can make it harder for the patient, nor that they are indifferent to that. Rather it is that this slips their mind when deciding what to do (as we saw in chapter one, it does not follow from the fact that someone knows something that that knowledge is readily available and incorporated in their decision making at all times). In other cases, while the people involved are trying to help, and may to some extent actually be helping, in the long run their actions make things worse. An example will help to make this clearer.[1] Suppose that to counteract the effects of his chronic illness a patient should keep active. But doing so is difficult. His children, let us suppose, do not like to see their father struggle so either do his shopping for him or take him in the car instead of letting him walk to the shops himself. In the short term this is helpful, it usefully counteracts the effects of the patient's illness on his ability to live his life. But, in the long term (and if this develops into a long term pattern, as it may well do) it is not. The patient needs to keep active, and his children's actions means that he is not doing things he was doing before. As such his strength deteriorates and it becomes harder for him to do things, and so his children provide more help. In this example the patient's children are usefully counteracting the effects of their father's illness on his ability to live his life in the short term, but are perhaps preventing him from doing the things that would help counteract its effects on his ability to live his life in the long term.

As already noted, it may in practice be very difficult for healthcare professionals to tell that any of this is happening, or that that it is happening explains why the patient's treatment is not going as well as it could. The extent to which they can do so will vary depending on the details of the case. For the moment I want to put this issue to one side, and look at what healthcare professionals' obligations are in cases of this type. Much of what we looked at in the case of non-intentional patient non-adherence (problems with paternalism, and the patient's responsibility for his own health) is not relevant here. But two things we looked at there are: the idea of joint action or working together (rather than each person being treated as an individual doing their own thing), and the need to treat those with whom one is working with respect.

In many, but not all, cases family members and other carers can appropriately be seen as working with the patient and healthcare professional in a shared activity (as described in chapter six). This is most apparent where 1. their role is significant—for example, where the patient has dementia and his spouse delivers his care—or 2. they are employed by other services to support the patient. In such cases their involvement is likely to be preceded an agreement to do so (though this may not be explicit). But other people, whose role may be more limited, can also sometimes be part of the collective 'we' who are engaged in a shared activity. Conceptualising things in this way, rather than seeing those involved as individuals each pursuing their own projects (projects that just happen to coincide), affects how we think about what is ethically required. To begin with it usefully highlights that many of those involved (such as, healthcare professionals, patient, family members, or social service professionals) have a shared aim or intention—counteracting the negative effects of the patient's illness on his ability to live his life.[2] Though it must be acknowledged that this is not an aim or intention shared by everyone. It would be unusual, for example, for it to be an aim shared by either the local shopkeepers whose decisions affect a diabetic's ability to manage her illness (to return to an earlier example), or those actively harming the patient. Such people are not among those with whom healthcare professionals and patient are acting. That will affect how it is appropriate to respond to what they are doing.

Recognising that those who are not, or are no longer, doing what was expected of them have this shared aim or intention matters. Their omissions should not be seen merely as a failure to benefit the patient, but as a failure to fulfil their own intentions and achieve their own ends. They are not, at least in the cases we are concerned with here, indifferent to the patient, or his wellbeing. They want to help him and have formed an intention to do so. As such, there is no need to impose on them, or to persuade them to do something they may not want to do. Instead what is needed is to bring the activity or project of which they are a part back on track. Doing this effectively requires an understanding of what the difficulty is, but also a willingness to adjust the plan to take account of their needs—where this adjustment could require changes in what either the healthcare professional or the patient does. We should not think of treatment as something done by healthcare professionals and/or patients that other people must just fit in with. To the extent that those people are essential to the treatment's success they are also part of the treatment team and adjustments may need to be made both to enable them to remain part of that team, and to perform their role within it well. Working out how to do that is likely to require the active engagement of all involved, and open lines of communication between them. It also requires that everyone be treated with respect, both as a person and as someone with whom healthcare professional and patient are acting to achieve something of value. Here we are not concerned with respect for autonomy, as that is usually conceptualised in healthcare ethics, but with the form of respect I highlighted at the end of chapter four—ensuring that those involved are not belittled, demeaned, or treated as incompetent. Something that, in turn, requires sensitivity to the details of their position and the pressures on them.

Another feature of shared activities is also relevant here. As we saw in chapter six, it is appropriate for those acting together to hold one another accountable for any failures that set back their shared activity. It might be thought that this is not really the healthcare professional's job, it is the patient's. He is both better placed to do it, and the one most seriously affected. Often that will be right. But it cannot be the whole story. It is not always reasonable to expect the patient to play this role. One case where it would not be reasonable is where the patient is incompetent. But even where he is competent, relationship dynamics (including within the family) may make it inappropriate to expect him to take the lead. Think, for example, of a case where an older patient is dependent on his son or daughter for help. They are failing to provide that help regularly or effectively (perhaps for very good reasons). In this situation it may not always be realistic to expect the patient to hold his child to account. Finally, we may doubt that the patient should always take the lead where the person not doing what is required is someone outside the family (for example, someone working, in either a professional or volunteer role, for a support service).

Having said that, in most cases it would be wrong for a healthcare professional to intervene with a patient's family and friends, or with professionals from a different service, without at least discussing it with him. Where he is competent, going behind his back in this way would be inimical with treating him with the respect he is owed. As such, even where it is not reasonable to expect the patient to act, or to take responsibility for addressing the failures of others, he should have a say in whether an intervention takes place, and if it does who performs it. When exploring the reasons for giving patients decisions about their treatment in earlier chapters two things turned out to be important: 1. the patient can have relevant expertise or knowledge that the healthcare professional lacks, and 2. where other people are given this opportunity, denying it to a patient would be to treat him as if he were incompetent or as if his views are less important than anyone else's. Both these reasons will play a role in the current case as well.

Particularly where the other people involved are family members or friends the patient will generally know more about their personalities, their relationships to each other, and how they are likely to react to any intervention than the healthcare professionals treating him. These are all things that might well affect what needs to be done to get his treatment back on track. In addition, the patient's relationships with his family and friends are likely to be among his most important commitments. As such, interventions that disrupt or undermine those relationships would be problematic given the aims of treatment for chronic illness. Even if they successfully counteract the negative effects of the patient's illness, their overall effect may be to leave the patient worse off. Assessing all this is not something healthcare professionals are likely to be able to do well unless they have the patient's input. It follows that if they are to do what is best for their patients, they need to consult with them before intervening.

That, however, is not the only thing that is important here. In many cases intervening without involving the patient will also be disrespectful. To see this, put yourself in his position. Your doctor has talked to your family about how better to help you, or has discussed with the local shopkeepers the possibility of stocking food that would be beneficial for you. But she did not let you know she was going to do this. Even if she meant well, and even if her intervention proves beneficial, you are likely to feel that she should not have acted as she did. Things would be different if she had no opportunity to consult with you, but usually she has. The doctor's failure here is a failure of respect (in the sense of recognition respect). But in saying that I do not mean that it is a failure to respect your autonomy, at least as that is usually characterised in healthcare. Her actions need not constitute a failure to respect your autonomous choices. You may never even have considered the matter, let alone made a choice about it. Neither can they realistically be thought of as a failure to respect your sovereignty. The realm over which a person is sovereign cannot extend to cover what other people do in their dealings with each other. It might, however, be thought that her intervention is a failure to respect your autonomy in the sense that it sets back, or interferes with, your ability to shape your own life—returning to Berlin (Berlin, 1969, p. 131), something has been done for you, you have not done it for yourself. By acting as she does, she diminishes your opportunity to be the agent who shapes how your life goes. At first sight that sounds right, but it does not show why your doctor has done anything wrong. It is not always wrong for other people to make decisions, and act on them, in ways that prevent you from doing so—even where those decisions affect your life. Nor is it always wrong for them to intervene to do things for you, meaning you cannot do them for yourself. Clearing a neighbour's path of snow means she cannot do it for herself, but is not wrong for that reason. It is important here that your doctor's actions are not a direct intervention in your life, they are an intervention that attempts to change what other people do in a way that helps you. While intervening in this way may sometimes be inappropriate it is hard to see it as a case of wrongfully setting back your personal autonomy. If it were, then any attempt to help someone else would be wrong on the grounds of failing to respect their autonomy unless they agreed in advance.

To explain why decisions about intervening with third parties are the patient's to make something else is needed. That something else is (as it was in chapter four) the fact that being the one to choose has symbolic value. In this context to be denied a say, or to have no opportunity to choose what happens, is to be treated in a way that is potentially demeaning. It is to be treated as someone who is not able, or cannot be trusted, to make a good choice; someone whose input is not important or does not matter. It is this that explains why there is a difference between two cases that might otherwise seem similar: those where a patient acts without consulting his doctor, and those where a doctor acts without consulting her patient. Given the context, a patient who challenges his family's failure to do what they said they would, without telling his doctor he is going to do this, does not in any way reflect on his doctor's competence or skill. He is simply doing what people regularly do in their relationships with family members—talking to them about what is happening, holding them to what they said they would do, and appealing to them for help where they can, all without consulting outsiders. In contrast, outsiders would not normally intervene on someone's behalf without consulting them in advance. As such, were a patient's doctor to do this it would send a message about how the patient is seen. It is that message that is the problem. That is, the different relationships that exist here affect what is communicated by consulting or failing to consult with others before acting.

The position just outlined is ambiguous. On the one hand, it could be interpreted as saying that it would be wrong for a healthcare professional to intervene with third parties unless she has consulted her patient beforehand. On the other, it could be interpreted as saying that it would be wrong for a healthcare professional to intervene unless her patient has chosen that she do so (that is, the choice about whether to intervene or not, and what should be done, is one the patient should make). It might be thought that in the situation we are concerned with here the latter interpretation is to be preferred. The patient's choices should be shown what I earlier called, following Uniacke, compliance respect (the healthcare professional should do what the patient has chosen). That, however, would be a mistake. While in chapter four I argued that when it comes to treatment patients' choices should sometimes be shown compliance respect, that is only the case where the choice is limited to things that would normally be made available to someone in the patient's situation. The reason for this limitation was that a more general requirement to show compliance respect for patients' choices would place positive demands on healthcare professionals that we should reject. Refusing to do what a patient wants does not always involve a failure to respect him, nor is it always to treat him in a way that is demeaning. The same kind of consideration applies here. To respect a patient and to acknowledge his standing does not require that he should be the one to choose, so that if he wants one of the healthcare professionals treating him to intervene in a certain way (perhaps a way that she thinks would be futile or harmful) she has an obligation to do so. The requirement to respect the patient is not a requirement to obey him. What this means is that in the context we are concerned with here a healthcare professional's obligation to respect her patients has two parts. First, the healthcare professional should not act without consulting her patient, and seeking his input. Second, she should show his preferences, and any choices he makes, consideration respect (she should take account of them and give them appropriate weight when deciding what to do). What the appropriate weight is will depend on the details of the situation, and may even depend on the content of the patient's preferences (a preference that the healthcare professional not do anything may be more weighty in this sense than one that she do something). In saying this I am not denying that sometimes the appropriate response is to defer to the patient. While I have characterised compliance respect and consideration respect as two different things (following Uniacke, 2013), the former should really be seen as a special case of the latter. Sometimes the appropriate weight to give to a patient's choices or preferences is to treat them as decisive. In that case consideration respect requires that those choices or preferences be shown compliance respect.

Many of these same considerations are important when we turn to the last type of case identified in the introduction—those where someone is intentionally setting back the patient's treatment. When thinking about such cases it is natural to home in on the most serious ones, such as deliberate interference with a patient's medication. In some countries there will be a legal requirement to report cases like this to the appropriate authorities, and healthcare professionals have an obligation to comply with such requirements. But not all cases will be as serious as this, and not all countries have the same laws concerning them. It would take us too far from the aims of this book to go into the details of how to address harms caused to patients by those caring for them, a topic that requires extensive investigation in its own right. There are, however, three general points we can make on the basis of the argument above. First, as already noted, healthcare professionals face a problem in determining what is happening and why. While they may be able to determine that something is not right, there could be lots of reasons for that and intentional interference by a third party is not likely to be the first thing that comes to mind. Furthermore, even where a healthcare professional suspects that this is happening, she may not have proof that it is. Second, where she has such suspicions she needs to consider whether there is anything she can effectively do about it. Perhaps she can challenge the person involved and persuade him or her to desist. Perhaps, particularly in more serious cases, the best that she can do is to speak to someone who is better placed to intervene. Perhaps if the person involved is a fellow professional there are internal process that can, and should, be followed. But there is also the potential for any of these options to backfire, leading to a worse situation for the patient. As such, particularly perhaps in the less serious cases, involving the patient in deciding what to do will be important (at least where he is a competent person). Third, when the only effective way to deal with the problem is to pass it on to others, this involves telling them about the patient's illness and treatment. Because that information is typically either confidential or private, it should not in general be passed on without the patient's consent (Bennett, 2007; Beauchamp and Childress, 2009, pp. 296–310). This is another reason for consulting with him before any action is taken. Of course, he may not consent (and in some cases will not be able to consent). In that situation those involved have a judgment to make: would it be justified to breach confidence or pass on private data given the harm being caused? In some cases it will, in others it will not. To make such judgments a proper account of the obligation not to breach confidentiality or pass on private information is needed. It is to this that we now turn.

7.3 Privacy and Confidentiality

Medical information (information about a patient's illness and its treatment) is generally either private or confidential. As such, passing it to on other people is generally, but not always, wrong. One situation where it would not be wrong is where the patient has consented. Another is where there are weightier reasons to disclose the information than reasons not to—examples might be where disclosure is needed to prevent serious harm to another person, or where disclosure would be in the public interest (for an argument that disclosure in such cases is never permissible see Kottow, 1986; Kipnis, 2006). Much of the discussion of privacy and confidentiality in healthcare concerns these exceptions (see, for example, Bennett, 2007; Beauchamp and Childress, 2009, pp. 307–310). Getting clear about them has become particularly pressing with the increased availability of genetic information, which by its nature can reveal facts about people other than the person from whom it was obtained. While much of the focus of this work concerns potential harms to third parties, it is important to remember that passing on information about a patient can also be necessary to prevent harm to the patient himself (as we saw at the end of the previous section). Furthermore, in order to benefit a patient those helping him need to know something about him and his illness—for example, that he has a certain illness, what needs to be done to manage it, the signs that things are going wrong, and what to do if they are. As such, healthcare professionals have a reason to provide this information to those involved in their patient's care (a reason stemming from their obligation to benefit their patients). Who they have a reason to provide this information to will vary from case to case, but where the patient has a chronic illness there is no reason to think it will be restricted to fellow healthcare professionals. There is thus a tension between what is needed to benefit the patient and the obligation to maintain confidentiality (Siegler, 1982). For example, where a patient refuses to allow information to be given to those who need it, complying with his refusal can mean he will not be able to get good quality care—something that needs to be explained to him (General Medical Council, 2017, p. 32). It is this tension that I want to focus on here.

To do so it is useful to start with an anomaly. While medical information is generally protected in healthcare, it is routinely passed on without the patient's explicit consent in two situations: 1. those where the recipient is a fellow healthcare professional directly involved in the patient's treatment (including supporting that treatment),[3] and 2. those where the patient is a young child and the person being given the information is their parent or guardian. None of this is thought to be morally wrong. The puzzle is to explain why it is not wrong in these cases, while holding onto the idea that it would be wrong in other cases. More specifically, the puzzle is to explain why it is morally permissible to pass medical information about a patient to family members in some cases (where he is a young child), but not others (where he is an adult); and why it is morally permissible to pass this information to some of those directly involved in his care (those employed as healthcare professionals), but not others (such as family members and other volunteers). The solution to this puzzle cannot rest on the idea that some people need information if the patient is to be effectively treated. That would draw the line in the wrong place. As we have seen, in the case of chronic illness those directly involved in caring for a patient can include both non-professionals (such as family or friends)[4] and professionals working outside the healthcare system. The role played by these non-professionals can be significant and comparable in extent and importance to the role played by parents caring for an ill child. As such, they, as much as those working within the healthcare system, may need information if the treatment is to be effective.

One response to this puzzle would be to turn to the laws (or other forms of regulation) that govern what can be done with medical information. While the legal and regulatory regime varies in detail from country to country, it often treats passing information to some people differently from passing it to others. Assessing the extent to which this is the case would take us too far from the aims of this book—it is not a book on medical law. And even if it is the case, it is not obvious that this captures everything that is morally important. For this reason it will be useful to look at the moral obligations of healthcare professionals independently of the law. In doing this we are returning to the topic of consent. In chapter five I addressed what was needed for something to be consent (to change the normative landscape such that an act that would otherwise have been wrong for some reason is no longer wrong for that reason), as well as looking at when consent is needed for treatment. But in that chapter we did not look at when consent is needed to avoid acting wrongly when passing on information about a patient's illness or medical treatment. Just as with consent for treatment, it is important to bear in mind that the normative landscape here is complex. It frequently includes, as just pointed out, legal and regulatory requirements that impose a need to obtain consent before passing on information about patients (what I called in chapter five 'regulatory consent'). This consent is needed to avoid the wrong of failing to comply with laws and regulations that healthcare professionals should comply with. It also includes a need to obtain consent to avoid acting wrongly in ways that are independent of, or pre-exist, those regulations (what I called 'non-regulatory consent'). It is the latter that will be our focus here.

In doing this the aim, as was the case in chapter five, is not to assess the adequacy of the law (or other regulations). My concern is with what healthcare professionals, as healthcare professionals, should do, not with what the regulations governing them should say. While the latter is undoubtedly connected to the former, for two reasons it is not the same. First, there may be good reasons to have laws protecting privacy or confidentiality that are not directly related to the moral obligations of individual healthcare professionals. One of the main arguments for having strict controls on what can be done with medical information, for example, is the broadly consequentialist one that such prohibitions are necessary to ensure public trust in the health service (see Beauchamp and Childress, 2009, pp. 305–306). The underlying thought here is that if medical information is routinely disclosed, people will be reluctant to be completely open with their doctors. That in turn would be bad for the health of society as a whole. This argument is not claiming that doctors passing on information about their patients without consent would wrong those patients. Instead it focuses on the consequences for society, and for the effectiveness of the health service, were it permissible for them to do so. Second, from the fact that healthcare professionals have a moral obligation not to pass on information, it does not necessarily follow that the law should enforce that obligation. To argue that it should requires an additional step—showing that it is justifiable to impose a penalty on those who do not do what, in this case, they morally ought to do.

Bearing this in mind, we can identify three main lines of argument for the conclusion that passing on information about a patient or his illness would be wrong if done without his consent. First, doing so would be a failure to respect the patient's autonomy. Second, doing so might have bad consequences for the patient. Third, doing so would involve breaching a duty of confidentiality. These arguments are not in conflict with each other, though they may cover different cases (for example, not every disclosure that breaches a duty of confidentiality will be bad for the patient). Setting things out in this way may seem problematic because confidentiality itself might be thought to be required in order to respect autonomy or to avoid harm (see Bennett, 2007). It would not then be a requirement that is independent of the other two reasons.[5] Before continuing therefore it is worth saying a bit more about what I mean by the duty of confidentiality. As I am conceptualising it the duty of confidentiality does not place any limitations on how healthcare professionals may obtain information, something that is required to respect patients' privacy. Instead it is a duty not to disclose information where that information was obtained on the understanding, accepted by the recipient of the information, that it would not be passed on without consent (Beauchamp and Childress, 2009, p. 304). In this situation the recipient is bound by her prior commitment to the patient. Were she to disclose that information to anyone else she would be breaking her word, and that is something she should not do. It is important to see that the wrong here is not a failure to respect the patient's autonomy—a failure, that is, to treat him (or his choices) in the way that is called for by the fact that he is autonomous. The source of the obligation lies not in the patient's autonomy, but in the healthcare professional's voluntary agreement. Having agreed, she ought not to disclose the information simply because she has at least implicitly said that she will not do so. The agreement here does not need to be explicit because it is built into the relationship between healthcare professional and patient that information provided by the latter is given on the understanding that it will not be passed on (unless stated otherwise). The reason it is built into the relationship in this way is, at least in part, something we have already seen. In order to benefit a patient those treating him need him to be forthcoming about all aspects of his condition. Patients may be reluctant to do that if they do not trust healthcare professionals to keep the information to themselves. By undertaking not to pass it on, those seeking to help the patient can overcome this reluctance (Brazier and Cave, 2007, p. 69). The reason for taking on the duty of confidentiality is thus to benefit the patient, but the obligation not to pass it on is not directly connected to protecting the patient's welfare. It would be at least *pro tanto* wrong to pass on any information obtained in this way even if doing so would benefit the patient.

In assessing these three lines of argument I want to start with the idea that it would be wrong to disclose information about a patient because this would constitute a failure to respect his autonomy. Despite its initial plausibility, as an explanation it faces considerable problems. To begin with, an autonomy-based account of why disclosing patient's medical information without consent is wrong cannot explain why disclosure is permissible in the cases where this is standard practice. It will not allow us to draw the lines in the right place. If it would be wrong on the grounds of failing to respect a patient's autonomy to disclose information about him without his consent, it would be wrong to disclose that information to other healthcare professionals without his consent—even if they are involved in caring for him. As such, there would be no moral difference between disclosing information about a competent patient to fellow healthcare professionals and disclosing it to those members of his family involved in his care. In both cases doing so would be a failure to respect the patient's autonomy, and in both cases disclosure would benefit the patient by enabling more effective treatment.

One possible response here is to argue that the patient has in fact consented—albeit implicitly, rather than explicitly—to the sharing of information between healthcare professionals directly involved in his care (see General Medical Council, 2017, pp. 22–23). But he has not consented, even implicitly, to that information being shared with anyone else. In that case it would not be wrong on the grounds of failing to respect her patient's autonomy for a healthcare professional to disclose information to other relevant healthcare professionals, but it would be wrong to disclose that information to other people. This response rests on an assumption about what the patient is doing. As we saw in chapter five for an act to constitute consent, to make permissible what would otherwise have been wrong, it must meet certain conditions. One of these is that the person consenting must have acted with the right intention. As such, it will only be permissible for a healthcare professional to share patient information with her colleagues if that patient has acted with the intention of making it permissible for her to do so. That in turn means that for the response we are considering here to succeed every competent patient (in every encounter with a healthcare professional) must have the same intention—to make it permissible for that healthcare professional to share information about him with, and only with, other healthcare professionals involved in his care. On the face of it that does not look particularly plausible. But we need to remember the context in which patients are engaging with these healthcare professionals. I said above that that context is one in which the healthcare professional accepts information on the understanding that she will not disclose it. But what if the context is one in which the mutual understanding between healthcare professional and patient is more fine grained than that? Suppose, for example, that the context is one in which patients provide information on the understanding that this information will be shared with other healthcare professionals where that is necessary for the success of their treatment. In that situation, when a healthcare professional accepts information she does so on the understanding that she will not disclose it to anyone other than those healthcare professionals. As such, it would be reasonable for her to take it that her patient has given her permission to share information about him with those of her colleagues directly involved in his care. If he does not want her to do this he would need to make this explicit (see General Medical Council, 2017, pp. 23–24). On the other hand it would not be reasonable for her to think that she has permission to share that information with anyone else. If he wants her to do that, he would need to explicitly give permission for her to do so.

The idea that the patient has given implicit consent to limited sharing of his information thus rests on the plausibility of this account of the context in which patients and healthcare professionals engage with each other. However, as an account it faces two problems. First, it will at best only cover some medical information. Consider information contained in an adult patient's medical record, but obtained when he was a young child—either from his parents or from samples taken at that time. Or consider information provided by other people, or obtained from tests on samples taken, when the patient was temporarily unconscious. In these cases the patient did not voluntarily supply this information to the healthcare professionals treating him, and hence did not voluntarily supply it on the understanding that it would be shared with others involved in his care. As such, there is no reason to think that he has implicitly consented to it being shared with them. He is, however, autonomous. If disclosing medical information is wrong on the grounds of failing to respect autonomy, it would thus be wrong to share this information with anyone (including healthcare professionals involved in his care). This conclusion cannot be avoided by arguing that he was not autonomous at the time the information was provided, and hence disclosure does not fail to respect his autonomy. Were that the case, there would be nothing wrong with disclosing this information to anyone—which at least intuitively there is.

Second, it is not at all clear that every patient has the understanding imputed to them on this account. Ascertaining whether they do is an empirical question, the answer to which is likely to vary from case to case. There is, however, reason to think that in at least some cases patients are unaware of just how widely their information will be shared. In a widely cited paper Mark Siegler estimated that between 25 and 100 people had access to, and a legitimate reason to view, the medical record of a patient with mild obstructive pulmonary disease (Siegler, 1982). This was a surprise both to him and to the patient concerned. While this number included 15 medical students, the rest were all either directly involved, or supporting those directly involved, in the patient's treatment. Siegler points out that the patient's treatment was relatively straightforward, and that in more complex cases further staff would have had legitimate reason to view the patient's record. On the basis of this he argues that medical confidentiality is a 'decrepit concept'. We will return to confidentiality below, but here I want to make a different point. If the patient does not know that information about him will be shared with all these people, can we reasonably claim that he acted with the intention of making it permissible to share that information with them? If we cannot, then we will need to conclude that this patient has not implicitly consented to his information being shared in this way. As such, it would appear that his doctor (in this case Siegler) has acted wrongly by failing to respect his, the patient's, autonomy. There is, however, nothing particularly special about this example. Given the complexity of much medical treatment it would not be surprising if other patients are also unaware of who might have access to their medical record—even if we restrict this to those who are directly involved in the patient's treatment.

At this point it is useful to return to the account of consent developed in chapter five. When we do so we can see that, in principle Siegler's patient, or those like him, could have consented to the wide sharing of his medical record. Because that account allows for broad consent, a patient does not need to know exactly who will have access to his data for him to consent to them having access to it. If, for example, he voluntarily acts with the intention of making it permissible for his nurse to share his medical data with any healthcare professional (or other health service employee) directly involved in his treatment, it will be permissible for her to share it with anyone who fits that description. The problem is that we have no good reason to think that every patient does act with that intention. If they do not, they will not have consented to their medical information being shared with all those directly involved in their treatment. Relying on implicit broad consent thus looks problematic.[6] It would be better not to do so if it can be avoided.

There is, however, a more fundamental problem with the idea that disclosing a patient's medical information without consent is wrong because it is a failure to respect his autonomy. To see why, we need to get clearer about what 'autonomy' means here. The basic idea is that the patient and the patient alone can make disclosure permissible (that is what it means to say that disclosure would always be wrong without his consent). As such, the relevant account of autonomy would seem to be one that characterises it in terms of sovereignty—information about a patient's health (including his diagnosis and any treatment he is on) falls within the realm over which he is sovereign (see Feinberg, 1986, pp. 52–57). The problem is in explaining why we should accept this claim. Doing so is much harder in the case of information than in the parallel case of a person's sovereignty over their body (which was discussed in chapter five). With the latter we could start with an account of internal sovereignty, something that according to Feinberg must be absolute (Feinberg, 1986). An individual is sovereign in this sense if he can do whatever he wants to his body (including inserting things into it, or modifying it). He must also have the authority to determine what it is permissible for anyone else to do his body (what I called, using the analogy with states, external sovereignty). If he did not, his internal sovereignty would not be absolute. That is, the reason for thinking that it would be wrong to do something to a competent adult's body without his consent is that he is sovereign (in the sense of internal sovereignty) over his body—though as we saw in chapter five this is not the only possible account.

No parallel of this argument is available when it comes to information about a person's health or medical treatment. The idea of internal sovereignty over this information makes little sense, and as such the metaphor with states breaks down at this point. A person can of course do what they want with information about their own health, or the treatment they are on. But that is not because it falls within a realm over which they, and they alone, are sovereign. It is because they have it—just as they might have information about things that are not private such as how to bake a cake, and the quickest route from their house to the station. Furthermore, limiting what other people can permissibly do with information about a patient's health is not needed to protect the patient's ability to do what they want with that information. While it would be needed to protect their ability to control what other people do with it, that is to move away from considerations of internal sovereignty to considerations of external sovereignty (what they have the authority to make it permissible for other people to do). As such, saying that a person's medical information falls into the realm over which he is sovereign turns out to be another way of saying that it should be up to him what other people can permissibly do with that information. It does not explain why it would be wrong to pass information on without consent; it is merely another way of saying that doing so would be wrong.

What this means is that we still have no explanation of why it would be wrong to disclose a patient's medical information without his consent. That does not, of course, undermine the idea that it would be wrong. But it does suggest that something other than the need to respect autonomy (in the sense of sovereignty) is doing the work. The only way to avoid that suggestion is to change our account of sovereignty. Drawing on the analogy with states (see Philpott, 2010), the realm over which an individual is sovereign could be conceptualised, not in terms of qualities he possesses, but in terms of what others recognise him as sovereign over. As such, if other people (or the state) treat a person's medical information as falling within the realm over which he is sovereign, it falls within the realm over which he is sovereign. By passing laws that protect medical information the state could in this way give people *de facto* sovereignty over what is done with that information. There may, as we saw earlier, be good reasons to do so—treating people as sovereign in this way protects a social good (trust in the health service). However, such an approach is unlikely to be satisfactory. In part this is because we have here moved from considerations of non-regulatory consent, to an account solely in terms of regulatory consent. In part it is because we have also moved from an account that says a person is sovereign (and so autonomous) in virtue of his attributes, to an account that says he is sovereign (and so autonomous) just to the extent that the state treats him as being autonomous. For these reasons some other explanation of why it would be wrong, independently of what the law requires, to disclose medical information without consent is needed. There are different ways we might try to provide that explanation, and I will explore three in what follows. As we will see each provides part, but only part, of the story.

The first explanation starts from the fact that typically the information a healthcare professional has about a person came from that person. He may have given it to her (by telling her something private), allowed her to access it (by giving her permission to look at his records), or acted in a way that enabled her to infer it (by describing his symptoms and/or giving her samples to analyse from which she works out a diagnosis). Assume that, as will usually be the case he did these things voluntarily. What needs to be explained is why, despite this, he retains control over what may be done with that information. This might be particularly puzzling in the case where the healthcare professional has inferred it, because in that case it is not something he had before she did her work. What would make it the case that that information (uncovered by her, but about him) is something that he has control over, so that he alone can make it permissible for her to do anything with it?

The obvious answer is that a healthcare professional in this situation has a duty of confidentiality. Her patient has made the information available to her, or given her the means to work it out, on the understanding that she would only do certain things with it—in particular that she would not pass it on to others without his agreement. As we have already seen, explaining why it is wrong to disclose or share patient information in this way has nothing to do with the need to respect autonomy. It is wrong because the healthcare professional accepted the relevant information (or sample) from her patient on the basis that she would not disclose or share it (or anything she infers from it) with other people. For her to do so would thus be for her to break her word, to go back on an agreement or commitment she voluntarily entered into, and that would be wrong.

This explanation is right as far as it goes but it has two limitations, both of which we have already seen. First, the agreement here, the conditions on which the information was provided, is standardly implicit. As such, healthcare professional and patient may understand it differently. The healthcare professional, for example, may think that this implicit, unspoken, agreement allows her to pass relevant information to fellow healthcare professionals involved in the patient's treatment, but not to anyone else. The patient, on the other hand, may think it does not—either because he does not think it allows her to share information about him so widely, or because he thinks it allows her to share it more widely. At least in principle there is an easy way to resolve this problem. This is to make explicit what is currently implicit so that healthcare professional and patient have the same understanding. Doing so does not require any detailed explanation of who exactly will see the information (something that may in any case not be known at that time). All that is required is that the healthcare professional makes clear at the start of any consultation that she will share relevant information with those of her colleagues who need it in order to provide, or facilitate, effective treatment—in some cases it might also be necessary, as Siegler argues, to make clear that that could be a large number of people (see Siegler, 1982). With that understanding in place she would not be in breach of her duty of confidentiality were she to share information with them, whoever they are. It is important to see that this account, unlike that outlined earlier, does not rely on the idea that the patient has given implicit consent for his information to be shared. That is because the healthcare professional in this case would not be breaking her word, or any commitment she has made, were she to share information with other healthcare professionals involved in treating her patient. She obtained that information on the basis that it would not be shared more broadly than that, not on the basis that it would not be shared at all. As such, no consent is needed to avoid the wrong of breaking her commitment to the patient. Because of that, this account (unlike accounts relying on implied consent) does not require any assumptions about what patients intend to make permissible when sharing information with the healthcare professionals treating them. It thus avoids the difficulties that stem from relying on such assumptions.

The second problem is that the duty of confidentiality will not necessarily cover all a patient's medical information. As we saw earlier there are two reasons for this: 1. some of that information may not have come from him in the first place, but have been provided by someone else (for example, by his parents when he was a child), and 2. in some cases, while the samples from which that information was obtained came from him, they were not provided by him (for example, they were obtained at a time when he was unconscious). In these cases there is not even an implicit agreement that the patient provided the information (or sample) on the understanding that it (or information derived from it) would not be passed on without his consent. As such, something else is needed to explain why it would be wrong to disclose, or share, this information. In saying that, it is important to remember that because the duty of confidentiality does not explain everything, it does not follow that it explains nothing. The options that we will look at below supplement it, they do not replace it. As with other areas of healthcare, the normative requirements when it comes to disclosing patient information are made up of a mosaic of different (at times overlapping) obligations. They are not something that can be captured by a single principle.

An alternative way of seeking to explain why disclosing medical information without consent is wrong sticks to the idea that doing so is a failure to respect autonomy, but moves to a different account of 'autonomy'—personal autonomy as described in chapter four (see Bennett, 2007). For a person to shape his life, to bring it about that it is at least roughly in accordance with his values, aims, and commitments, requires that he manage the information others have about him (or at least is easier if he can do so). By controlling what people know about him he can affect how they see him and that in turn can affect how they treat him (whether they help him, or put obstacles in his way). Think in this context of the problems that can result if a patient's diagnosis becomes available to his insurers or potential employers. Having control over information about themselves, including information about their health and medical treatments, thus enables people to live more autonomously. It gives them more control over their own lives and what happens in them.

However, that it gives them this control does not necessarily explain why healthcare professionals would be acting wrongly if they were to share information about a patient without his consent. There are three reasons for this. First, as we saw in chapter four acting in ways that frustrate a person's plans, or that make it harder for him to shape his life in the way he chooses, is not always wrong. As such, merely pointing out that disclosing medical information can have this effect is not enough. A doctor telling a potential employer about his patient's illness might mean the patient does not get the job. But a colleague telling that employer about the patient's past involvement in a racist organisation might have the same effect, as might an honest but bad reference from a former employer. In these latter cases we would not think that anyone has acted wrongly by failing to respect the patient's autonomy (they do not look like cases where anyone has failed to treat him in the way called for by the fact that he is autonomous). Thus, if the medical case is different, it cannot simply be because it sets back the patient's ability to shape his life.

Second, people sometimes attempt to control information, including information about themselves, as a way to influence how others live their lives. To see this consider the following case.[7] A man discovers he has Huntington's disease, and refuses to allow his doctors to disclose this information to his pregnant daughter. His reason for doing so is that he thinks she may, on the basis of this information, choose to have an abortion—something he objects to. In this case the man values control over his diagnosis, not because of what people might do to him if they learn it, but because it enables him to keep his daughter in the dark. His aim is to ensure that she cannot make informed choices about her own life. In this way he seeks to restrict her personal autonomy. Saying that it would be wrong to tell his daughter his diagnosis is to say that it would be wrong to thwart him in this attempt. While doing so may well be wrong, it is hard to see how appeals to the need to respect personal autonomy could show that it is wrong. Disclosure would not set back his ability to live *his* life in accordance with his aims, values, and commitments. What it would do is set back his ability to ensure that someone else, his daughter, lives *her* life according to his values. Setting back that ability, however, does not look as if it would be wrong on the grounds of failing to respect a person's (personal) autonomy.

Third, and following on from this, passing on medical information will not always interfere with a person's ability to shape his life (even where it is done without his consent). Suppose that Joe has just had a medical check-up and received a clean bill of health. Knowing that Joe has applied for a job, his doctor reveals the results of this check-up to his potential employer. When Joe finds out what she has done, he is glad (it helped him get the job). In acting as she does Joe's doctor has broken the law and acted contrary to professional codes of conduct. But it does not look as if she has set back or frustrated Joe's ability to live his life on his own terms. On the contrary she has helped facilitate his plans. If she has acted wrongly, and she has, a failure to treat him as is called for by the fact that he is living his own life cannot be the explanation for why it was wrong. She has helped him get the job he wants. In doing so her actions are no different from those of an ex-colleague of Joe's, now working for the firm Joe is applying to, who without telling Joe provides a glowing account of his work. If this ex-colleague has not acted wrongly by failing to respect Joe's autonomy, and he has not, then neither has Joe's doctor. Of course, a doctor has different obligations than an ex-colleague, and we should expect different things of her. But that does not require us to think that she has failed to respect Joe's personal autonomy. There are other ways to explain that difference—unlike the ex-colleague she has both legal obligations and a duty of confidentiality that she has failed to live up to.

For these three reasons it does not look as if all disclosure of medical information would be wrong on the grounds of failing to respect personal autonomy, and we do not yet have any reason to think that it would ever be wrong for that reason. How then do we explain why disclosure would be wrong in those cases where it seems clear that it is wrong (such as disclosing details of a patient's illness to his employer or insurer without his consent)? In the remainder of this section I want to consider two ways of answering this question, both of which move us away from a focus on respecting personal autonomy. The first starts from something that distinguishes these cases from others we have looked at—what the recipients of the information can reasonably be expected to do with it. In the case of the employer or insurer, the concern is that they will use it to wrongfully harm or unfairly discriminate against the patient. By giving them relevant information the patient's doctor would be complicit in that wrongdoing (at least where she can reasonably be expected to foresee it). Were it not for her, it would not have happened. That gives her a reason not to provide it. It might also provide a reason to introduce regulations restricting employers' and insurers' access to certain types of information. These reasons are consequentialist ones, not ones that rely on the idea that disclosing information would fail to respect anyone's autonomy. As such, they move us to a different type of explanation for why disclosing information without consent is wrong.

Moving to that account enables us to explain why there is a moral difference between passing information to some people (such as insurers) and passing it to others (such as fellow professionals involved in the patient's treatment). What matters is what these people can reasonably be expected to do with the information. That, in turn, affects what healthcare professionals should do (because they should not do things that could harm their patients, and should do things that could benefit them). This way of dividing things up, however, does not allow us to explain why Joe's doctor has done anything wrong, nor does it allow us to make a distinction between passing information to healthcare professionals directly involved in a patient's treatment, and passing it to members of their family who are also part of the treatment team. In most cases it is not reasonably foreseeable that family members will use that information in ways that harm the patient. That is not to deny that sometimes family members do use it in that way. Nor is it to deny that this is sometimes foreseeable. Where it is, healthcare professionals should not (for the reasons just considered) disclose the relevant information to them. But that some family members will use information to harm their ill relatives, does not support a general restriction on sharing information with members of the patient's family on consequentialist grounds. We do not conclude from the fact that some parents use medical information to harm their children, that parents in general should not be given this information. And we do not conclude from the fact that some healthcare professionals use information to harm patients, that information should not be shared with fellow healthcare professionals. While abuse within families, and by carers, should be taken seriously, we should not treat every person who cares for a relative as if they were an abuser.

Given these limitations of the consequentialist account, it would be useful to see if there is an alternative that can fill in the gaps. One option is an account based on a person's permissive interests (as introduced in chapter five). In developing his account of permissive interests Owens focuses on the body (Owens, 2011, 2012, pp. 164–182). He argues that the following two things would be bad for a person: 1. if other people were *always* allowed to do what they wanted to his body, and 2. if other people were *never* allowed to do what they want to his body. The former would make it permissible for someone to give him surgery, or have sex with him, even where he does not want them to; the latter would make their performing such acts impermissible even where he does want them to. Being able to control what it is permissible for others to do to his body is the only way to avoid both these bad options. Each competent person, therefore, has an interest in having that control (one that is potentially grounded in their interests in their own well-being and/or exercising their personal autonomy). Acting without their consent would set back that interest, and for that reason would be wrong. In this way we can explain why individuals are sovereign (in the sense of external sovereignty) over their bodies without drawing on an analogy with sovereign states. Given that that analogy broke down in the case of private information, it is worth exploring whether a similar explanation can be given here.

At first sight it appears that it can. It would be bad for a competent person if other people were *always* allowed to disclose information about his health—doing so could expose him to discrimination and harm. But it would also be bad for him if other people were *never* allowed to do so. That would prevent his doctor sharing information with those who need it. The only way to avoid these two bad outcomes is for him to have control over when disclosure is permissible. As such, each competent person has an interest in having that control (what Owens' refers to as a permissive interest). Were someone, a patient's doctor say, to reveal that he has a certain illness (or something from which that could be inferred) without his consent they would be setting back this interest. That would be wrong. In this way we can see why, in our earlier example, it is wrong for Joe's doctor to reveal his test results. By doing so she sets back Joe's permissive interests. Of course, by helping him get the job he wants she also promotes his interests. To navigate this clash all that is required is for Joe's doctor to check with him before passing on the information. Given the way I described the situation he is likely to consent to her doing so. If he does not, she will need to decide what to do. That requires taking account of all the reasons on both sides. Disclosing without consent would set back Joe's permissive interests. But in most cases it will also breach a duty of confidentiality, break the law, and be a failure to comply with professional or institutional codes she should comply with. Only rarely will a healthcare professional's reasons to disclose be weightier than this combination of reasons for not doing so.

However, does this account enable us to resolve the puzzles with which we started this section? To assess that we need to keep in mind all the reasons disclosing medical information without consent might be wrong (not all of which apply in each case): 1. it would breach a duty of confidentiality, 2. it would set back the patient's permissive interests, 3. it would breach regulations healthcare professionals ought to comply with, and 4. it is reasonably foreseeable that it would enable others to harm the patient. Let us start by looking at the difference between giving information to the parents of a young child, and giving it to the carer of an adult. As we saw in chapter five, young children do not have the same permissive interests as older children and adults—they have no interest in it being them, and only them, who can make things permissible. As such, sharing information with a child's parents would not set back his permissive interests, but sharing information with a competent adult's carer would. That does not mean it is always permissible to share information about a young child. Doing so may expose the child to harm, and that is something healthcare professionals should not do. Things are a bit more complicated when it comes to sharing information with the carers of incompetent adults. Like young children, and for similar reasons, those who are incompetent may not have an interest in controlling what it is permissible for others to do. But in this case healthcare professionals may have a duty of confidentiality that means it would be at least *pro tanto* wrong to disclose relevant information without consent (consent that the incompetent person cannot give). However, that duty can only apply to information provided by the patient when he was competent (as only then will he have provided it with the relevant understanding). Because of this there is no moral reason (independent of existing laws and regulations) why information obtained later, or from other people, cannot be disclosed to those caring for the patient, except where it is foreseeable they may use it to harm him.

We now need to turn to the second puzzle, explaining why disclosing information to some of those involved in a patient's care (healthcare professionals) is different from disclosing it to others involved in his care (such as family members). As we saw earlier, this explanation cannot rely on assumptions about what patients have implicitly consented to. For information covered by the duty of confidentiality we can only explain this difference on the assumption that the conditions under which information is provided and accepted were made clear. If the recipient accepts the information on the understanding that it will not be shared with anyone except healthcare professionals involved in the patient's care, then it can be shared with those healthcare professionals (but no-one else) without consent. When it comes to information in which a patient has a permissive interest a different kind of explanation is needed—one that involves a more nuanced account of that interest. To see why, consider whether it really would be bad for a patient if healthcare professionals involved in his treatment were always allowed to share relevant information with fellow healthcare professionals involved in his care (remembering that they are all bound by regulations that prohibit them from disclosing this information to anyone else). If it would not, and it does not look as if it would, then this is a limitation to the idea that he has an interest in controlling what it is permissible to do with information about his health. That limitation is tightly constrained. It would not, for example, extend to sharing information with family members—given that it may be bad for patients if relatives were always allowed access to that information. If that is right, then it would not be wrong on the grounds of setting back a patient's permissive interests for healthcare professionals to share information among themselves (so consent is not needed to avoid that wrong). But it would be wrong on those grounds for them to disclose it to anyone else unless they have his consent.

This conclusion is perhaps unsurprising. For the most part the argument in this section supports current best practice when it comes to sharing patient information. What is different is the argument itself. First, as in other areas we have looked at, the normative landscape here turns out to be complex. There are a number of reasons it might be wrong for healthcare professionals to share information about patients with chronic illness, not all of which apply in each case. Second, with one exception, the need to respect autonomy has fallen out of the picture. While this has standardly been presented as one of the principle reasons grounding an obligation not to disclose patient information, close examination of what is meant by 'autonomy' shows that it is not. The exception occurs when a person's medical information (information about his health, any illnesses he may have, and his treatment) falls into a realm over which the state, or other people collectively, have made him sovereign. By treating him as having sole authority to determine what it is permissible to do with this information, they have effectively brought it about that he alone has that authority. But in this case their collective actions (or the laws and regulations they have made) do not treat the individual as sovereign because he is sovereign (and hence autonomous). It is the other way around—he is sovereign because he is treated as sovereign.

7.4 Conclusion

The success of medical treatment is not solely determined by healthcare professionals and their patients. It can be affected for good or ill by other people. This chapter has focused on how that fact affects what healthcare professionals should do. Its starting point, as in chapter six, was that because healthcare professionals have an obligation to benefit their patients they cannot sit idly by when treatment is not working. In working through the implications of this we have had to think in terms of interactions over time. But we have done so in a limited way, for the most part assuming an unchanging world. In practice, however, the world in which healthcare professionals and patients live is constantly changing. While that can safely be ignored when thinking about discrete medical interventions—such as performing surgery, or giving an injection—it is inappropriate to do so when thinking about chronic illness. It is to this that we turn in the next chapter.

This chapter has also looked at what healthcare professionals can permissibly do with information about a patient. This was necessary because those helping to manage a patient's illness can normally do so more effectively if they know something about that illness and its treatment. That information, however, is often either confidential or private. As such, it would be wrong to pass it on without the patient's consent. This places a barrier in the way of healthcare professionals doing what is necessary to benefit their patients. In practice that barrier only seems to preclude sharing information with some of those involved. Section 7.3 investigated why this should be. I argued there that the explanation cannot rest on the assumption that patients have implicitly consented to their information being shared with some people but not others. Instead we have to look at what it would be permissible to do even in the absence of consent. That, it turns out, depends on why disclosing medical information would be wrong. One reason it might be wrong is that it is covered by a duty of confidentiality. The patient provided that information (or the samples from which it was obtained) on the understanding that it would not be shared without his consent. It matters here what, exactly, that understanding is—is it that it will not be shared with anyone, that it will not be shared with anyone except healthcare professionals involved in the patient's treatment, or something else? Problems will arise where the patient and those treating him understand this differently. The only way to avoid this is to make explicit what is often left implicit. The duty of confidentiality, however, is not the only reason disclosing information about a patient might be wrong if done without consent. It might be wrong because it potentially harms a patient, something that healthcare professionals should not do, or because it sets back his permissive interests. Not all sharing of information would be wrong for these reasons. As such, limited sharing of patient information can be permissible even in the absence of consent. Finally, it would often be wrong to share information about a patient because doing so is forbidden by the law or by other regulations that healthcare professionals should comply with. I have had little to say about this here. The details vary from country to country, and assessing what exactly is permitted, and what is not, requires detailed analysis of the appropriate regulations—something that would take us too far from the aims of this book.

Notes

1 This example is based on one from Muir Grey available at www.bbc.co.uk/programmes/articles/5s0W25SpthkpRlpckTCB73S/three-top-tips-from-an-nhs-expert-to-help-you-stay-fit-as-you-get-older (last accessed 01/03/2018)
2 This is the case even if the patient is unable to do very much for himself, or is unable to play a leading role because of his physical or cognitive condition. All that is required is that he understand enough to have the relevant intention, and in fact has that intention. To see this think of a non-medical example: a couple and their daughter are painting a room together. If the daughter is very young her role may be limited. But it would be wrong to deny that she is one of the people with whom her parents are painting the room.
3 It is sometimes argued that the patient in these cases has given implicit consent. I will assess that claim below. It should be noted that if this is consent, patients do not need to understand much to be able to consent. That too requires some explanation.
4 As in chapter one when referring to non-professionals I mean to include those who work in healthcare but are not acting in that role—for example, a nurse looking after her husband who has Parkinson's disease.
5 In part this is a terminological issue—Bennett is using the term 'confidentiality' in a broader way than I do here.
6 It would be even more problematic if only acts performed with substantial understanding of what is proposed can constitute consent (as many accounts of informed consent insist). On those accounts if the patient does not understand who the information might be given to, he cannot have consented to it being disclosed to them.
7 This example is based on a legal case: *ABC vs St George's NHS Trust* [2015] EWHC 1394 QB.

8 Changes Over Time

8.1 Introduction

Treatment for chronic illness can continue over many months or years. A type 1 diabetic, for example, must take insulin every day for the rest of her life, and a patient with asthma might need her inhaler with her at all times. The world in which this treatment occurs is constantly changing—new medicines are developed, the weather turns cold, the patient retires, the bus she relied on to get to her appointments is cancelled, her son has to work extra hours and can no longer help her, she decides the time is right to have a child. Many of these changes will not affect how well a patient's treatment works, but some will. That creates a problem. I argued earlier that healthcare professionals ought to do what (of the things they can do given their expertise and the available resources) is prospectively best for their patients. As the world changes what that requires sometimes changes with it. The development of new medicines, for instance, changes what resources are available, and developing an additional illness (something that is not unusual among older patients with chronic illness) might affect what treatment is best for the patient (even where the available resources remain unchanged). By continuing with an existing treatment in the face of these changes a healthcare professional could end up failing to fulfil his obligations. The obvious response in these cases is for the treatment to be changed to fit the new circumstances. But it is not as simple as that. Explaining why, and the implications of this for healthcare professionals' obligations, is the aim of this chapter.

We can start by identifying three broad types of change. First, there are changes in what treatments are available: new ones are developed, or old ones are discontinued. While keeping on top of such changes can be challenging, particularly for the general practitioner, there may be a professional obligation to do so. Second, there are changes that happen to the patient or her environment (broadly construed). A healthcare professional can be fairly confident some of these will happen (though may be less sure about the timing). High pollen levels, for example, can affect what is needed to control a patient's asthma, and it is predictable that these will happen at certain times of the year. Parkinson's disease will get worse over time, though how quickly that happens will vary from patient to patient. Other changes are less predictable—including changes to the patient's working life, her support network, and the local transport system. Determining that these changes have occurred, and whether they are significant, is not always easy. Some are gradual, and it can be difficult to pick up that gradual change is occurring (particularly for those close to it). Some are things that a healthcare professional will only realise if his patient tells him (while she may know her bus has been cancelled, or her son has had to take on more work, he will not). Finally, there are changes initiated by the patient—for example, she retires, decides to have a child, or starts drinking more heavily. Some of these things will affect either her illness or its treatment. The patient will know what she is doing, but may not realise its significance. Those treating her, in contrast, may know it is significant, but not that she is going to do it. The ethical issues raised by these three types of change are different. As such, we will look at them in turn over the following three sections. In doing that, however, it is important to bear in mind both that the boundaries between types are sometimes blurred, and that not all changes fall neatly into one category.

8.2 When What Healthcare Professionals Can Do Changes

At its most simple changes in this category come in one of two forms: a treatment either becomes available or becomes unavailable. At first sight neither seems particularly morally problematic. Where what becomes available would be better for a patient than her current treatment, she should be given it (if it is not, no change should be made). Where what ceases to be available is the patient's current treatment, she should be transferred to whichever of the remaining options would be prospectively best for her (if it is not, then again no change should be made). Determining what to do here may seem to require no more than deciding which of the newly expanded or contracted range of options would be prospectively best for the patient. That is something we have already examined in some detail (in chapters two to four). Things are not, however, quite as straightforward as this might suggest.

There are two reasons for this. First, because chronic illness can last for many years the patent on a patient's medication can expire, and generic versions become available, during the course of her treatment. Switching to a generic medication would not affect the efficacy of the treatment, but it would be cheaper. As such, particularly perhaps where the treatment is being funded by the state, healthcare professionals have good reason to make that switch. Doing so will not be better for the patient, but it will make more effective use of scarce resources. The arguments in previous chapters do not support giving patients a choice in this matter. Any special expertise the patient has in determining what is best for her as a person (given her goals, values, and commitments) is irrelevant. The two options, brand name and generic version, do not differ on that. That does not mean she will not prefer one over the other. It is not unusual for people to have clear preferences between things that are effectively identical, and to erroneously attribute that preference to features of the preferred option (Nisbett and Wilson, 1977). But there is no reason for healthcare professionals to think that a patient's preferences in this situation indicate what is best for her (except where her preference is so strong it affects what she will do). Equally, denying a patient choice in this case would not treat her differently than other people, and so would not send a message that is demeaning or belittling. Recognising this reveals an ambiguity in the argument in chapter four that now needs to be removed. I argued there that healthcare professionals ought to allow their patients to choose between those locally available treatments they (the healthcare professionals) think would be beneficial. We can now see that this is only correct if medications are characterised in terms of their composition, not what their manufacturer calls them. This did not matter for that earlier argument because a new patient would generally not be given a choice between two versions of the same drug (one a brand name and the other a generic). When we are talking about changing treatment, however, this is sometimes precisely what is at stake.

Second, as we saw in chapter one treatments affect different patients in different ways. A patient's current treatment will be at least somewhat effective (if it were not, she would not be on it). A newly available treatment may be better for her, but it may also be worse. New treatments typically come with negative side effects for at least some people. Were she to experience those side effects the new treatment may leave her worse off than her current treatment. That raises a question: in these circumstances would it be morally permissible for a healthcare professional to change his patient onto the new treatment? While that question has not been addressed in the literature on clinical ethics, it is very similar to one that has received considerable attention in the literature on research ethics (see, for example, Ashcroft, 1999; Foster, 2001; Freedman, 1987; Gifford, 2000; London, 2001; Miller and Weijer, 2003; Veatch, 2002). There the concern is with the ethics of recruiting patients, who are currently being treated, into trials of new treatments for their condition—particularly where this might mean they do not get their current treatment. Given that doctors have an obligation to do what is best for their patients, the challenge is whether this is consistent with fulfilling that obligation. While our concern is not with research ethics, at first sight this challenge seems very similar to the one we are considering here.

That might be challenged. In research there is often considerable uncertainty about whether the new drug is better than those that already exist. The aim of research is, at least in part, to reduce this uncertainty. As such, once a treatment has been approved we are in a different situation. However, while that is right as far as it goes, research is unlikely to totally eliminate uncertainty about what is best for a particular patient. It will have shown that the new treatment is safe and effective. It may also have shown that it is, in general, better for patients than what was available before (though whether it does this will depend on how the research was carried out). But it does not follow that it will be better for the individual patient who is her doctor's current concern. What would be best for most people is not necessarily best for her. As an individual she could fall anywhere on the spectrum of possibilities for the new treatment—including those where it leaves the patient worse off. For this reason there will still be some uncertainty about whether moving *this* patient to the new treatment would benefit her (uncertainty that will be increased if she belongs to a category of people not included in the research—as may be the case if she is old, a child, or pregnant). Thus the challenge faced by the researcher, determining whether acting is compatible with his obligation to do what is best for his patients, can also arise in this case.

However, while the challenge is broadly the same, the solution will need to be different. In research ethics the focus has been on randomised control trials, and it is randomisation that has been the main problem. Equipoise has thus been a key concept. A researcher (or healthcare professional) is in equipoise when he is genuinely uncertain which arm of a trial—for example, getting the new treatment or getting the existing one—would be best for his patient. In that case whatever treatment the patient gets there is no available alternative that he judges would be better for her. In the case we are concerned with here, however, equipoise is of no help. If a doctor is in equipoise between a new treatment and the existing one, he has no reason to change his patient onto the new treatment (and, as we will see below, some reason not to do so). Similar considerations apply when we turn to the main alternatives to equipoise discussed in the literature—group equipoise (see Freedman, 1987) and patient indifference (see Veatch, 2002). In both cases being in the specified state would mean there is no reason to change the patient's treatment.

While patient indifference is not the relevant issue, however, it might be thought that patient choice is. What the healthcare professional should do is give his patient the option of changing to the new treatment, and treat that choice as decisive. That cannot be argued for on the grounds that it is necessary to respect the patient's autonomy, for the reasons set out in chapter four. But there are other ways we might do so. It might be argued, for example, that this is a situation where the patient (once informed about the new option) is likely to be a better judge that the healthcare professional of what is prospectively best for her. As such, telling her about the new treatment and letting her choose is the most reliable way for him to work out what he should do. Alternatively, it might be argued that the patient is the appropriate judge of whether to move to the new treatment (even if there is no good reason to think she is the best judge). She is the one who runs any risks involved in switching, and she is the one who foregoes any benefits in not doing so. We assessed these arguments in chapters two and three, and saw there that in at least some cases they support giving the choice to the patient.

However, changing treatments is not the same as initiating treatment, and this introduces a limitation on the applicability of these arguments. Specifically, this limitation occurs where taking the new treatment requires the patient to change what she is doing. Where the patient has been following a given treatment for some time the actions required are likely to have become habits—she does not need to think about them anymore because she knows what she is doing. In this they are no different from any new skill. Switching to a new treatment may mean that these habits are no longer the right ones. But habits are hard to change (see, for example, Neal, Wood, and Wu, 2011; Neal, Wood, and Drolet, 2013). It is easy for people to fall back into doing what they are used to doing, particularly in moments of pressure or stress. That can be dangerous.

That there is this tendency (at least for a time) to revert to old habits in times of stress is well-established (Barthol and Ku, 1959; Lustig, Konkel, and Jacoby, 2004). It has been a factor in air accidents (see, for example, Weick, 1990), and is a known problem for coaches seeking to improve athletic performance (see Maschette, 1985; Crampton and Adams, 1995). The basic problem is that falling back into the old habit is cognitively easier than sticking to the new requirements, particularly in the presence of cues that trigger those habits (ones the patient needs to remember *not* to act on). Where someone is under pressure or in a stressful situation they may not remember what they need to do differently, but instead act automatically in the way they have become used to. The lives of those with chronic illness are frequently like this. In some cases stress is caused by the very features of their illness that mean they must act now (for example, the shortness of breath that requires an asthmatic patient to use her new reliever inhaler). More commonly, perhaps, people with chronic illness are (like everyone else) busy—they have looming work deadlines, difficult people to deal with, a lack of money, and not enough time to fit everything in. Like everyone else things crowd in on them, they get distracted, and have other problems on their minds. As such, we should expect them at times to relapse into old habits. A diabetic trying to stick to a new diet will not always succeed, and nor will a patient trying to switch to a new way of managing her illness. Those relapses may be temporary, but it would be surprising if they did not occur. Where they do, the patient is at least temporarily non-adherent. She is not sticking to her new treatment plan; she is adhering to the old, no longer relevant, one. Even if the new treatment is better than the old one, that may leave her worse off.

None of this may be apparent, however, to the patient faced with a decision about whether to switch to a new treatment. What she needs to do is not likely to look difficult at the time she makes that decision, particularly where this is done in the cool of her doctor's office. The circumstances in which a decision to change is made are likely to be very different from those in which it must be implemented. If, in this situation, the patient attempts to decide what to do by using simulation—imagining herself using the treatment—she is unlikely to do so well (simply because she is unlikely to take adequate account of how hard it is to implement changes in the midst of a busy life). As such, the decision about whether to switch to a new treatment is similar to those cases (discussed in chapter three) where other people have been through a change the patient has not been through. Indeed, in many cases other people will have done exactly this. As we saw in that earlier chapter this is a situation where a different method of deciding what is best for the patient—surrogation (basing the decision on what others have experienced in the patient's situation)—can be more accurate. In that case, however, healthcare professionals have no good reason to think that their patients are the best judges of their own interests.

The easy way to avoid these problems is to avoid making changes that require the patient to do something different. The safe option is the status quo. That does not mean that changing treatments should always be avoided. But it does mean the default should be against change, at least in those cases where change requires the patient to act differently. If the new medication must be taken on an empty stomach to be effective and the patient's current medication is taken after meals, that is a potential problem. If the new medication cannot be safely taken with alcohol but the existing medication can, that is also a potential problem. Making decisions about what would be best for a patient who is not currently receiving treatment is different from making decisions about what would be best for her if she is currently receiving treatment. The latter requires more things to be taken into account. The costs and risks associated with the process of changing need to be incorporated into the decision, along with an assessment of the end state of any particular change. None of this is to deny that patients can change what they do, of course they can. And sometimes that is what will be best for them. It is rather to point out that the transition period while the patient gets used to the new way of doing things comes with risks of its own. Those risks are ones healthcare professionals need to take into account if they are to do what is prospectively best for their patients.

8.3 When the Patient's World Changes

The changes we have just been looking at concern what healthcare professionals can do, in particular the treatments available to them. But these are not the only changes that matter. Like everyone else, patients live in a changing world. While most of those changes will not affect how well their treatment works, some will. If healthcare professionals are to do what is prospectively best for their patients, they must both identify when such a change has occurred and realise its significance. Failing to do so risks failing to fulfil their obligation to do what (of the things they can do) is prospectively best for those patients. Given the changed circumstances that may no longer be the current treatment. In assessing the implications of this for what healthcare professionals should do, it will be useful to split these changes into two categories: those that are reasonably foreseeable, and those that are not.

In this context changes that are reasonably foreseeable have two features: healthcare professionals can reasonably be expected to know 1. that they will occur and 2. that when they occur they are likely to require a change to the patient's treatment. Changes that result from the ways illness develops over time will generally fall into this category. It is reasonably foreseeable that a patient's Parkinson's disease will become more serious, and that what treatment is best for her will change as it does. When exactly those changes will occur cannot be known, but that they will occur can. Some changes to the patient's environment are also foreseeable in this way. Where the patient has asthma high pollen levels or a period of cold weather can require adjustments to their treatment. It is foreseeable that pollen levels will be high in the spring or early summer, and that cold weather will occur in the winter.

At first sight, changes that are foreseeable do not pose any particular moral problems. The healthcare professionals concerned know how the patient's treatment will need to be adjusted if it is to continue to be what is best for her. They also know what will trigger the need to make that adjustment. In principle this can all be agreed in advance and written into the patient's treatment plan (even if only to indicate the circumstances in which the plan needs to be reviewed). However, in practice that may not be enough. To see why, think about the asthma example. The patient and her healthcare professional agree that because high pollen levels trigger the patient's asthma a change in medication is needed when they occur. They also agree what that involves: the patient must adjust her medication. For that to be done successfully she must notice pollen levels are rising, remember that this means she has to adjust her medication, and remember what that adjustment is and how to do it. Not only that, but the last time she did this was about a year ago, and a lot is likely to have happened in that year. In these circumstances it would be unsurprising if the changes are not always made. But what if her healthcare provider were to remind her she needs to act by sending her a text message when high pollen is forecast (these kinds of automated text reminder are available in some places, though often provided by charities, such as Asthma UK, rather than by the health service). That would benefit the patient, it would help her to do what is needed to counteract the effects of her illness on her ability to live her life. Reminding patients of what they need to do in this way is also being investigated as a way to improve patient adherence (for a review of the evidence in the case of asthma, see Tran et al., 2014). In at least some cases there is evidence that it does, though the exact method used matters (see Wald, Butt, and Bestwick, 2015). Where that is the case, and it is something healthcare professionals can do, then it is something they should do—it is required by their obligation to do what (of those things they can do given their expertise and the available resources) is prospectively best for their patients. That might not be have been obvious at first sight. When we think about benefiting patients it is easy to assume that this means providing treatment. But here it requires going beyond that.

All else being equal sending reminders where doing so is both possible and would increase adherence is something healthcare professionals should do. But it is important to recognise that reminders are not always morally innocuous. They can sometimes involve a failure of respect. To see why, suppose that you are prescribed a course of medication to be taken three times a day with meals. Every meal time, day after day, you get a text from your doctor reminding you that you need to take your medication. Not only is this likely to be annoying, it conveys (perhaps unintentionally) a message about how your doctor sees you—you cannot remember, or are not sufficiently in control of your life, to do something as simple as take a pill with meals. That, as we saw in chapter four, is something healthcare professionals should not do. Even fairly young children may take it as a failure to recognise that they are able to do things for themselves. And, as we saw earlier, it may be a message to which those struggling to take, or maintain, control over their own lives (such as some older people) are particularly sensitive. Avoiding this problem is not hard. In cases of chronic illness healthcare professional and patient are working together to manage the latter's illness. That joint action is standardly initiated by an agreement. Where changes are foreseeable, what is required to deal with them can be discussed at the time this agreement is made. Doing so helps ensure that healthcare professional and patient achieve their shared goal in a way both are comfortable with (though it does not guarantee that this will happen). If the patient voluntarily agrees at that time that it would be helpful for her doctor to send her a reminder, then his doing so will not involve any failure of respect. He is doing what they have agreed should be done to help achieve their common goal.

The example we have just looked at is somewhat unusual because what needs to be done when the environment changes can be determined in advance. Even where the change itself is foreseeable, that is not always the case. While it is perhaps foreseeable that something will need to be done, what that is will vary with the details of the case (something that is not itself foreseeable). Identifying that a change has occurred should thus prompt a review of the patient's treatment. However, healthcare professionals may not be well placed to see that this is needed. Their interaction with patients is limited. The patient is likely to be in a better position to notice the change, but may not recognise its significance. For that reason those treating the patient should tell her what to look for, and what to do when she sees it (Walker, 2017). Providing this information is not a way of ensuring informed consent, and is not really about enhancing the patient's autonomy as that is usually conceptualised within healthcare ethics.[1] It is instead rooted in the idea of a shared activity. It is a way of working together to identify when adjustments need to be made if the aim of that shared activity (counteracting the effects of the patient's illness on her ability to live her life) are to be met.

The obligation here extends beyond telling patients about what changes in their environment they should look out for. Other things could also reveal that something needs to be done and healthcare professionals ought to tell their patients about these too. A couple of examples will help to make this clearer. First, as we have seen, type 1 diabetics can sometimes take too much insulin leading to hypoglycaemia (very low blood glucose levels). If not dealt with this can lead to confusion or loss of consciousness—both harmful to the patient. Healthcare professionals are not likely to be around to notice that hypoglycaemia is occurring. But they can let the patient know what the symptoms are (typically feeling weak, confused, shaky, or irritable) and what to do to combat it (eating or drinking something sugary).[2] Second, some medications cause serious side effects in some people. Where these occur it will not always be obvious to the patient that what is happening is caused by her medication, not her illness. In this situation she can only accurately identify the source of the problem if she has been told about possible side effects (Walker, 2017). While there may be nothing the patient can do to alleviate those side effects, their occurrence may indicate that the treatment she is on is not what is best for her. As such, if the healthcare professionals treating her are to continue to do what is prospectively best for their patient, they need a way of picking up what side effects she is experiencing. That in turn means they need to ensure that their patient knows what to look out for. Where the patient does experience these side effects a reconsideration of her treatment plan will be needed. At that point we are back to the topics discussed in chapters two to four above.

A healthcare professional who does not tell his diabetic patients how to spot and respond to hypoglycaemia has acted wrongly. As has a healthcare professional who does not tell his patients about serious side effects of their medication. That is not because his omissions constitute a wrongful failure to respect his patients' autonomy. Seeing this is straightforward where autonomy is conceptualised as sovereignty. As we saw in chapter five a patient's external sovereignty only gives her authority over what it is permissible for others to do to her, not what they in fact do. If we conceptualise autonomy as a capacity, things are a bit more complex. The healthcare professional here has failed to do something that would enable his patients to be more autonomous (in this sense of autonomy). As such, if respecting a person's autonomy requires enabling them to be more autonomous, he has failed to respect his patients' autonomy. Whether that is required to respect autonomy is a significant question, one that will be the main topic of the next section. I will argue there that it is not. Before we get to that argument, however, we can already see that characterising the wrong here in terms of a failure to respect autonomy would miss something important. To see why, consider the case where the patient, who is living at home with her family, has both diabetes and advanced dementia. Intuitively the healthcare professionals treating her should tell her family about the risks of hypoglycaemia, how to spot it, and what to do about it. That cannot be because doing so is needed to respect either the patient's autonomy or that of her family. It is straightforwardly about protecting the patient's wellbeing. Something similar is the case where the patient is a young child. In that case her parents need to know what to do, and when to do it, if the patient is to be protected from harm. In these cases the patient's well-being gives healthcare professionals sufficient reason to tell those best placed to notice hypoglycaemia how to spot it and what to do about it. Similar reasons will apply in cases where the patient is competent, though here she herself is likely to be best placed to notice what is happening. Healthcare professionals have obligations to benefit, and not harm, their patients irrespective of whether or not the patient is competent (though her being competent may mean they have additional obligations as well). Making sure that their patients understand what might go wrong, how to spot it is going wrong, and what to do about it if it does go wrong, is something healthcare professionals need to do if they are to fulfil those obligations.

This is not to say that competence is irrelevant for determining healthcare professionals' obligations in these cases. It is instead to say that whatever the patient's level of competence healthcare professionals are not usually well placed to notice that something is going wrong. Other people are—but only where they both know what to look for and can act on that knowledge. Typically a patient who lacks competence cannot do this, whereas a patient who is competent can (indeed most of the time she is better placed to do so than anyone else). That, however, is not always the case. Think back to the diabetic with hypoglycaemia, one symptom of which is confusion. In this case the very thing that shows action is needed potentially interferes with the ability to perform that action. For this reason it would be beneficial if those around the patient—her family, friends, and colleagues—know what to look for and what to do. However, while this gives healthcare professionals some reason to disclose this information, it is important to remember that they also have reasons not to do so—given their obligations to respect confidentiality and privacy.

So far in this section we have been concerned with changes that are, at least to some extent, foreseeable. Not all changes are. There are lots of things that affect how well patients, or those helping them, can manage the patient's illness. These include: what other illnesses the patient develops (does her arthritis make it harder to use her asthma inhaler?), the local transport system (has the bus that took the patient to the shops stopped running?), what their family are able to do (has the patient's daughter had to take on more work, has her husband's ability to help diminished given his own ill health?), or the actions of planners or shop managers (have the seats in the local park been removed, have the shops stopped stocking fresh food?). While in some cases the healthcare professionals treating a patient may be aware of these changes, in others they will not (unless the patient, or someone close to her, tells them). This creates a problem. Healthcare professionals ought to do what, of the things available to them, is prospectively best for their patients. They also have an obligation not to waste resources, particularly where these are scarce. Even if a patient's current treatment fulfilled these obligations at the time it was initiated, in a changing world that may no longer be the case. What was beneficial then is not as beneficial now. Steps that could have been taken to adjust for this have perhaps not been taken. Because of this the healthcare professionals involved are no longer fulfilling their obligation to do what is prospectively best for their patient given the resources and expertise available to them. Dealing with these changes effectively is thus morally required. They cannot simply be ignored by those involved.

However, responding effectively to unforeseeable changes is hard. Someone needs to notice both that the change has occurred, and that it is potentially significant. The patient may be well placed to do the first (indeed in most of the examples I have used there is no difficulty in her doing so), but not the second. In contrast, the healthcare professionals treating her may be better placed to recognise the significance of what is happening, but not well placed to notice that it is happening. To overcome these difficulties three things are required. First, lines of communication between healthcare professionals and patients (and their families) need to be kept open. Second, all those involved need to work to see the patient as a person, rather than simply as someone with a particular illness. That is, they need to see her as an agent not simply as a patient (something familiar from the discussion in chapter six). Third, time needs to be taken to find out about the patient's life, and what is happening in it, not just about her illness and what is happening with that.

None of this is new. To those working in healthcare, however, it may appear idealistic. In practice the time available for each patient is frequently limited. Patients do not always see the same person when attending appointments. Things that a patient tells one person may not be passed on to others involved in their care. These are features of many modern healthcare systems worldwide. The argument here suggests that they are features that get in the way of healthcare professionals doing what is best for their patients. As such, there is at least some reason to think they should be changed. Assessing whether that reason should be decisive would take us too far from our aims (particularly as the details will vary depending on which country we are concerned with). Our concern is with what healthcare professionals should do in the world in which they work, not with how that world should be organised. Given that concern, however, the features we have just been considering are relevant for a different reason—they affect the scope of healthcare professionals' obligations. At first sight the argument in this section may seem to require healthcare professionals to do things they cannot in practice do. That is not surprising. In setting out the problem I did not specify the context in which it occurs (that of frequently busy and time constrained contemporary healthcare systems). But when thinking about what healthcare professionals ought to do we need to take that context into account. Healthcare professionals cannot have an obligation to do things they cannot in fact do (from the principle that ought implies can). Furthermore, in setting out healthcare professionals' obligations in chapter two I argued that their obligation is to do what (of those things they can do given their expertise and the available resources) is prospectively best for the patient. Although this was not highlighted there, time is one such resource. It is the scarcity of this resource that the argument in this section has bumped up against. Because of this the argument above needs to be modified. Healthcare professionals do have an obligation to do the things set out in the previous paragraph, but only to the extent that that is possible given the available resources (including time). This may be less than ideal, and less than might be thought from the perspective of a theorist looking in. But we should not expect those working in non-ideal conditions to do what they would have a moral obligation to do if they were in ideal conditions. Our account of healthcare professionals' obligations must take account of the circumstances in which they work. In the case we are concerned with here that means their obligations are more limited than might have first appeared.

8.4 When the Patient Plans to Do Something Different

The final type of change I want to consider in this chapter are those made by the patient. People with chronic illness make many decisions about what to do (and what not to do), most of which are not decisions about treatment. They plan for the future and are active in bringing about both short and long term changes in their life. A patient might, for example, decide to retire, to start a family, or to go out drinking at the weekend. Some, but not all, of these changes will affect what is needed to manage her illness effectively (though she may be unaware of this). There may also be things a patient is currently doing that she would stop doing were she aware of the risks they pose to her future health. In this patients with chronic illness are no different from anyone else. There are things that anyone might start doing if unaware of the risks involved, but which they would not do if aware of those risks. Similarly, for anyone there may be things they would stop doing if they learnt about the associated risks to their health, and things they might start doing if they became aware of the health benefits of doing so. Though, of course, merely knowing about the risks or benefits might not in fact change their behaviour.

Intuitively, where a healthcare professional both knows about these risks and benefits, and has reason to believe this is relevant given his patient's situation, he should tell her about them. But what are the limits of his obligations here? To answer that question we need to look at their source. There are, broadly, two options (leaving aside for the moment any contractual obligations healthcare professionals may have). The first rests on the idea that providing relevant information enables the patient to be more autonomous, in one sense of that term.[3] Being better informed means she is better placed to ensure her actions align with her goals, her values, and her commitments. She is thus in a better position to shape her life on her own terms (even if she does not in fact do so). As such, if healthcare professionals' obligations to respect autonomy incorporate an obligation to enable patients to be more autonomous, they should give their patients any relevant information they possess. As we have seen, according to at least some accounts the obligation to respect autonomy does incorporate such a requirement (see Beauchamp, 2010b, p. 37; Levy, 2014).[4] The other option rests on the idea that giving patients relevant information is a way to either benefit them or protect them from harm. As such, healthcare professionals should provide this information. In this case, while they have an obligation to do things that enable their patients to be more autonomous, the source of this obligation is not the requirement to respect autonomy. Which option we take matters because, as we will see, the first would impose much greater obligations on healthcare professionals than the second. That first account, however, is one we should reject.

That may be both surprising and controversial. The idea that respecting autonomy requires enabling patients to be more autonomous plays a central role in two important arguments: the argument that it is wrong for healthcare professionals to withhold information from patients, and the argument that healthcare professionals have a positive obligation to provide information to patients before obtaining consent (see Beauchamp and Childress, 2009, pp. 104–105). In the first part of this section I will argue that it is not needed in these cases. As such, we have no good reason to think that the obligation to respect autonomy incorporates a requirement to enable patients to be more autonomous. We do, however, have good reason to think that it does not (or so I will argue). That means we need a different kind of account to explain healthcare professionals' obligations to tell patients about the risks and benefits of the things they are doing, or may choose to do. Providing that account is the aim of the last part of this section. In doing all this I will not be challenging the idea that healthcare professionals have an obligation to respect their patients' autonomy, only one interpretation of what that obligation requires. I will also not be challenging the idea that healthcare professionals should do things that enable their patients to be more autonomous. They should, but the reason they should is independent of the obligation to respect autonomy.

Let us start by considering why it is wrong to withhold information from patients. The case I want to consider (because it is familiar from the existing literature) is one where a patient has been diagnosed with a terminal illness. Her doctors withhold this diagnosis because they judge it would be better for her if she does not know—she would find it too distressing or would not be able to handle the information well (for discussion of this case see Harris, 1985, pp. 208–212; Beauchamp and Childress, 2009, p. 105). In doing so the doctors act wrongly. At first sight this is because they fail to respect their patient's autonomy. On some (but not all) accounts of paternalism they have acted paternalistically because, while they aim to benefit their patient, they 1. do not have her consent to act as they do, and 2. either bring it about that her opportunity to make important choices is denied (Bullock, 2015) or interfere with her autonomy (Dworkin, 2017). Were the patient in this scenario informed about her diagnosis she would be able to shape the remainder of her life in accordance with her values, commitments, and goals. As such, she would be able to live more autonomously (in the sense familiar from chapter four) in the time she has left. She would also be able to make more autonomous choices about what she wants to happen. Withholding information about her diagnosis prevents her from being able to do any of this. If this is right, and the doctors in this example have acted wrongly by failing to respect their patient's autonomy, the requirement to respect autonomy is not simply negative (restricting what can be done). It also has a positive element. To adequately respect autonomy healthcare professionals would need to provide information that enables their patients either to be more autonomous or to make more autonomous choices.

While this is perhaps the standard way of explaining why withholding a terminal diagnosis is wrong, it is not the only way to do so. An alternative would be to start by noting that withholding information is something that people do, and do for a reason. It is not the same as merely failing to provide that information—which may be an omission, rather than an action. To say that Bill withheld information from Mary, is not the same as saying he did not give that information to Mary. People might withhold information for many reasons. In the case we are concerned with here the doctors' reason is a judgment about their patient—she is not able to handle the information, or it would be too distressing for her. Where that judgment evidences a lack of respect, it would itself make withholding the diagnosis wrong. Given that patients are standardly told their diagnosis, this patient is being treated differently from other people. And the reason she is being treated differently is a negative judgment about her as a competent agent (one that is not warranted by the circumstances). Her doctors would want this information if they were in her place, but they refuse to give it to her. They do not, therefore, treat her as an equal (something they ought to do). They choose for her, where others get to choose for themselves. And we saw in chapter four that that is wrong.

This explanation of why the doctors in this example have acted wrongly does not imply that there are any positive obligations to provide information to patients. It locates the wrong in the action of withholding the information, not in a failure to provide that information. Withholding information, it argues, is sometimes wrong because it shows a lack of respect for the person from whom it is withheld. Were a healthcare professional to forget to tell his patient something important he may have acted wrongly, but we would need a different explanation to show why. Unlike the previous explanation, therefore, this account allows us to draw a moral distinction between withholding information and failing to provide it.[5] It also allows us to make moral distinctions between different cases of withholding information. A person's reasons for withholding information seem to make a difference to how we assess their actions. To see why, think back to the case (introduced in chapter seven) of a man who does not want his pregnant daughter to know he has Huntington's disease because he thinks knowing that information would cause her to have an abortion.[6] If his reason for withholding his diagnosis is that he thinks his daughter is an incompetent or poor decision maker, his doing so is a failure of respect (and wrong for that reason). But, if his sole reason is that, while he judges that she is a competent decision maker, he thinks she is misguided about whether abortion is morally permissible, it is not. In that case his reason for withholding his diagnosis is that he does not want to assist, or do something that might lead to, an act he sincerely believes is morally wrong. Some people will disagree with him about whether abortion is wrong, but that should not affect their assessment here. It is not morally wrong (though it may be misguided) to refuse to do things you sincerely believe will assist, or provoke, moral wrongdoing on the basis that they would assist or provoke moral wrongdoing. Indeed it would appear to be morally required to withhold information in such cases.[7]

Explaining why it is wrong to withhold a diagnosis of terminal illness does not require incorporating an obligation to enable autonomy into the obligation to respect autonomy. There is, as we have just seen, an alternative explanation, one that has the advantage of allowing a more fine-grained approach. That alternative explanation, however, may seem less useful because it cannot deal with other cases where respecting autonomy may seem to require enabling patients to be more autonomous. Consider the case of consent. If we take it that 1. consent is needed to respect autonomy and 2. healthcare professionals should give patients relevant information as part of obtaining consent, it is easy to conclude that respecting autonomy requires enabling patients to be more autonomous. Such a conclusion would, however, be problematic for two reasons. First, the argument here involves an equivocation on the meaning of 'autonomy'. When we say 'giving patients information enables them to be more autonomous' we are using 'autonomy' to refer to a capacity that people have (as we saw in chapter four). But when we say 'consent is needed to avoid the wrong of failing to respect autonomy' we are using 'autonomy' to refer to the patient's authority to determine what is permissible (as we saw in chapter five). Second, the argument here takes it that consent is needed to respect autonomy. While that is not necessarily wrong, as we saw in chapter five it is not the whole story. Healthcare professionals only need consent where they have good reason to do something that would be wrong if done without it, and there are different reasons it might be wrong if done without consent. As such, the situation is better described like this:

1. In order to benefit their patients healthcare professionals sometimes need to do things that would be wrong if done without consent.
2. In order to consent patients need to know something about what is proposed.
3. Therefore, healthcare professionals should tell their patients about what is proposed—unless they do this they cannot get the consent they need if they are to benefit their patients without at the same time acting wrongly.

On this account, while providing information enables patients to be more autonomous, that it does so is not the reason healthcare professionals should provide it. Once again, therefore, there is no reason to think that the obligation to respect autonomy incorporates an obligation to enable patients to be more autonomous (or to make more autonomous decisions).

Given all this we do not appear to have any reason to think that enabling patients to be more autonomous is required if healthcare professionals are to avoid the wrong of failing to respect autonomy—particularly in the absence of any positive argument for that claim. We do, however, have good reason to think it is not. This is not because there is something problematic about the idea that a person's life goes better if she is in a position to be more autonomous, in the sense of 'autonomous' being used here. To say that it does, is merely to say that her life goes better to the extent that she is able to shape it in light of the things that matter to her (her goals, her values, her commitments). As we saw in chapter six accepting this is required if we are to make sense of many of the treatments given for chronic illness. The problem is rather with the idea that healthcare professionals have an obligation to enable their patients to live more autonomously.

To see why, it will be useful to start by noting a tension in the idea that they have such an obligation. This is that enabling others to live more autonomously can come into conflict with living autonomously. There are two reasons for this. First, there are lots of ways in which one person could enable another to be more autonomous—the former could, for example, provide resources that help the latter fulfil his or her aims, or provide the latter with information relevant to each and every one of his or her commitments. As such, fulfilling an obligation to enable others to live more autonomously would leave little time for anyone to achieve their own goals, or to do the things needed to fulfil their own commitments. This is related to the problem of demandingness that Bernard Williams raised for act utilitarianism (Williams, 1973). But in this case it is even worse because, if people are not able to pursue their own goals and commitments, they are not able to live autonomously themselves and it is the value of living autonomously that we are concerned with here. Second, those whose ability to be autonomous a person could enhance may have goals and values that are incompatible with their own. As such, doing things that enable the other person to be more autonomous may require doing things that are inimical with achieving the actor's own goals (for example where the actor is in competition with the other person). Or it may require acting in ways that are incompatible with the actor's values. Think back to the man who wants to prevent his daughter knowing his diagnosis. Suppose that he does so purely because he thinks she will (on the basis of that knowledge) have an abortion and he sincerely believes abortion is morally wrong. He also, let us suppose, believes that acting in ways that would lead other people to act wrongly is itself wrong. In this situation requiring him to do what would enable his daughter to be more autonomous is to require him to do something incompatible with his values. For these two reasons doing what is needed to enable others to live more autonomously can get in the way of living autonomously. Indeed, it may make it impossible to live autonomously in the relevant sense. That is hard to square with the idea that living autonomously is something valuable that should be enhanced.[8]

It might be objected that this ignores the fact that our concern is with the obligations of healthcare professionals, not those of people in general. And, just as healthcare professionals have obligations to benefit their patients stemming from their role, their obligation to respect their patients' autonomy may also be different from (and more demanding than) people's general obligation to do so. Suppose, for example, that it is not the woman's father in our earlier example who withholds information, but her doctor. He does so because he believes providing that information (in this case information about how to access an abortion) may lead her to have an abortion, something he sincerely believes is morally wrong. Many people would say both that this doctor does something wrong and that the reason it is wrong is that he is inappropriately imposing his moral views on his patient. That looks like the wrong of failing to respect her autonomy. If that is right, then healthcare professionals' obligation to respect their patients' autonomy would include a requirement to provide information that enables the patient to be more autonomous.

There is something right about this. There are things that healthcare professionals ought to do to enable their patients to be more autonomous that are specific to them (stemming from their role as healthcare professionals). We have already seen that this follows from their obligation to do what is prospectively best for their patient (as well as from their distinct legal and contractual obligations). But that healthcare professionals ought to enable their patients to be more autonomous, does not, in itself, support the idea that doing so is required in order to respect autonomy. To do that we would need some reason to think that being a healthcare professional brings with it a more demanding obligation to respect autonomy (one that has a positive aspect). No such reason has been provided. Furthermore, the idea that healthcare professionals have such an obligation has implausible implications for what they should do. These I will argue give us good reason to reject it.

Before doing so, however, I need to deal with the example just given (a doctor withholding information about how to access an abortion). The issue is not whether in withholding this information he has acted wrongly. We do not need the idea that healthcare professionals should enable their patients to be more autonomous to explain that. Where abortion is provided by the health service, he has intentionally prevented his patient from accessing a service to which she is entitled. That is something he should not do. The issue is rather whether by withholding this information he has acted wrongly by failing to respect his patient's autonomy. According to the argument presented above whether he has depends on his reasons for withholding the information. Where his sole reason for withholding information is that he thinks his patient would, or might, use it to do something he sincerely believes is morally wrong, his action is not a wrongful failure to respect her (or her autonomy). You may (as I do) think he is wrong about the morality of abortion. But that does not alter the situation. In withholding information he is not imposing his moral views on her.[9] He is refusing to help, or enable, her do something he believes to be morally wrong. That would usually be commendable. People ought not to collaborate with, or enable, wrongdoing. Whether we in fact find it commendable will depend on whether we agree that the proposed act is morally wrong. But even if we do not, we should not think that the obligation to respect autonomy requires anyone (including healthcare professionals) to act in ways they sincerely believe are morally wrong. To do so would be to say that healthcare professionals who are in this doctor's position should compromise their own autonomy by going against their values. While there will be situations where they should—such as where the patient is entitled to the service her doctor objects to—we cannot argue to that conclusion on the grounds that living autonomously is valuable.

The idea that healthcare professionals' obligation to respect their patients' autonomy includes an obligation to enable them to be more autonomous is thus problematic. It implies that healthcare professionals sometimes have a moral obligation to do things they sincerely believe are morally wrong simply because this will help a patient achieve her goals. But it is also problematic for other reasons. Two examples will help to show why. First, while healthcare professionals know about medical treatments and the effects of people's choices on their health, that is not all they know. They may well know, and be aware that they know, things that would help a particular patient make more informed choices about her career, her holiday plans, or her relationship with her partner. If their obligation to respect autonomy means they should enable their patients to be more autonomous, then in these circumstances they have an obligation to disclose this information (whatever it may be). A failure to do so would be a wrong of exactly the same kind as a failure to disclose information directly relevant to the patient's health. At least intuitively, however, it is not. Suppose my nurse knows I am planning a holiday, has information that would help me make a more informed choice about where to go, but does not give it to me (perhaps it just does not occur to him to do so). In this situation it does not look as if he has acted wrongly by failing to respect my autonomy. If that is right, healthcare professionals' obligation to respect their patients' autonomy cannot include an obligation to enable their patients to be more autonomous (or to enable them to make more informed choices). This conclusion cannot be avoided by stipulating that healthcare professionals' obligations to enable their patients to make more informed (and hence autonomous) choices is limited to choices about medical treatment, or choices about things that might affect their future health. The focus on respect for autonomy does not allow for such a restriction. Introducing it moves us to a different type of account—one that grounds the obligation to enable patients to be more autonomous (or make more autonomous choices) in the obligation to promote or enhance their health.

Second, there is a difference between what healthcare professionals do in different aspects of their role. It is well-established that healthcare professionals should tell their patients about both the risks and benefits of treatment. Doing so enables the patient to make a more informed (and hence more autonomous) choice. I argued earlier that we do not need to posit an obligation to enable patients to be more autonomous to explain this. But if there were such an obligation, this is what it would require.

By giving their patients balanced information, healthcare professionals enable those patients to be more autonomous (in the relevant sense of 'autonomous'). When it comes to prevention, however, this is not typically what healthcare professionals do. They tell patients about the risks of things like smoking, heavy drinking, and unsafe sex. But they do not tell patients about the potential benefits of doing these things (such as the pleasure they might give). If the obligation to enable patients to be more autonomous requires providing balanced information in the treatment case, it should also require providing balanced information in the prevention case. Healthcare professionals do not, in general, enable someone to live more autonomously (to better shape their life according to their goals, values, and commitments) by giving them a biased account of the consequences that might follow certain choices.

Two objections are likely to be raised at this point. One is that healthcare professionals may not know much about the potential benefits. As such, they are not in a position to give a balanced picture. While that may be right in some cases, it will not be right in all. There are cases where healthcare professionals do have the relevant information and we can restrict our attention to them. The other, and more important, objection rests on the idea that patients already know about the benefits, but do not know about the risks. As such, healthcare professionals are filling in the gaps in what is already a biased picture. In some, perhaps many, cases that will be right. But where healthcare professionals are telling patients about the risks involved in activities those patients might take up (as opposed to things they are currently doing) it cannot be assumed that it is. It is not reasonable to assume that a person not currently engaging in some activity already knows everything in favour of engaging in it, but nothing about what counts against doing it. At the very least in this situation an obligation to enable patients to be more autonomous would require healthcare professionals to check their patients' knowledge of the potential benefits, and fill in any gaps they find. That is not something they usually do. One of two things follows: 1. in their health promotion work healthcare professionals are systematically acting wrongly by failing to respect their patients' autonomy, or 2. healthcare professionals' obligation to respect autonomy does not include an obligation to enable their patients to be more autonomous. Given this choice we should take the latter option. The idea that healthcare professionals should tell patients about the benefits of unhealthy behaviour is intuitively implausible. Furthermore, we have been given no good reason to think that the obligation to respect autonomy does include an obligation to enable patients to be more autonomous. In the absence of any such reason we should not conclude that healthcare professionals are systematically acting wrongly. Such a claim requires support, and that support has not been given.

For these reasons we should reject the idea that healthcare professionals' obligation to respect autonomy includes an obligation to enable their patients to be more autonomous. Doing so does not mean rejecting the idea that healthcare professionals should sometimes act so as to enhance patients' autonomy (by, for example, providing relevant information). As we have seen, this is sometimes required for other reasons (to do what is prospectively best for their patients, or to comply with regulations they ought to comply with). But it does mean that we need a different approach if we are to explain why healthcare professionals have an obligation to give patients information about the risks and benefits to their health of different lifestyle choices. That involves turning away from considerations of the patient's autonomy to considerations of her wellbeing.

Doing so is not straightforward. At first sight it might seem that giving patients information that is relevant given the choices they face (or may face) benefits them. There are, however, two ways of filling out such a claim, and both face problems. The first starts from the point that taking one option—say not doing X—would be better for the patient than the other. In that case providing information about the risks of doing X makes it more likely that the patient will do what is best for her. She may not. She may still do X despite being told of the risks. In which case providing the information does not affect her wellbeing. But if it leads her to avoid X, it does. The problems with this should be apparent from earlier chapters. As we saw in chapter two, to determine which option is best for a patient requires an assessment of how each will affect her as a person (with her own goals, commitments, and values). That is a tricky epistemic task, one that healthcare professionals have no special expertise in performing. They may know that one option involves a risk to the patient's future health. But that does not necessarily mean it would be worse for her, all things considered, than the alternatives. What is best for most people is not necessarily best for her. To assume that it is would be similar to assuming that because a particular treatment is best for most people it is also best for this patient. We saw in chapter three that in the case of treatment this is sometimes a reasonable assumption. The same may also be true in some cases involving prevention. But it is unlikely that all cases will be like this. As such, it is not clear that healthcare professionals know enough to determine what will benefit their patients. Furthermore, there is another problem with this proposal. A healthcare professional giving his patient partial information (telling her about the risks but not the benefits) with the aim of leading her to choose what he (the healthcare professional) thinks is best for her is attempting to manipulate her into doing what he wants. That is something he should not do.

The second way of filling out the claim that 'giving patients relevant information benefits them', rests on the idea that informed patients are more likely to choose what will in fact benefit them than uninformed patients. This is not the idea, familiar from Mill (1859/1974), that an individual is the best judge of her own interests. It is rather the idea that people are better judges of their own interests the more relevant information they have.[10] As such, healthcare professionals might seem to have an obligation to give this information (whatever it is) to their patients—doing so is a way to benefit the patient, and healthcare professionals ought to benefit their patients. That, however, would take us straight back to the problems confronting the idea that healthcare professionals ought to enable their patients to be more autonomous. First, where healthcare professionals have information relevant to a patient's business, holiday plans, or relationships they would have an obligation to pass it on. Doing so would put the patient in a position to make more informed choices, and so (according to this account) would benefit her. Second, we would be unable to distinguish between the treatment and prevention cases. Telling patients about the risks, but not the benefits, of doing something is not, in general, a way to enable them to make more informed choices about what is best for them. The exception here is where they already know about the benefits but not the risks. But as we have seen healthcare professionals cannot always assume this is the case.

These problems arise because healthcare professionals have been assumed to have an obligation to benefit their patients. I argued in chapter two, however, that that is not quite right. The relevant obligation is better characterised as an obligation to do what of the things they can do (given their expertise and available resources) is prospectively best for their patients. With a slight tweak to make explicit something that was only implicit in that earlier discussion, this enables us to avoid the first of the two problems just identified. The tweak is to clarify that the expertise referred to here is what we might call medical expertise (expertise about things like how to treat illness, or protect oneself against it). Characterising healthcare professionals' obligations in this way limits the kinds of information they have an obligation to pass on to patients. In particular it means that they will not have any obligation to disclose information unrelated to the patient's illness, medical treatment, or future health. That information falls outside the scope of their expertise as healthcare professionals, and hence of their obligation *qua* healthcare professional.

At first sight this does not seem to help with the second problem. If a more informed patient is in a better position to choose the option that is prospectively best for her, healthcare professionals might seem to have an obligation to give patients as much relevant information as possible (including information about both risks and benefits). And it is true that it would give them such an obligation if patients were fully rational and made use of everything they know when deciding what to do. But, as we saw in chapter three, they are not. As such, the situation is more complex than it first appears. An example will help to make this clearer. So consider this situation. A healthcare professional knows that engaging in a particular activity, call it X, carries an increased risk of developing serious illness. He also knows that many people receive some benefit from doing X, at least in the short term. He has some evidence that for most people the risk outweighs the benefit (though as we have seen it does not follow that it will do so for this patient). He does not know whether his patient will do X if he says nothing about it (though he may have some idea how likely this is from historical data). What should he do if he is to do what is prospectively best for his patient? Telling her about the risks may make it less likely she does X. That is something that he has some, but not decisive, reason to think will be best for her. Telling her about both the risks and benefits may make it more likely she will do X than if she was only told about the risks.[11] He has some (but not decisive) reason to think that would not be best for her, but also some (but not decisive) reason to think that it would (being more informed means she is likely to be making better choices). What he should do in this situation will depend on the strength of the various reasons he has. We should not assume that these will always come down in favour of providing more information. Whether or not they do will depend on the details of the case. As such, healthcare professionals will not always have an obligation to tell patients about the benefits of things they (the patients) may do when telling them about the risks. That does not mean there are no problems here. Working out what is prospectively best is hard (Zimmerman, 2014). As such, what they should do may be entirely unclear to healthcare professionals in the midst of a busy surgery or ward.

Fortunately they do not need to work all this out to determine what they should tell their patients. Two things matter here (both of which risk being overlooked if we ignore the context). One is that much of the information we are concerned with in this section is about harms that might occur were the patient to make certain choices—for example, were she to increase her alcohol consumption, skip exercise, or fail to control her blood glucose levels. It is the information that acting in certain ways increases her chances of developing serious illness, makes it more likely that any existing illnesses will get worse, or will potentially shorten her life. I have argued elsewhere that where healthcare professionals have such information they, like everyone else, have a 'duty to warn' their patients (see Walker, 2017). The basic idea can be illustrated with an example from J.S. Mill (1859/1974, for further discussion see Hanna, 2012). Suppose you see a man walking towards a footbridge that, if he attempts to cross it, will collapse sending him to his death. In this scenario you have good reason to think that the man is unaware that the bridge will collapse in this way. Mill argues that stopping the man to tell him about the dangers is morally permissible. But saying it is morally permissible seems too weak (even on Mill's own account). Were you to watch him proceed towards the bridge unaware of the risks of serious injury or death involved and do nothing, it would display a troubling lack of concern for his wellbeing. Indeed, it might suggest you are indifferent to his well-being.

Healthcare professionals, however, ought not to be indifferent to their patients' well-being. They have an obligation to help their patients, not merely to avoid harming them (though they should do that too). Warning about avoidable risks is one way to fulfil that obligation. As such, healthcare professionals should tell their patients about the risks involved where they have reasonable grounds to think the patient is doing, or may start doing, something that either increases her chances of becoming ill, or is likely to exacerbate her existing condition. That will include telling patients about the risks involved in things like smoking and unsafe sex. It will also include giving those with chronic illness information specific to their illness. For example, it will include telling patients with type 2 diabetes that failing to control their diet both risks their condition getting worse, and increases their risk of heart disease, stroke, and foot ulcers (along with all the other things that are more likely if diabetes is poorly controlled). This obligation falls on healthcare professionals because they are uniquely placed epistemically. They know more than other people about what will increase the patient's chances of becoming ill, or make her existing illness worse. They are also in a position to know something about what their patients are doing or may be thinking about doing. As such, when it comes to health risks the duty to warn falls squarely on them.

It is important to note three things about this argument. First, the duty is a duty to warn, to ensure that the patient is aware of the risks she may be running. As such, healthcare professionals do not need to determine whether the patient would be better off, all things considered, acting in one way rather than another (something it is hard for them to do). Second, while the obligation only requires telling patients about the risks (not about the benefits) it does not involve manipulation. The healthcare professional is not trying to bring it about that his patient does what he thinks would be best for her. He is warning her of the risks so that she can decide for herself whether these are, for her, risks worth taking. Third, while the duty to warn means healthcare professionals should sometimes enable patients to make more informed decisions, this is not rooted in their obligation to respect autonomy. Because of this its scope is severely limited (something we have seen is not possible for accounts that base the obligation to enable autonomy on the obligation to respect it). It requires healthcare professionals to treat their patients as autonomous, as people who can decide for themselves what to do. But it also recognises that those patients are not omniscient (there are relevant things they do not know but that other people do).

The other contextual feature that matters is that when treating chronic illness healthcare professional and patient are engaged in a shared activity (as discussed in chapter six). They are working together to manage the patient's illness and increase (to the extent possible) her effective freedom to live life on her own terms despite being ill. When acting together in this way those involved have at least some obligation to share information where this is relevant to the success of their shared activity. Failing to do so would be irrational given their own aims. Furthermore, healthcare professionals participate in this kind of shared activity because that is what, of the things they can do given their expertise and the resources available, is prospectively best for their patient. As such, failing to maximise its chances of success would be inconsistent with their obligations. This all affects what information healthcare professionals should give their patients. It also makes it easier to determine what they should do. What matters is not whether providing certain information would be prospectively best for a patient in its own right; it is whether providing that information would help or hinder the success of the shared activity they are engaged in with that patient. For example, where a doctor is working with his diabetic patient to manage her glucose levels the relevant question is what he should tell her to help her do that well (not what he should tell her to benefit her, where that is considered in isolation from everything else). Similarly, if healthcare professional and patient have agreed to a treatment plan that requires the patient to cut down her alcohol consumption, and reminding her of the risks associated with heavy drinking will help her do so, that is something he should do. If reminding her about the pleasure some people get from heavy drinking would make it harder to cut back, that is something he should not do. In this case it is providing a biased account (focusing only on the risks) that helps the patient be more autonomous (that is, to shape her life in accordance with her aims, values, and commitments).[12] Healthcare professionals ought to enable their patients to be more autonomous in this way. But that is not because doing so is part of respecting the patient's autonomy. It is because it is required by the shared activity healthcare professional and patient are engaged in. That limits the scope of what healthcare professionals are required to do. They only need to provide information where doing so will help a patient do his or her own part in their shared project of managing the patient's illness as effectively as they can.

The arguments we have just looked at (focusing on a duty to warn and the nature of shared activities) mean healthcare professionals have an obligation to give patients information in some cases. But the scope of that obligation is limited. That enables us to avoid the counterintuitive consequences of accounts that ground an obligation to enable patients to be more autonomous in the obligation to respect autonomy. For example, on this account my nurse does nothing wrong if he fails to pass on information that might help me make more informed holiday choices, but does if he fails to tell me about serious risks to my health. He will also have done nothing wrong if he does not balance that information about risks with information about benefits. That does not mean that there is no requirement to provided balanced information when a patient needs either to choose what treatment to have or to consent to that treatment. As we have seen in earlier chapters there are other moral considerations that apply in those cases.

8.5 Conclusion

Treatment of chronic illness takes place over relatively long periods of time in a world that is constantly changing. In this chapter we have been considering how that affects healthcare professionals' obligations. Working in a changing, rather than a static, world creates challenges of its own. Sometimes, such as with one-off treatments for patients with acute illness, these can safely be ignored. But they cannot be ignored when it comes to the treatment of chronic illness. In thinking about how change affects what healthcare professionals should do we have had to take account of different types of change: changes in what treatments are available, changes in the patient's environment, and changes that might be initiated by the patient. These raise different problems. In each case responding to those problems has meant modifying some of the positions reached in earlier chapters to fully capture the ethical implications of acting in a dynamic world. In the last section in particular we have also seen that characterising healthcare professionals' obligations in broad terms—an obligation to respect autonomy, or to benefit patients—can create problems. These may not be apparent if we restrict ourselves to a relatively narrow range of examples, indeed they may seem to capture everything needed. But as the range of examples is expanded they quickly run into difficulties, leading to implausible results in some cases. To avoid these problems a more nuanced account of healthcare professionals' obligations is needed, one that takes seriously the context in which they work.

Notes

1 As such, the obligation to provide it does not fit easily into standard accounts of healthcare professionals' obligations to share information with their patients. It is not unusual in general healthcare ethics texts to find the entire discussion of information disclosure within a chapter devoted to autonomy (the bulk of which is in turn devoted to informed consent; see, for example, Beauchamp and Childress, 2009, ch.4; Harris, 1985, ch.10), or to be entirely contained in a chapter on consent (see, for example, Gert, Culver, and Clouser, 2006, ch.9).
2 Sometimes consuming something sugary is not enough (or not possible) and a hormone, glucagon, needs to be injected into the bloodstream. Healthcare professionals will thus also need to make sure the patient has a supply of glucagon. They or the patient will then need to ensure that those around her know both when it is needed and how to give it.
3 It will not enable them to be more autonomous on other ways of interpreting 'autonomy'. As we have already seen, becoming better informed does not affect a person's sovereignty or authority to determine what it is permissible for others to do.
4 The relationship between enabling someone to be more autonomous and respecting their autonomy could be cashed out in two different ways, and it is not always clear which is meant. One option is that the term 'respect' is here being given an extended meaning that incorporates enabling. The other is that in order to respect someone's autonomy—to treat it in the way that

is called for by the type of thing it is—one ought to enable them to be more autonomous. That is, enabling someone to be more autonomous is a way in which we respect their autonomy. This difference will not affect the argument in this section.

5 The earlier explanation cannot do this because it locates the wrong in the failure to provide information. It is this that means the doctor has not enabled his patient to be more autonomous.
6 Your intuitions about this example are likely to vary depending on your views about the morality of abortion. It is this that makes it a hard case for the position I am defending here.
7 We will return to this example below.
8 It is also incompatible with Ronald Dworkin's argument (that we looked at briefly in chapter five) that respecting autonomy does not preclude people setting back the interests of those they are in competition with (Dworkin, 2011, pp. 285–299).
9 Were he to do so by, for example, forcibly preventing her from accessing an abortion, this would be a failure to respect her autonomy.
10 While that may not always be correct (see Walker, 2017) for our purposes here we can assume that it is.
11 It may not. For example, if she uses a 'stopping rule' such as 'if an option could lead to serious harm, don't do it' when making decisions, telling her about the benefits will not affect what she does (for further discussion, see Walker, 2017).
12 Doing so is not necessarily manipulative. This is not a case of the doctor manipulating the patient to achieve his, the doctor's, aims. The ends being pursued here are the ones shared by doctor and patient. What he is going to do can all be agreed as part of the shared treatment plan.

9 Conclusion

We started this investigation by imagining someone looking at healthcare ethics as a way to learn what healthcare professionals do, and what they should do. They would, or so I argued, receive a distorted picture. Some areas of healthcare would be both brightly lit and picked out in great detail—including interventions at the start and end of life, medical research, consent, public health policy, and treatments for acute illness. Others, such as the treatment of patients with chronic illness, would be at best roughly sketched and remain largely in the shadows. The aim of this book has been to throw light onto these areas. It does so by providing an account of the normative landscape in which treatment for chronic illness occurs.

As we have seen, that landscape is irreducibly complex. Healthcare professionals' moral obligations in this area overlap those that exist in other areas of healthcare. But they also go beyond what is required in those other areas. Even where obligations are broadly the same, they are not exactly the same. Consent, for example, is something that has been dealt with extensively in healthcare ethics, normally in the context of informed consent for medical interventions that do something to the body, for participating in research, or for disclosing patient data. That is all relevant when it comes to some treatments for chronic illness, but it does not capture everything that is important (for example, it does not capture what is required when entering a patient's home).

The distinct moral challenges raised when treating patients with chronic illnesses stem from two features. First, because treatment extends over many months or years there is a need to take account of the fact that the world changes—something that can safely be ignored when considering one off interventions for acute conditions. Those changes can come in a variety of forms. For example, the medications available to healthcare professionals, and the support available from the patient's family, can change during the course of treatment. As a consequence what was best for a patient when treatment started may not be what is best for them at some later time. How to manage and effectively respond to such changes raises moral questions of its own (as we saw in chapter eight). A full account of healthcare professionals' moral obligations must take these into account. But these are not the only changes that are important when thinking about the treatment of chronic illness. The illness itself can both get worse over time and cause other health problems. Treatment is frequently aimed, at least in part, at reducing the chances that this happens. As such, when thinking about healthcare professionals' obligations in the context of chronic illness we need to blur the distinction between treatment (studied by clinical ethics) and prevention (studied by public health ethics). Healthcare professionals treating patients with chronic illness are often engaged in both treatment and prevention at the same time. That affects what they should do.

Second, while some treatments for chronic illness are provided directly by healthcare professionals, most are not. Instead treatment is delivered on a day to day basis either by patients themselves or by those close to them. In these cases healthcare professionals play an enabling and supporting role. Once a treatment plan is in place the patient, healthcare professionals, and others (such as members of the patient's family) work together to achieve a common goal (exactly who is included here will vary considerably from case to case). In practice this does not always work as well as it might, simply because the people involved do not always do their part well. When investigating this in chapters six and seven I did not consider cases where the person who does not do their part well is a healthcare professional (in most cases that will be covered by institutional procedures). Instead my focus was on cases where it is either the patient or a member of their family—that is, on cases of non-adherence.

What healthcare professionals should do in such cases depends on why the patient (or the person helping them) is not adhering. Sometimes it is because they cannot—despite having been given relevant resources and information. A person's capability to be healthy depends in part on their ability to convert the resources provided into improved functioning, and not every patient has that ability. Where this is the reason for non-adherence, steps should be taken to enable the patient (or care provider) to adhere to the extent that that is possible. In other cases the person concerned can adhere despite not doing so. Determining what healthcare professionals' obligations are in such cases takes us into the area of patient responsibility. I have argued that where patients are an integral part of the treatment team, where they are working together with healthcare professionals, it would be wrong to deny that they are responsible in this way. Doing so would fail to treat them as moral agents, people who can take responsibility for their own life and for completing tasks they have agreed to do. That would be both a failure to show them the respect they are due, and to treat them in way that is belittling. However, I have also argued that given the context in which healthcare professional and patient interact it does not follow from this that non-adherent patients should have lower priority for treatment. What treatment patients are owed is not normally dependent on their responsibility in that way.

Conclusion 223

The perspective on all these matters that I have been adopting in this book is that of the healthcare professional in the world in which they work. My concern has been to determine what they should do when treating patients with chronic illness in that world. In doing so, certain values, familiar from work in other areas of healthcare, have been important—principally benefiting the patient, avoiding harm, and respecting the patient's autonomy. But it turns out that the way these values have been conceptualised in healthcare ethics creates problems in this context. We have thus had to investigate what exactly they require. For example, it might have been thought that healthcare professionals benefit their patients by curing them. While that is true in the case of many acute illnesses, with chronic illness it is not. As such, we have had to rethink what benefits healthcare professionals can, and should be, aiming at.

I have argued that when it comes to chronic illness the benefit healthcare professionals provide is one, or both, of two things. They can either 1. alleviate or prevent unpleasant sensations caused by the illness, or 2. counteract the ways a patient's illness negatively effects their ability, either now or in the future, to live their life according to their own goals, values, and commitments. Given the way that personal autonomy has been characterised in healthcare ethics, the latter could be described as counteracting the negative effects of the illness on the patient's autonomy. 'Autonomy' here does not refer to complete independence. It refers to a person's capacity to make their life their own, by, for example, making important decisions for themselves rather than having decisions imposed on them. That people have this capacity does not mean that they will always use it. Sometimes they may prefer not to make decisions for themselves, but to either collaborate with others or defer to their expertise. In most cases there is nothing wrong with that. With one exception, when describing the benefit of treatment as counteracting the illness's negative effects on a person's autonomy I mean only that it puts them in a better position to shape their life according to what is important to them should they choose to do so. The exception occurs where treatment aims to enhance a patient's capacity to manage their illness. In that case those treating the patient have reason to be concerned not only with ensuring that the patient has that capacity, but also with how well they use it. Finally on this point, it is important to see that autonomy in this sense is a range property. People can have it to a greater or lesser extent. Some people are able to shape their life according to a long term plan. Others are constantly firefighting from one crisis to the next. But all competent people have the capacity to shape their lives to some extent. It is this capacity that healthcare professionals should respect and protect, not the extent to which it is used to live well planned lives. In this context, what matters is recognition respect, not appraisal respect.

At first sight, characterising the benefits of treatment in this way challenges a widely held position in healthcare ethics (exemplified by the four principles approach)—the position that the values of beneficence and respect for autonomy are independent. When our concern is with the treatment of chronic illness there is no way to avoid that. However, this link between autonomy and beneficence only occurs if autonomy is conceptualised as a capacity. That is not the only way 'autonomy' is used in healthcare. There are other values that may be picked out using that word which we need to keep separate from both autonomy (as a capacity) and beneficence. Three in particular are important when dealing with chronic illness.

The first is that an individual typically has authority over what it is permissible to do to them, their body, their property, or their data. Benefitting a patient sometimes involves doing things that would be wrong unless they have exercised this authority to make those acts permissible. That is, they would be wrong unless the patient has consented to them. There are, as we have seen, often several reasons for this, each connected to a different wrong that would be done in the absence of consent. The patient's authority here is sometimes described as their sovereignty, something which in turn can be captured using the language of autonomy. There is nothing wrong with that. Having this authority is both an important part of what it is to be self-governing, and something healthcare professionals must respect. But autonomy (in this sense) is not the same as the personal autonomy described above. It does not, for example, come in degrees. A competent patient has absolute authority over whether it would violate their bodily integrity to stick a needle into them irrespective of their level of understanding or ability to act on their choices. It is also not something that treatment for chronic illness would normally aim at enhancing. Most of those with chronic illness, whatever their age, are already fully autonomous in this sense before they receive any treatment. It is unfortunate that there are two distinct and important values picked out in English by the same term. That cannot be helped. But it does mean we need to be careful when thinking about autonomy in the context of chronic illness. We should not let the linguistic fact that two things have the same name blur the distinction between them.

The second is that not allowing a person to choose what will happen to them, particularly where others are allowed to do so, is disrespectful. It marks them out as different from, and less important than, others in the same situation. For healthcare professionals to treat their patients in this way would be wrong. But that is not because it would constitute a failure to respect their autonomy in either of the two senses we have just examined (autonomy as either capacity or sovereignty). It is true that what is important here could, if we chose, be captured using the concept of autonomy. However, doing so would incorporate yet another important and distinct value under a concept already being used to pick out two different and equally important ones. That would create even more room for confusion. Instead it is clearer to characterise what is important here in terms of the respect owed to patients because they are persons. That has the added advantage of not restricting those to whom this respect is owed to those who count as autonomous in any rich sense. Being treated with respect in this way is something that children, even young children, are likely to be concerned about. At the other end of life, those whose abilities (particular those whose cognitive abilities) are in decline may also be particularly sensitive to failures of this form of respect. Given that many people with chronic illnesses fall into this age range, that makes it a particularly important consideration in the treatment of chronic illness.

The third value in this vicinity is that of respecting patient choice. That is because in healthcare ethics considerable attention has been paid to the need to respect autonomous choices—that is, the need to respect the voluntary choices of competent people who have substantial understanding of what is proposed. In the context of chronic illness this focus turned out to be problematic. This is in part because it tells us nothing about how healthcare professionals should treat choices that are not autonomous (for example those made by people without the required level of understanding). But it is also because if we assume that what is required to respect a person's choice is to comply with it, there is little reason to think patients' choices should always be respected. It would be unreasonable to think healthcare professionals should comply with any choice, however uninformed, of their patients. But, as we have seen, it is equally unreasonable to think that healthcare professionals should always comply with the autonomous choices of their patients. The thought that they should may be a consequence of blurring the distinction between choosing and consenting. For example, a competent patient's autonomous refusal of treatment must be complied with. That may lead one to infer that respecting patients' choices requires complying with them. However, once we separate out choice and consent we can see that this does not follow. The patient's refusal must be respected, not because they have made an autonomous choice, but because they have not exercised their authority to make acting permissible. This becomes clearer when we consider refusals that are not autonomous (such as those made with little understanding). In such cases it would still be wrong to act, but that cannot be because to do so would fail to respect the patient's autonomous choice. A better way to think about what is required to respect patient choice in cases of chronic illness is to characterise respect in terms of consideration— the patient's choices should be given due weight when deciding what to do. What that weight is requires judgment. Those choices that are well thought out and based on substantial understanding will typically carry more weight than those that are rushed and made on the basis of very little understanding. In some cases the appropriate weight will be to treat the choice as decisive and comply with it. But the appropriate weight to give to a patient's choice is not solely determined by features of that choice. If other people's choices are treated as decisive, there would need to be very good reasons to treat this patient's choice differently (given the respect owed to them as a person).

Finally, as already pointed out the focus of this book has been on healthcare professionals' obligations when treating patients with chronic illness in the world as it is. It has not considered what the institutional, legal, or regulatory regimes that govern that world should be. At various points this is something we have bumped up against. Sometimes that has happened in ways that suggest there are problems with the existing regimes governing healthcare in some places. There has been no space here to assess these. Given the differences between chronic and acute illnesses, however, this is an area that would benefit from more detailed investigation. It has also not been possible to provide clear and simple guidelines for healthcare professionals treating patients with chronic illness. We have repeatedly seen that a one size fits all approach can neither capture the range of moral considerations involved, nor the ways in which what is morally important varies from case to case (depending on the specific illness, the stage of treatment, and the patient). Having said that, it should be possible to draw up clear guidelines for particular types of encounter based on the work presented here. Where that is possible it would be advantageous to those working in healthcare. This is something else that would benefit from more detailed investigation.

References

Altham, J. (1985), 'Wicked Promises', in J. Hacking (ed.), *Exercises in Analysis: Essays by Students of Casimir Lewy*, Cambridge: Cambridge University Press, pp. 1–22.
Anderson, Elizabeth S. (1999), 'What is the Point of Equality?', *Ethics*, 109(2): pp. 287–337.
Andreou, Chrioula. (2008), 'Making a Clean Break: Addiction and Ulysses Contracts', *Bioethics*, 22(1): pp. 25–31.
Archard, David. (1990), 'Paternalism Defined', *Analysis*, 50(1): pp. 36–42.
Archard, David. (2008), 'Informed Consent: Autonomy and Self-Ownership', *Journal of Applied Philosophy*, 25(1): pp. 19–34.
Archard, David W. (2007), 'Children's Consent to Medical Treatment', in Richard Ashcroft, Angus Dawson, Heather Draper, and John McMillan (eds.), *Principles of Health Care Ethics* (2nd Edition), Chichester: John Wiley and Sons Ltd, pp. 311–317.
Arneson, Richard J. (1999), 'Egalitarianism and Responsibility', *Journal of Ethics*, 3: pp. 225–247.
Arneson, Richard J. (2001), 'Luck and Equality', *Proceedings of the Aristotelian Society*, 75: pp. 73–90.
Arpaly, Nomy. (2003), *Unprincipled Virtue: An Inquiry into Moral Agency*, Oxford: Oxford University Press.
Ashcroft, Richard. (1999), 'Equipoise, Knowledge and Ethics in Clinical Research and Practice', *Bioethics*, 13: pp. 214–326.
Audi, Robert. (2004), *The Good in the Right: A Theory of Intuition and Intrinsic Value*, Princeton, NJ: Princeton University Press.
Bach, Kent. (1995), 'Terms of Agreement', *Ethics*, 105: pp. 604–612.
Barthol, R. P. and Ku, N. D. (1959), 'Regression Under Stress to First Learned Behavior', *Journal of Abnormal and Social Psychology*, 59: pp. 134–136.
Batson, Daniel C. (1991), *The Altruism Question: Toward a Social Psychological Answer*, Hillsdale NJ: Lawrence Erlbaum Associates Inc.
Beauchamp, Tom L. (2005), 'Who Deserves Autonomy, and Whose Autonomy Deserves Respect?', in James Stacey Taylor (ed.), *Personal Autonomy: New Essays on Personal Autonomy and Its Role in Contemporary Moral Philosophy*, Cambridge: Cambridge University Press, pp. 310–329.
Beauchamp, Tom L. (2010a), 'Informed Consent: Its History and Meaning', in Tom L. Beauchamp (ed.), *Standing on Principles: Collected Essays*, Oxford: Oxford University Press, pp. 50–78.

Beauchamp, Tom L. (2010b), 'The Four Principles Approach to Health Care Ethics', in Tom L. Beauchamp (ed.), *Standing on Principles: Collected Essays*, Oxford: Oxford University Press, pp. 35–49.
Beauchamp, Tom L. (2010c), 'The Origins and Evolution of the *Belmont Report*', in Tom L. Beauchamp (ed.), *Standing on Principles: Collected Essays*, Oxford: Oxford University Press, pp. 3–17.
Beauchamp, Tom L. (2011), 'Informed Consent: Its History, Meaning, and Present Challenges', *Cambridge Quarterly of Healthcare Ethics*, 20: pp. 515–523.
Beauchamp, Tom L. and Childress, James F. (2009), *Principles of Biomedical Ethics* (6th Edition), Oxford: Oxford University Press.
Bennett, Rebecca. (2007), 'Confidentiality', in Richard Ashcroft, Angus Dawson, Heather Draper, and John McMillan (eds.), *Principles of Health Care Ethics* (2nd Edition), Chichester: John Wiley and Sons Ltd, pp. 325–332.
Berlin, Isaiah. (1969), *Four Essays on Liberty*, Oxford: Oxford University Press.
Bernell, S. and Howard, S. W. (2016), 'Use Your Words Carefully: What Is a Chronic Disease?', *Frontiers in Public Health*, 4: p. 159, available online at: http://doi.org/10.3389/fpubh.2016.00159 (last accessed August 2, 2017).
Berofsky, Bernard. (1995), *Liberation From Self: A Theory of Personal Autonomy*, Cambridge: Cambridge University Press.
Bieri, Peter. (2017), *Human Dignity: A Way of Living* (translated by Diana Siclovan), Cambridge: Polity Press.
Black, Jeremy. (2008), *George III: America's Last King*, New Haven, CT: Yale University Press.
Blackburn, Simon. (1998), *Ruling Passions: A Theory of Practical Reasoning*, Oxford: Oxford University Press.
Boorse, Christopher. (1977), 'Health as a Theoretical Concept', *Philosophy of Science*, 44: pp. 542–573.
Boorse, Christopher. (1997), 'A Rebuttal on Health', in J. M. Humber and R. F. Almeder (eds.), *What is Disease?*, Totowa NJ: Humana Press, pp. 3–134.
Boorse, Christopher. (2011), 'Concepts of Health and Disease', in F. Gifford (ed.), *Handbook of the Philosophy of Science (Vol.16: Philosophy of Medicine)*, Oxford: Elsevier, pp. 13–64.
Brannan, J., Moss, P., and Mooney, A. (2004), *Working and Caring in the Twentieth Century: Change and Continuity in Four Generation Families*, Basingstoke: Palgrave Macmillan.
Bratman, Michael. (1993), 'Shared Intentions', *Ethics*, 104: pp. 97–113.
Bratman, Michael. (1999), 'Shared Intention and Mutual Obligation', in Michael Bratman (ed.), *Faces of Intention*, Cambridge: Cambridge University Press, pp. 130–141.
Bratman, Michael E. (2014), *Shared Agency: A Planning Theory of Acting Together*, Oxford: Oxford University Press.
Brazier, Margaret and Cave, Emma. (2007), *Medicine, Patients and the Law* (4th Edition), London: Penguin Books.
British Thoracic Society (BTS) and Scottish Intercollegiate Guidelines Network (SIGN). (2016), *British Guideline on the Management of Asthma. A National Clinical Guideline*, available online at: www.sign.ac.uk/assets/sign153.pdf (last accessed January 27, 2018).
Broad, C. D. (1950), 'Egoism as a Theory of Human Motivation', in David R. Cheney (ed.), *Broad's Critical Essays in Moral Philosophy*, London: George Allen and Unwin Ltd., pp. 247–261.

Brock, Dan W. (2003), 'Precommitments in Bioethics: Some Theoretical Issues', *Texas Law Review*, 81: pp. 1805–1821.
Brocklebank, D., Ram, F., Wright, J., Barry, P., Cates, C., Davies, L., Douglas, G., Muers, M., Smith, D., and White, J. (2001), 'Comparison of the Effectiveness of Inhaler Devices in Asthma and Chronic Obstructive Airways Disease: A Systematic Review of the Literature', *Health Technology Assessment*, 5(26): pp. 1–149.
Brudney, Daniel. (2007), 'Are Alcoholics Less Deserving of Liver Transplants?', *Hastings Center Report*, 37(1): pp. 41–47.
Buetow, S. and Elwyn, G. (2006), 'Are Patients Morally Responsible for Their Errors?', *Journal of Medical Ethics*, 32: pp. 260–262.
Bullock, Emma C. (2015), 'A Normatively Neutral Definition of Paternalism', *The Philosophical Quarterly*, 65: pp. 1–21.
Butler, Joseph. (1726), 'Fifteen Sermons Preached in the Rolls Chapel', in D. D. Raphael (ed.), *British Moralists 1650–1800: Volume I. Hobbes—Gay*, Indianapolis IN: Hackett Publishing Company Inc., pp. 325–377.
Cappelan, A. W. and Norheim, O. F. (2005), 'Responsibility in Health Care: A Liberal Egalitarian Approach', *Journal of Medical Ethics*, 31: pp. 476–480.
Cave, Eric M. (2007), 'What's Wrong with Motive Manipulation', *Ethical Theory and Moral Practice*, 10: pp. 129–144.
Charland, L. C. (2002), 'Cynthia's Dilemma: Consenting to Heroin Prescription', *American Journal of Bioethics*, 2(2): pp. 37–47.
Christman, John and Anderson, Joel. (2005), 'Introduction', in John Christman and Joel Anderson (eds.), *Autonomy and the Challenges to Liberalism*, Cambridge: Cambridge University Press, pp. 1–23.
Coggon, John and Miola, Jose. (2011), 'Autonomy, Liberty, and Medical Decision-Making', *The Cambridge Law Journal*, 70(3): pp. 523–547.
Cohen, G. A. (2011), *On the Currency of Egalitarian Justice: And Other Essays in Political Philosophy*, Princeton NJ: Princeton University Press.
Commission on the Social Determinants of Health. (2008), *Closing the Gap in a Generation: Health Equity through Action on the Social Determinants of Health. Final Report of the Commission on Social Determinants of Health*, Geneva: World Health Organization.
Coons, Christopher and Weber, Michael. (2013), 'Introduction: Paternalism—Issues and Trends', in Christian Coons and Michael Weber (eds.), *Paternalism: Theory and Practice*, Cambridge: Cambridge University Press, pp. 1–24.
Corrigan, Oonagh. (2003), 'Empty Ethics: The Problem With Informed Consent', *Sociology of Health and Illness*, 25(3): pp. 768–792.
Coulter, Anne and Collins, Alf. (2011), *Making Shared Decision-Making a Reality: No Decision About Me, Without Me*, London: The King's Fund.
Crampton, J. and Adams, R. (1995), 'Expert Errors', *Sports Coach*, 18: pp. 28–30.
Cribbs, Alan and Donetto, Sara. (2013), 'Patient Involvement and Shared Decision-Making: An Analysis of Components, Models and Practical Knowledge', *European Journal for Person Centered Healthcare*, 1(1): pp. 41–49.
Cullity, Garrett. (2007), 'Beneficence', in Richard Ashcroft, Angus Dawson, Heather Draper, and John McMillan (eds.), *Principles of Health Care Ethics* (2nd Edition), Chichester: John Wiley and Sons Ltd, pp. 19–26.
Daniels, Norman. (2008), *Just Health*, Cambridge: Cambridge University Press.
Darwall, Stephen. (1977), 'Two Kinds of Respect', *Ethics*, 88(1): pp. 36–49.
Davis, John K. (2002), 'The Concept of Precedent Autonomy', *Bioethics*, 16(2): pp. 114–133.

References

Davis, John K. (2008), 'How to Justify Enforcing a Ulysses Contract When Ulysses is Competent to Refuse', *Kennedy Institute of Ethics Journal*, 18(1): pp. 87–106.

Dawson, A. (2004), 'What Should We Do About It? Implications of the Empirical Evidence in Relation to Comprehension and Acceptability of Randomisation', in Soren Holm and Monique Jonas (eds.), *Engaging the World: The Use of Empirical Research in Bioethics and the Regulation of Biotechnology*, Amsterdam, Netherlands: IOS Press, pp. 41–52.

Dawson, A. and Garrard, E. (2006), 'In Defence of Moral Imperialism: Four Equal and Universal Prima Facie Principles', *Journal of Medical Ethics*, 32: pp. 200–204.

Department of Health. (2010), 'Improving the Health and Wellbeing of People with Long Term Condition', available online at: http://webarchive.nationalarchives.gov.uk/20130124052951/www.dh.gov.uk/prod_consum_dh/groups/dh_digitalassets/@dh/@en/@ps/documents/digitalasset/dh_111187.pdf (last accessed August 1, 2017).

Dickenson, Donna. (1994), 'Children's Informed Consent to Treatment: Is the Law an Ass?', *Journal of Medical Ethics*, 20(4): pp. 205–207.

Dietrich, Frank. (2002), 'Causal Responsibility and Rationing in Medicine', *Ethical Theory and Moral Practice*, 5: pp. 113–131.

Draper, Heather and Sorell, Tom. (2002), 'Patients' Responsibilities in Medical Ethics', *Bioethics*, 16(4): pp. 335–352.

Dresser, Rebecca S. (1982), 'Ulysses and the Psychiatrists: A Legal and Policy Analysis of the Voluntary Commitment Contract', *Harvard Civil Rights—Civil Liberties Review*, 16: pp. 777–854.

Dworkin, Gerald. (1988), *The Theory and Practice of Autonomy*, Cambridge: Cambridge University Press.

Dworkin, Gerald. (2017), 'Paternalism', in Edward N. Zalta (ed.), *The Stanford Encyclopedia of Philosophy* (Winter 2017 Edition), available online at: https://plato.stanford.edu/archives/win2017/entries/paternalism/ (last accessed April 16, 2018).

Dworkin, Ronald. (1981a), 'What is Equality? Part 1: Equality of Welfare', *Philosophy and Public Affairs*, 10(3): pp. 185–246.

Dworkin, Ronald. (1981b), 'What is Equality? Part 2: Equality of Resources', *Philosophy and Public Affairs*, 10(4): pp. 283–345.

Dworkin, Ronald. (2002), *Sovereign Virtue: The Theory and Practice of Equality*, Cambridge: Harvard University Press.

Dworkin, Ronald. (2006), 'Life Past Reason', in Helga Kuhse and Peter Singer (eds.), *Bioethics: An Anthology* (2nd edition), Oxford: Blackwell Publishing Limited, pp. 357–364.

Dworkin, Ronald. (2011), *Justice for Hedgehogs*, Cambridge: The Belknap Press of Harvard University Press.

Edwards, A. and Elwyn, G. (eds.) (2009), *Shared Decision Making in Health Care: Achieving Evidence-Based Patient Choice*, Oxford: Oxford University Press.

Elster, Jon. (2003), 'Don't Burn Your Bridge Before You Come To It: Some Ambiguities and Complexities of Precommitment', *Texas Law Review*, 81: pp. 1751–1787.

Elwyn, G., Tilburt, J., and Montori, V. (2013), 'The Ethical Imperative for Shared Decision Making', *European Journal for Person Centered Healthcare*, 1(1): pp. 129–131.

Evans, Richard J. (2016), *The Pursuit of Power: Europe 1815–1914*, London: Penguin Books.
Faden, Ruth R. and Beauchamp, Tom L. (1986), *A History and Theory of Informed Consent*, Oxford: Oxford University Press.
Feinberg, Joel. (1965), 'Psychological Egoism', in Joel Feinberg and Russ Shafer-Landau (eds.), *Reason and Responsibility: Readings in Some Basic Problems in Philosophy* (10th Edition), Princeton NJ: Princeton University Press, pp. 272–292.
Feinberg, Joel. (1971), 'Legal Paternalism', *Canadian Journal of Philosophy*, 1: pp. 105–124.
Feinberg, Joel. (1984), *Harm to Others: The Moral Limits of the Criminal Law*, Oxford: Oxford University Press.
Feinberg, Joel. (1986), *Harm to Self: The Moral Limits of the Criminal Law*, Oxford: Oxford University Press.
Feiring, E. (2008), 'Lifestyle, Responsibility and Justice', *Journal of Medical Ethics*, 34: pp. 33–36.
Felson, G. and Reiner, P. B. (2011), 'How the Neuroscience of Decision Making Informs Our Conception of Autonomy', *AJOB Neuroscience*, 2(3): pp. 3–14.
Flanagan, Owen. (1991), *Varieties of Moral Personality: Ethics and Psychological Realism*, Cambridge: The MIT Press.
Foddy, B. and Savulescu, J. (2006), 'Addiction and Autonomy: Can Addicted People Consent to the Prescription of Their Drug of Choice', *Bioethics*, 20(1): pp. 1–15.
Foster, C. (2001), *The Ethics of Medical Research on Humans*, Cambridge: Cambridge University Press.
Frankfurt, Harry G. (1988), 'Freedom of the Will and the Concept of a Person', in Harry G. Frankfurt (ed.), *The Importance of What We Care About*, Cambridge: Cambridge University Press.
Freedman, B. (1987), 'Equipoise and the Ethics of Clinical Research', *New England Journal of Medicine*, 317(3): pp. 141–145.
Friesen-Storms, J. H. H. M., Bours, G. J. J. W, van der Weijden, T., and Beurskens, A. J. H. M. (2015), 'Shared Decision Making in Chronic Care in the Context of Evidence Based Practice in Nursing', *International Journal of Nursing Studies*, 52: pp. 393–402.
Galvin, Rose. (2002), 'Disturbing Notions of Chronic Illness and Individual Responsibility: Towards a Genealogy of Morals', *Health: An Interdisciplinary Journal for the Social Study of Health, Illness and Medicine*, 6(2): pp. 107–137.
Gaus, Gerald. (2016), *The Tyranny of the Ideal: Justice in a Diverse Society*, Princeton NJ: Princeton University Press.
Gawande, Atul. (2014), *Being Mortal: Illness, Medicine and What Matters in the End*, London: Profile Books Ltd.
General Medical Council. (2017), *Confidentiality: Good Practice in Handling Patient Information*, London: General Medical Council, available online at: Confidentiality_good_practice_in_handling_patient_information_-_English_0417.pdf (last accessed March 7, 2018).
Gert, Bernard, Culver, Charles M., and Clouser, K. Danner. (2006), *Bioethics: A Systematic Approach* (2nd Edition), Oxford: Oxford University Press.
Gifford, F. (2000), 'Freedman's 'Clinical Equipoise' and 'Sliding-Scale All-Dimensions-Considered Equipoise'', *Journal of Medicine and Philosophy*, 25(4): pp. 399–426.

Gigerenzer, Gerd. (2000), *Adaptive Thinking: Rationality in the Real World*, Oxford: Oxford University Press.
Gigerenzer, Gerd. (2008), *Rationality for Mortals: How People Cope with Uncertainty*, Oxford: Oxford University Press.
Gigerenzer, Gerd. (2015), 'On the Supposed Evidence for Libertarian Paternalism', *Review of Philosophy and Psychology*, 6: pp. 361–383.
Gigerenzer, Gert and Selten, Reinhard. (eds.) (2001), *Bounded Rationality: The Adaptive Toolbox*, London: The MIT Press.
Gilbert, Daniel. (2006), *Stumbling on Happiness*, London: Harper Press.
Gilbert, Daniel T., Killingsworth, M. A., Eyre, R. N., and Wilson, T. D. (2009), 'The Surprising Power of Neighborly Advice', *Science*, 323: pp. 1617–1619.
Gilbert, Daniel T. and Wilson, Timothy D. (2009), 'Why the Brain Talks to Itself: Sources of Error in Affective Forecasting', *Philosophical Transactions of the Royal Society B*, 364: pp. 1335–1341.
Gilbert, Margaret. (2014), *Joint Commitment: How We Make the Social World*, Oxford: Oxford University Press.
Gilboa, Itzhak. (2010), *Rational Choice*, Cambridge: The MIT Press.
Gillon, Raanan. (1986), *Philosophical Medical Ethics*, Chichester: Wiley.
Gillon, Raanan. (2003), 'Ethics Needs Principles—Four Can Encompass the Rest—and Respect for Autonomy Should be "First Among Equals"', *Journal of Medical Ethics*, 29: pp. 307–312.
Glannon, Walter. (1998), 'Responsibility, Alcoholism, and Liver Transplants', *Journal of Medicine and Philosophy*, 23(1): pp. 31–49.
Godolphin, W. (2009), 'Shared Decision-Making', *Healthcare Quarterly*, 12: pp. e186–e190.
Goldman, Alan H. (2009), *Reasons from within: Desires and Values*, Oxford: Oxford University Press.
Grimm, Dieter. (2015), *Sovereignty: The Origin and Future of a Political Concept*, New York: Columbia University Press.
Hanna, Jason. (2012), 'Paternalism and the Ill-informed Agent', *Journal of Ethics*, 16: pp. 421–439.
Hansson, Sven Ove. (2013), *The Ethics of Risk: Ethical Analysis in an Uncertain World*, Basingstoke: Palgrave Macmillan.
Hardwig, John. (1990), 'What about the Family?', *Hastings Center Report*, 20(2): pp. 5–10.
Harris, John. (1985), *The Value of Life: An Introduction to Medical Ethics*, Abingdon Oxon: Routledge.
Harris, John. (1995), 'Could We Hold People Responsible for Their Own Adverse Health', *The Journal of Contemporary Health Law and Policy*, 12: pp. 147–153.
Hausman, Daniel M. (2012), *Preference, Value, Choice, and Welfare*, Cambridge: Cambridge University Press.
Higgs, Roger. (2006), 'On Telling Patients the Truth', in Helga Kuhse and Peter Singer (eds.), *Bioethics: An Anthology* (2nd Edition), Oxford: Blackwell Publishing Limited, pp. 611–617.
Ho, Dien. (2008), 'When Good Organs Go to Bad People', *Bioethics*, 22(2): pp. 77–83.
Ho, P. Michael, Bryson, Chris L., and Rumsfeld, John S. (2009), 'Medication Adherence: Its Importance in Cardiovascular Outcomes', *Circulation*, 119: pp. 3028–3035.

Hobbes, Thomas. (1650), 'Human Nature', in D. D. Raphael (ed.), *British Moralists 1650–1800: Volume I. Hobbes—Gay*, Indianapolis IN: Hackett Publishing Company Inc., pp. 3–17.
Hoffman, Tammy C. and Del Mar, Chris. (2015), 'Patient's Expectations of the Benefits and Harms of Treatments, Screening, and Tests: A Systematic Review', *JAMA Internal Medicine*, 175(2): pp. 274–286.
Iltis, Ana. (2006), 'Lay Concepts of Informed Consent to Biomedical Research: The Capacity to Understand and Appreciate Risk', *Bioethics*, 20(4): pp. 180–190.
Jackevicius, C. A., Li, P., and Tu, J. V. (2008), 'Prevalence, Predictors, and Outcomes of Primary Nonadherence After Acute Myocardial Infarction', *Circulation*, 117: pp. 1028–1036.
Jackson, Emily. (2012), *Law and the Regulation of Medicines*, Oxford: Hart Publishing Ltd.
Jackson, Frank. (1991), 'Decision-theoretic Consequentialism and the Nearest and Dearest Objection', *Ethics*, 101: pp. 461–482.
Jonson, A. R. (1998), *The Birth of Bioethics*, Oxford: Oxford University Press.
Jonson, A. R., Siegler, M., and Winslade, W. J. (2002), *Clinical Ethics* (5th Edition), New York: McGraw Hill.
Kahneman, Daniel. (2011), *Thinking, Fast and Slow*, London: Penguin Books.
Kant, Immanuel. (2005), *The Moral Law*, London: Routledge.
Kay, John. (2010), *Obliquity*, London: Profile Books Ltd.
Kelleher, J. Paul. (2014), 'Beneficence, Justice and Health Care', *Kennedy Institute of Ethics Journal*, 24(1): pp. 27–49.
Kipnis, Kenneth. (2006), 'A Defense of Unqualified Medical Confidentiality', *The American Journal of Bioethics*, 6(2): pp. 7–18.
Kottow, Michael H. (1986), 'Medical Confidentiality: An Intransigent and Absolute Obligation', *Journal of Medical Ethics*, 12: pp. 117–122.
Levy, Neil. (2006), 'Autonomy and Addiction', *Canadian Journal of Philosophy*, 36(3): pp. 427–448.
Levy, Neil. (2014), 'Forced to be Free? Increasing Patient Autonomy by Constraining It', *Journal of Medical Ethics*, 40: pp. 293–300.
Lewens, Tim. (2015), *The Biological Foundations of Bioethics*, Oxford: Oxford University Press.
Loewenstein, George. (1996), 'Out of Control: Visceral Influences on Behavior', *Organizational Behavior and Human Decision Processes*, 65(3): pp. 272–292.
London, A. J. (2001), 'Equipoise and International Human-Subjects Research', *Bioethics*, 15(4): pp. 312–332.
Lustig, C., Konkel, A., and Jacoby, L. L. (2004), 'Which Route to Recovery? Controlled Retrieval and Accessibility Bias in Retroactive Interference', *Psychological Science*, 15(11): pp. 729–735.
Lysaught, M. Therese. (2004), 'Respect: Or, How Respect for Persons Became Respect for Autonomy', *The Journal of Medicine and Philosophy*, 29(6): pp. 665–680.
Manson, Neil C. (2007), 'Consent and Informed Consent', in Richard Ashcroft, Angus Dawson, Heather Draper, and John McMillan (eds.), *Principles of Health Care Ethics* (2nd Edition), Chichester: John Wiley and Sons Ltd, pp. 297–303.
Manson, Neil C. (2015), 'Transitional Paternalism: How Shared Normative Powers Give Rise to the Asymmetry of Adolescent Consent and Refusal', *Bioethics*, 29(2): pp. 66–73.

Manson, Neil C. and O'Neill, Onora. (2007), *Rethinking Informed Consent in Bioethics*, Cambridge: Cambridge University Press.

Marmot, Michael and Wilkinson, Richard G. (eds.) (2005), *Social Determinants of Health* (2nd Edition), Oxford: Oxford University Press.

Martin, J. A. and Buckwalter, J. A. (2002), 'Aging, Articular Cartilage Chondrocyte Senesecence and Osteoarthritis', *Biogerontology*, 3(5): pp. 257–264.

Martin, Mike W. (2001), 'Responsibility for Health and Blaming Victims', *Journal of Medical Humanities*, 22(2): pp. 95–114.

Maschette, W. (1985), 'Correcting Technique Problems of a Successful Junior Athlete', *Sports Coach*, 9: pp. 14–17.

May, Thomas. (2005), 'The Concept of Autonomy in Bioethics: An Unwarranted Fall from Grace', in James Stacey Taylor (Ed.), *Personal Autonomy: New Essays on Personal Autonomy and Its Role in Contemporary Moral Philosophy*, Cambridge: Cambridge University Press, pp. 299–309.

McCrum, Robert. (1998), *My Year Off*, London: Picador.

McCrum, Robert. (2017), *Every Third Thought: On Life, Death and the Endgame*, London: Picador.

McGregor, Joan. (1994), 'Force, Consent, and the Reasonable Woman', in James L. Coleman and Allen Buchanan (eds.), *In Harm's Way*, Cambridge: Cambridge University Press.

Mckenna, M. and Russell, P. (eds.) (2008), *Free Will and Reactive Attitudes: Perspectives on P.F. Strawson's "Freedom and Resentment"*, Farnham: Ashgate Publishing Ltd.

McNichol, Barbara, Pauker, Stephen G., Sox Jr, Harold C., and Tversky, Amos. (1982), 'On the Elicitation of Preferences for Alternative Therapies', *New England Journal of Medicine*, 306: pp. 1259–1262.

Melani, A. S., Bonavia, M., Cilenti, V., Cinti, C., Lodi, M., Martucci, P., Serra, M., Scichilone, N., Sestini, P., Aliani, M., Neri, M., on behalf of the Gruppo Educazionale Associazione Italiana Pneumologi Ospedalieri (AIPO). (2011), 'Inhaler Mishandling Remains Common in Real Life and is Associated with Reduced Disease Control', *Respiratory Medicine*, 105: pp. 930–938.

Mill, J. S. (1859/1974), *On Liberty*, Harmondsworth: Pelican Books.

Miller, P. B. and Weijer, C. (2003), 'Rehabilitating Equipoise', *Kennedy Institute of Ethics Journal*, 13: pp. 93–118.

Molyneux, D. (2009), 'Should Healthcare Professionals Respect Autonomy Just Because it Promotes Welfare?', *Journal of Medical Ethics*, 35: pp. 245–250.

Morreim, E. Haavi. (1995), 'Lifestyles of the Risky and Infamous', *Hastings Center Report*, 25(6): pp. 5–13.

Mounk, Yascha. (2017), *The Age of Responsibility: Luck, Choice, and the Welfare State*, Cambridge: Harvard University Press.

Nagel, Thomas. (1970), *The Possibility of Altruism*, Princeton NJ: Princeton University Press.

Nagel, Thomas. (1979), 'Death', in Thomas Nagel (ed.), *Mortal Questions*, Cambridge: Cambridge University Press, pp. 1–10.

Nagel, Thomas. (1986), *The View From Nowhere*, New York: Oxford University Press.

Neal, David T., Wood, Wendy, and Drolet, Aimee. (2013), 'How Do People Adhere to Goals When Willpower is Low? The Profits (and Pitfalls) of Strong Habits', *Journal of Personality and Social Psychology*, 104(6): pp. 959–975.

Neal, David T., Wood, Wendy, and Wu, Mengju. (2011), 'The Pull of the Past: When Do Habits Persist Despite Conflict with Motives?', *Personality and Social Psychology Bulletin*, 37(11): pp. 1428–1437.

Nickerson, Raymond S. (1998), 'Confirmation Bias: A Ubiquitous Phenomena in Many Guises', *Review of General Psychology*, 2: pp. 175–220.

Nisbett, Richard E. and Wilson, Timothy D. (1977), 'Telling More Than We Can Know: Verbal Reports on Mental Processes', *Psychological Review*, 84(3): pp. 231–259.

Nordenfelt, Lennart. (1987), *On the Nature of Health: An Action-Theoretic Approach*, Dordrecht: Kluwer Academic.

Nunes, V., Neilson, J., O'Flynn, N., Calvert, N., Kuntze, S., Smithson, H., Benson, J., Blair, J., Bowser, A., Clyne, W., Crome, P., Haddad, P., Hemingway, S., Horne, R., Johnson, S., Kelly, S., Packham, B., Patel, M., and Steel, J. (2009), *Clinical Guidelines and Evidence Review for Medicines Adherence: Involving Patients in Decisions about Prescribed Medicines and Supporting Adherence*, London: National Collaborating Centre for Primary Care and Royal College of General Practitioners.

Nussbaum, Martha C. (2006), *Frontiers of Justice: Disability, Nationality, Species Membership*, Cambridge: The Belknap Press.

O'Neill, Onora. (2002), *Autonomy and Trust in Bioethics*, Cambridge: Cambridge University Press.

O'Neill, Onora. (2003), 'Some Limits of Informed Consent', *Journal of Medical Ethics*, 29: pp. 4–7.

Osterberg, L. and Blaschke, T. (2005), 'Adherence in Medication', *New England Journal of Medicine*, 353: pp. 487–497.

Owens, David. (2011), 'The Possibility of Consent', *Ratio (New Series)*, 24(4): pp. 402–421.

Owens, David. (2012), *Shaping the Normative Landscape*, Oxford: Oxford University Press.

Owens, John and Cribb, Alan. (2013), 'Beyond Choice and Individualism', *Public Health Ethics*, 6(3): pp. 262–271.

Parekh, S. A. (2007), 'Child Consent and the Law: An Insight and Discussion into the Law Relating to Consent and Competence', *Child: Care, Health and Development*, 33(1): pp. 78–82.

Parens, Eric. (2017), 'Choosing Flourishing: Towards a More "Binocular" Way of Thinking about Disability', *Kennedy Institute of Ethics Journal*, 27(2): pp. 135–150.

Phillips, Anne. (2013), *Our Bodies, Whose Property?* Princeton NJ: Princeton University Press.

Philpott, Dan. (2010), 'Sovereignty', in Edward N. Zalta (ed.), *The Stanford Encyclopedia of Philosophy* (Summer 2010 edition), available online at: http://plato.stanford.edu/archives/sum2010/entries/sovereignty/ (last accessed March 03, 2014).

Rachels, J. (1999), *The Elements of Moral Philosophy* (3rd Edition), Singapore: McGraw-Hill College.

Rawls, John. (1971), *A Theory of Justice*, Cambridge: Harvard University Press.

Raz, Joseph. (1986), *The Morality of Freedom*, Oxford: Clarendon Press.

Raz, Joseph. (2009), *Between Authority and Interpretation*, Oxford: Oxford University Press.

Raz, Joseph. (2011), *From Normativity to Responsibility*, Oxford: Oxford University Press.
Resnik, D. B. (2007), 'Responsibility for Health: Personal, Social, and Environmental', *Journal of Medical Ethics*, 33: pp. 444–445.
Richman, Kenneth A. (2004), *Ethics and the Metaphysics of Medicine: Reflections on Health and Beneficence*, London: The MIT Press.
Ripstein, Arthur. (2006), 'Beyond the Harm Principle', *Philosophy and Public Affairs*, 34(3): pp. 215–245.
Robertson, John A. (2003), 'Precommitment Issues in Bioethics', *Texas Law Review*, 81: pp. 1849–1876.
Ross, James. (2016), *Henry VI*, London: Allen Lane.
Ross, James R., Capozzi, James D., and Matava, Matthew. (2012), 'Discussing Treatment with a Minor: The Conflicts Related to Autonomy, Beneficence, and Paternalism', *The Journal of Bone and Joint Surgery American Volume*, 94, pp. e3(1)–e3(4).
Ross, W. D. (1930), *The Right and the Good*, Oxford: Oxford University Press.
Ruger, Janet Prah. (2010), *Health and Social Justice*, Oxford: Oxford University Press.
Scanlon, Thomas M. (1986), 'The Significance of Choice', The Tanner Lectures on Human Values (Brasenose College, Oxford University), available online at: https://tannerlectures.utah.edu/_documents/a-to-z/s/scanlon88.pdf (last accessed February 16, 2018).
Scanlon, Thomas M. (1998), *What We Owe to Each Other*, London: The Belknap Press.
Searle, John. (1969), *Speech Acts: An Essay in the Philosophy of Language*, Cambridge: Cambridge University Press.
Searle, John. (1990), 'Collective Intentions and Actions', in P. Cohen, J. Morgan, and M. Pollack (eds.), *Intentions in Communication*, Cambridge: The MIT Press, pp. 401–415.
Searle, John. (2001), *Rationality in Action*, Cambridge: The MIT Press.
Segall, Shlomi. (2010), *Health, Luck, and Justice*, Oxford: Princeton University Press.
Sen, Amartya. (1979), 'Rational Fools: A Critique of the Behavioural Foundations of Economic Theory', in Frank Hahn and Martin Hollis (eds.), *Philosophy and Economic Theory*, Oxford: Oxford University Press, pp. 87–109.
Sen, Amartya. (1982), 'Equality of What?', in Amartya Sen (ed.), *Choice, Welfare, and Measurement*, Cambridge: The MIT Press.
Sen, Amartya. (1999), *Development as Freedom*, Oxford: Oxford University Press.
Sen, Amartya. (2009), *The Idea of Justice*, London: Allen Lane.
Shiffrin, Seana. (2011), 'Immoral, Conflicting and Redundant Promises', in J. Wallace, R. Kumar, and S. Freedman (eds.), *Reasons and Recognition: Essays on the Philosophy of T. M. Scanlon*, Oxford: Oxford University Press, pp. 155–178.
Siegler, Mark. (1982), 'Confidentiality in Medicine: A Decrepit Concept', *New England Journal of Medicine*, 307: pp. 1518–1521.
Simon, Herbert A. (1997), *Administrative Behavior: A Study of Decision-Making Processes in Administrative Organizations* (4th Edition), New York: The Free Press.
Singer, Peter. (1972), 'Famine, Affluence, and Morality', *Philosophy and Public Affairs*, 1(3): pp. 229–243.

Smart, Brian. (1994), 'Fault and the Allocation of Spare Organs', *Journal of Medical Ethics*, 20: pp. 26–30.
Smith, Holly M. (1997), 'A Paradox of Promising', *The Philosophical Review*, 106(2): pp. 153–196.
Sober, Elliott and Wilson, David Sloan. (1998), *Unto Others: The Evolution and Psychology of Unselfish Behavior*, Cambridge: Harvard University Press.
Sokal, Daniel K. (2009), 'Sweetening the Scent: Commentary of "What Principles Misses"', *Journal of Medical Ethics*, 35: pp. 232–233.
Spellecy, Ryan. (2003), 'Reviving Ulysses Contracts', *Kennedy Institute of Ethics Journal*, 13(4): pp. 373–392.
Stoljar, Natalie. (2007), 'Theories of Autonomy', in Richard Ashcroft, Angus Dawson, Heather Draper, and John McMillan (eds.), *Principles of Health Care Ethics* (2nd Edition), Chichester: John Wiley and Sons Ltd, pp. 11–17.
Strawson, Peter F. (1962), 'Freedom and Resentment', *Proceedings of the British Academy*, 48: pp. 187–211, reprinted in Mckenna, M. and Russell, P. (eds.) (2008), *Free Will and Reactive Attitudes: Perspectives on P.F. Strawson's "Freedom and Resentment"*, Farnham: Ashgate Publishing Ltd, pp. 19–36.
Sutrop, M. (2011), 'How to Avoid a Dichotomy between Autonomy and Beneficence: From Liberalism to Communitarianism and Beyond', *Journal of Internal Medicine*, 269: pp. 370–382.
Tamblyn, R., Tewodros, E., Huang, A., Winslade, N., and Doran, P. (2014), 'The Incidence and Determinants of Primary Nonadherence with Prescribed Medication in Primary Care; A Cohort Study', *Annals of Internal Medicine*, 160: pp. 441–450.
Taylor, James Stacey. (2005a), 'Autonomy and Informed Consent: A Much Misunderstood Relationship', *The Journal of Value Inquiry*, 38: pp. 383–391.
Taylor, James Stacy. (2005b), 'Introduction', in James Stacey Taylor (ed.), *Personal Autonomy: New Essays on Personal Autonomy and Its Role in Contemporary Moral Philosophy*, Cambridge: Cambridge University Press, pp. 1–29.
Taylor, S. E. (1983), 'Adjustment to Threatening Events: A Theory of Cognitive Adaptation', *American Psychologist*, 38: pp. 1161–1173.
Thaler, Richard H. (2015), *Misbehaving: The Making of Behavioural Economics*, London: Allen Lane.
Thaler, Richard H. and Sunstein, Cass R. (2008), *Nudge: Improving Decisions about Health, Wealth, and Happiness*, London: Yale University Press.
Thomson, Judith Jarvis. (1990), *The Realm of Rights*, Cambridge: Harvard University Press.
Tran, N., Coffman, J. M., Sumino, K., and Cabana, M. D. (2014), 'Patient Reminder Systems and Asthma Medication Adherence: A Systematic Review', *Journal of Asthma*, 51(5): pp. 536–543.
Unger, Peter. (1996), *Living High and Letting Die: Our Illusion of Innocence*, Oxford: Oxford University Press.
Uniacke, Suzanne. (2013), 'Respect for Autonomy in Medical Ethics', in David Archard, Monique Deveaux, Neil Manson, and Daniel Weinstock (eds.), *Reading Onora O'Neill*, Abingdon Oxon: Routledge, pp. 94–110.
Varelius, Jukka. (2006), 'On Taylor on Autonomy and Informed Consent', *The Journal of Value Inquiry*, 40: pp. 451–459.

Veatch, Robert M. (2002), 'Indifference of Subjects: An Alternative to Equipoise in Randomized Clinical Trials', *Social Philosophy and Policy*, 19(2): pp. 295–323.
Veatch, Robert M. (2006), 'Abandoning Informed Consent', in Helga Kuhse, and Peter Singer (eds.), *Bioethics: An Anthology* (2nd Edition), Oxford: Blackwell Publishing Limited, pp. 636–645.
Velleman, J. David. (2000), 'How to Share an Intention', in J. David Velleman (ed.), *The Possibility of Practical Reason*, Oxford: Oxford University Press, pp. 200–220.
Venkatapuram, Sridhar. (2011), *Health Justice*, Cambridge: Polity Press.
Vogel, Else. (2016), 'Clinical Specificities in Obesity Care: The Transformations and Dissolution of 'Will' and 'Drives'', *Health Care Analysis*, 24(4): pp. 321–337.
Voigt, Kristin. (2007), 'The Harshness Objection: Is Luck Egalitarianism Too Harsh on the Victims of Option Luck?', *Ethical Theory and Moral Practice*, 10: pp. 389–407.
Wald, D. S., Butt, S., and Bestwick, J.P. (2015), 'One-way Versus Two-way Text Messaging on Improving Medication Adherence: Meta-analysis of Randomized Trials', *The American Journal of Medicine*, 128(10): pp. 1139.e1–1139.e5.
Waldron, Jeremy. (2017), *One Another's Equals*, London: The Belknap Press.
Walker, Tom. (2008), 'Giving Addicts Their Drug of Choice: The Problem of Consent', *Bioethics*, 22(6): pp. 314–320.
Walker, Tom. (2010), 'Who Do We Treat First When Resources Are Scarce?', *Journal of Applied Philosophy*, 27(2): pp. 200–211.
Walker, Tom. (2012a), 'Ulysses Contracts in Medicine', *Law and Philosophy*, 31(1): pp. 77–98.
Walker, Tom. (2012b), 'Informed Consent and the Requirement to Ensure Understanding', *Journal of Applied Philosophy*, 29 (1): pp. 50–62.
Walker, Tom. (2016), 'Adolescent Consent and Refusal', in M. Donnelly and C. Murray (eds.), *Ethical and Legal Debates in Irish Healthcare: Confronting Complexities*, Manchester: Manchester University Press, pp. 71–83.
Walker, Tom. (2017), 'The Obligation to Provide Information When Valid Consent is not Needed', *Kennedy Institute of Ethics Journal*, 27(4): pp. 501–524.
Walker, Tom. (2018), 'Consent and Autonomy', in Andreas Müller and Peter Schaber (eds.), *The Routledge Handbook of the Ethics of Consent*, Abingdon Oxon: Routledge, pp. 131–139.
Walsh, E. and Ayton, P. (2009), 'My Imagination Versus Your Feelings: Can Personal Affective Forecasts be Improved by Knowing Other People's Emotions?', *Journal of Experimental Psychology: Applied*, 15(4): pp. 351–360.
Watson, Gary. (2009), 'Promises, Reasons and Normative Powers', in D. Sobel and S. Wall (eds.), *Reasons for Action*, Cambridge: Cambridge University Press, pp. 155–178.
Weick, Karl E. (1990), 'The Vulnerable System: An Analysis of the Tenerife Air Disaster', *Journal of Management*, 16(3): pp. 571–593.
Wikler, Daniel. (2002), 'Personal and Social Responsibility for Health', *Ethics and International Affairs*, 16(2): pp. 47–55.
Wilkinson, Stephen. (1999), 'Smoker's Rights to Healthcare: Why the "Restoration Argument" is a Moralising Wolf in a Liberal Sheep's Clothing', *Journal of Applied Philosophy*, 16(3): pp. 255–269.

Williams, Bernard. (1973), 'A Critique of Utilitarianism', in J. J. C. Smart and Bernard Williams (eds.), *Utilitarianism For and Against*, Cambridge: Cambridge University Press, pp. 77–150.

Williams, Bernard. (1981), 'Persons, Character, and Morality', in Bernard Williams (ed.), *Moral Luck*, Cambridge: Cambridge University Press, pp. 1–19.

Wilson, James. (2007), 'Is Respect for Autonomy Defensible?', *Journal of Medical Ethics*, 33: pp. 353–356.

Wilson, T. D. and Gilbert, D. T. (2003), 'Affective Forecasting', in M. Zanna (ed.), *Advances in Experimental Social Psychology* (Vol. 35), New York: Elsevier.

World Health Organization. (2014), *Global Status Report on Noncommunicable Diseases 2014*, Geneva: WHO Press, available online at: http://apps.who.int/iris/bitstream/handle/10665/148114/9789241564854_eng.pdf;jsessionid=5DB852A6E213047A2516BA8F17882E2F?sequence=1 (last accessed January 2019).

World Health Organization. (2015), *World Report on Ageing and Health*, Geneva: WHO Press, available online at: http://apps.who.int/iris/bitstream/10665/186463/1/978924094811_eng.pdf?ua=1 (last accessed March 2018).

World Health Organization. (2016), *Global Report on Diabetes*, Geneva: WHO Press, available online at: http://apps.who.int/iris/bitstream/handle/10665/204871/9789241565257_eng.pdf?sequence=1 (last accessed January 2019).

Wormald, Jenny. (1988), *Mary, Queen of Scots*, London: George Philip.

Young, Robert. (2008), 'John Stuart Mill, Ronald Dworkin, and Paternalism', in C. L. Ten (ed), *Mill's On Liberty*, Cambridge: Cambridge University Press.

Zimmerman, Michael J. (2008), *Living with Uncertainty: The Moral Significance of Ignorance*, Cambridge: Cambridge University Press.

Zimmerman, Michael J. (2014), *Ignorance and Moral Obligation*, Oxford: Oxford University Press.

Zweig, Stefan. (2009), *The World of Yesterday* (translated by Anthea Bell), London: Pushkin Press.

Index

advice 12, 28–30; *see also* prevention
ageism 25, 92–93, 156
agreement *see* voluntary agreement
arthritis 4–5, 138–139
asthma 4–7, 133, 139–140, 198, 200–201
autonomy 16–17, 74–76, 135, 143–144, 174, 180–184; as capacity 23–24, 78–80, 85, 186–188, 202–203, 207; as feature of choice 77–79; moral limits on exercise of 82–85, 87–88; obligation to promote 28–29, 85, 202–203, 206–214, 218; as sovereignty 21, 87–88, 109, 124–125, 183–184, 202–203; value of exercising 80–82; *see also* choice, living autonomously and; consent, respect for autonomy and

beneficence *see* benefit; best interests
benefit: determining what will 13–16, 34–36, 50–51, 195–199, 204–205; nature of obligation to 37–44, 132–136, 139–140, 158; providing information as way to 29–30, 202–203, 214–216; prospective account of 40–41, 67; *see also* best interests
Berlin, Isaiah 74–75, 81
best interests 38–44, 141, 204–205, 215; family as best judge of 35–36; patient as best judge of 35–36, 60–66, 135–136, 197–199; *see also* benefit; choice; decision making
bodily integrity 87, 109–111, 116–117, 124–125, 127
Bratman, Michael 25–26, 145, 147–148

capabilities 137–140, 142, 222
change 165, 221–222; in patient's environment 27, 199–205; patient initiated 205–207, 214–218; in treatments available 27, 195–199; in what patient can do 27, 56–59
children *see* consent, children and; decision making, children and; privacy, children and; transitional cases
choice 13–17; as different from consent 9–11, 74–75, 225; instrumental value of 16, 80, 89–90, 196; living autonomously and 16–17, 80–87, 207; respect for 77–79, 196, 225; symbolic value of 17, 77, 88–95, 174–176, 196; voluntary 49, 90, 94–95; *see also* best interests; decision making; informed choice
chronic illness: aims of treatment for 4–5, 23–24, 132–134, 223–224; definition of 3; distinctive features of 3–7; increasing prevalence of 1–2
competence 78–80, 92, 173, 203; *see also* consent, competence and; decision making, incompetent adults and
compliance respect 48, 50, 68–69, 77–78, 96, 175–176; *see also* choice, respect for
confidentiality 26, 47, 109, 126, 129, 164–165, 179–180, 185–186, 190–191
conflicting obligations 22–24, 44, 93–94, 97, 121, 126–127, 144, 190
consent 7–12, 17–22, 74–75, 77–78; children and 21, 124–127;

competence and 20–21, 100, 103, 123–128; constitutive rules for 100–101, 103–105, 108; patient's intention and 100, 114–115, 116–117, 123, 181–183; respect for autonomy and 12, 18–21, 107–109, 119–123, 209; standing to 101, 103; understanding and 101, 104–107, 115–123, 182; voluntariness and 100, 114–115; when needed 7–8, 10–11, 20–21, 99–100, 108–109, 112–113; *see also* implicit consent; informed consent; non-regulatory consent; regulatory consent

consideration respect 49–50, 64–66, 77, 97, 175–176; *see also* choice, respect for

Darwall, Stephen 76, 122
decision making: changing treatments and 195–199; children and 35–36, 48–49, 69, 92–94; different methods of 34–37, 45–49, 63–66, 89–90; incompetent adults and 35–36, 48–49, 69; involving risk 67–71; patients' task when 60–66; patient understanding and 69–71; significant changes and 56–59, 199–205; *see also* choice; shared decision making; transitional cases
diabetes 4–6, 10–11, 139–140, 167–168, 202–203
Dworkin, Gerald 78–79
Dworkin, Ronald 36, 111

equipoise 197
expected utility 40, 67

families: respect for 172; as treatment providers 26, 164–165, 166, 167–170, 171–176; *see also* consent, children and; decision making, children and; non-adherence, by family members; shared action, family involvement in
Feinberg, Joel 21, 87–88, 109, 125
functionings 137–139, 142

generic medications 195–196
Gilbert, Margaret 25–26, 102, 145, 147–148
guidelines 20; *see also* regulations

habits 198–199
harm: consent and 108–109, 111–112, 117, 188–189; determining what will 13–15, 34–36; by family members 165, 171, 176–177, 189; obligation to avoid 13, 37, 93–94, 127–129, 202–203; *see also* risk

implicit consent 181–183, 185–186; *see also* consent
incompetent adults *see* competence; consent, competence and; decision making, incompetent adults and; privacy, incompetent adults and
information, obligation to provide 104–107, 131–132, 168; *see also* advice; autonomy, obligation to promote; benefit, providing information as way to; prevention, providing information and
informed choice 46–47; *vs.* informed person 9, 64–66, 118–119; when not needed 94–95, 97; *see also* autonomy, as feature of choice; choice; decision making
informed consent: as autonomous authorisation 105, 108, 119–122; as regulation 8, 18–21, 69, 102–106, 117–118, 126–127; *see also* consent

justice 137–138, 151–159

mature minors *see* transitional cases
Mill, John Stuart 35, 72n1, 109, 216
Mounck, Yascha 152, 154, 156–157

non-adherence: capabilities and 137–140, 142, 167–169, 222; by family members 26, 132, 165, 167–176; intentional *vs.* non-intentional 11, 22, 137, 149–150, 169–170; paternalism and 140–141, 143–143, 150–151; patient responsibility and 141, 154–156, 173; by patients 11–12, 22–26, 198; resource allocation and 141, 151–159; shared action and 149–150, 171–176
non-maleficence *see* harm

non-regulatory consent 20–21, 107–109, 177–179, 180–184, 186–192; *see also* consent

O'Neill, Onora 18, 37, 66, 104, 116, 118
Owens, David 9, 87, 89, 110, 189

pain 56–57, 65, 133, 138
Parkinson's disease 4–5, 7, 133–134, 165, 167, 200
paternalism 25–26, 84, 127–128, 140–143, 150–151, 207; *see also* non-adherence, paternalism and
patient: respect for 89–91, 149–150, 155–156, 173–176, 201, 207–208; responsibilities of 24–25, 151–159; *see also* non-adherence, patient responsibility and
permissive interests 110, 111, 124, 189–191
personal autonomy *see* autonomy
prevention: as aim of treatment 5–6, 133–134, 222; providing information and 29, 212–213, 215–217
privacy 26, 47, 108–109, 164–165, 177–184, 186–192; children and 178, 190; consequentialist reasons and 179, 188–189; implicit consent and 181–183, 185–186; incompetent adults and 190–191; permissive interest in 189–191; regulation of 178–179; respect for autonomy and 180–184, 186–188
promises 100, 147, 148–149, 159
property 100–101, 110, 125

reasoning biases 53–54, 57–59, 64–66, 215–216
regulations 20–21, 102–103
regulatory consent 20–21, 101, 102–107, 126–127, 178–179, 184; *see also* consent
resource allocation *see* justice
risk: appropriate judge of 68–69, 197–199; different attitudes to 67–68; duty to warn of 30, 216–217; patient choice and 67–71, 206; *see also* decision making

Scanlon, Thomas M. 17, 88–89, 91, 156
Sen, Amartya 61, 137–139, 141, 157–158
shared action: family involvement in 26, 166, 171–176; initiation of 145–146; obligations created by 147–149, 158–159, 217–218; treatment as 24–26, 145–146, 149–151, 201–202
shared decision making 32n13, 144–145
Siegler, Mark 177, 182–183, 185
simulation 56–57, 199; *see also* decision making
surrogation 57–59, 199; *see also* decision making

transitional cases: consent and 126–127; decision making and 48–50, 92–94
treatment: indirect 5–7, 22–28, 131–132, 136–139, 222; moral objections to 60–62; as prevention 4–5, 12, 29, 222; *see also* shared action, treatment as

understanding 69–70; *see also* consent, understanding and; decision making, patient understanding and

values, conflict of *see* conflicting obligations
Veatch, Robert M. 16, 42, 46, 60–61
Velleman, David 25–26, 145
visceral factors 65, 133
voluntary agreement 18, 145–148, 180, 183, 185; *see also* choice, voluntary; consent, voluntariness and

withholding information 12, 28, 207–208

Zimmerman, Michael 40–41, 216